The Minor Illness and Beyond Handbook

MARGARET PERRY

Advanced Nurse Practitioner
Linkway Medical Practice
West Bromwich, West Midlands

Radcliffe Publishing
London • New York

Radcliffe Publishing Ltd
St Mark's House
Shepherdess Walk
London N1 7BQ
United Kingdom

www.radcliffehealth.com

British Library Cataloguing in Publication Data

A catalogue record for this book is available from the British Library.

ISBN-13: 978 184619 767 3

Typeset by Darkriver Design, Auckland, New Zealand
Printed and bound by Cadmus Communications, USA

Contents

About the author

Margaret Perry completed her registered general nurse training in 1984 and moved very quickly into general practice as a practice nurse, having already been married and had her first child. Her second daughter was born in 1988 and she continued to work in general practice where she began to enhance her knowledge with further training in various areas of nursing. She completed a Nurse Practitioner Diploma in 1998 and a BSc (Hons) in 2000. In 2001, she took a position as a trainee Advanced Nurse Practitioner and completed her Master's degree in 2004. As nurses completing this course were advised to develop more in-depth skills in a particular area, she worked for three years as a community respiratory nurse dealing with patients with chronic lung diseases. In 2007, she returned to general practice where she is now employed full-time in an advanced role which involves minor illness clinics and chronic disease management.

During her time in general practice she has had several articles published on a range of topics which fuelled her interest in writing this book, which, it is hoped, will be a source of information and learning for other nurses expanding their roles.

CHAPTER 1

Nurse practitioners and advanced nurse practitioners

ORIGINS OF THE ROLE

Nurses working at an advanced level has been credited to as long ago as the American Civil War where Catholic sisters served as nurses and assisted surgeons in the administration of chloroform. No training or formal qualifications existed at that time and it was not until the late nineteenth century that nursing became a trained profession, led by Florence Nightingale. Her influence saw the implementation of the first standards and regulations for nursing, and in 1897 the first professional body was formed in the United States in Maryland, with the purpose of regulating nursing colleges. During the First World War the need for nurses rose dramatically and training was implemented to enable those who undertook the role to cope with the horrific injuries they were required to treat. However, during the Great Depression, need for their skills declined and work became scarce. The need for nurses again became important during the Second World War when there was another surge in demand for those with nursing skills, with the American government offering incentives to entice nurses to again take up the profession. Further growth and development of the profession continued in the 1930s and 1940s with the emergence of nurse specialists in the United States and, in 1965, Loretta Ford and Henry Silver created the first training programme for nurse practitioners with a curriculum which focused on health promotion, disease prevention, and the health of children and families.[1]

Developments to nursing practice in the UK were influenced enormously by Barbara Stillwell, who introduced a nurse practitioner role in primary care in 1988. Her vision was one of experienced nurses using their existing nursing skills but in addition to health assessment and diagnostic skills in an autonomous working environment.[2] Her work saw the growth and development of nursing in primary care through the 1990s and beyond and although not without difficulties, nursing roles continued to progress. It was not until the 1990s, however, that the profession saw a real move towards regulation and standardisation of nurse practitioner education. The first formal training programme for the role in the UK was introduced by the Royal College of Nursing (RCN) and was designed to equip nurses with a range of competencies and skills to allow them to work autonomously. From then on universities around the country have developed courses which were initially at Diploma level but are now at Master's level, which is regarded as the necessary educational level for advanced practice.[3]

DEFINITION AND WHAT IS EXPECTED OF ADVANCED NURSE PRACTITIONERS

There are many definitions of the role of nurse practitioner (NP) and advanced nurse practitioner (ANP), but the one laid down by the Nursing and Midwifery Council (NMC) is as follows: 'Advanced Nurse Practitioners are highly experienced and educated members of the care team who are able to diagnose and treat your healthcare needs or refer you to an appropriate specialist if needed.'[4]

In 2005, the NMC proposed that the title 'Advanced Nurse Practitioner' should be registered and recorded on the nursing register. One of the key concerns has centred around the fact that the title itself has been used to such a varied degree and applied inconsistently across a range of different roles and clinical areas, which has led to a lack of clear definition and has resulted in confusion about the exact scope of the role and the level of skills and competence actually required to enable nurses to practice at this higher level.

DEPARTMENT OF HEALTH (DOH) GUIDANCE

In 2010, the DOH issued a position statement which echoed the need for nationally agreed standards for advanced level practice with the intention of protecting and supporting nurses, employers and the public. The statement incorporates a number of nationally agreed elements underpinned by emphasis on clinical care, leadership and collaborative practice, quality improvement and development of practice.[3]

Much of the guidance of the DOH mirrors and supports that of the NMC, focusing on a number of elements which are seen as key to providing quality care at an advanced level.

The main emphasis from both organisations centres on the ability to work autonomously, providing independent assessment of needs and providing care from initial consultation through to diagnosis, treatment, follow-up and referral if needed, ensuring best practice is adhered to at all times. Leadership skills and collaboration with other professionals and services is also advocated as well as the ability to play an active role in service development with the aim of further enhancing the service offered to patients. Following on from the original proposal from the NMC that the title of 'Advanced Nurse Practitioner' should be registered, further proposals have followed. In 2009, the Council for Healthcare Regulatory Excellence

(CHRE) published a report entitled *Advanced Practice: Report to the Four UK Health Departments*, which indicated that statutory regulation is unnecessary.[5] More recently, the Command paper *Enabling Excellence, Autonomy and Accountability for Healthcare Workers, Social Workers and Social Care Workers*[6] concluded regulation of healthcare workers should be targeted to safeguard the public yet maintain professional standards, but at the same time reduce the cost burden of regulation. It appears that formal regulation will not yet take place but instead emphasis will be placed on employers to take responsibility through governance processes.

THE FUTURE OF ADVANCED NURSE PRACTITIONERS

Advanced nursing roles now exist in several countries and in the UK the service demand for advanced nursing is growing, driven by a number of factors which have been cited as reductions in junior doctors' working hours, recruitment and retention problems in clinical specialties, substantial health service restructuring and workforce redesign demands.[7] Systematic reviews have shown positive patient outcomes[8] with evidence that advanced nurses can play an important role in resolving service issues, and if utilised correctly with appropriate training will continue to grow both in numbers and in value and will continue to improve patient care.

REFERENCES

1. Ford L. Nurse, nurse practitioners: the evolution of primary care. *Image J Nurs Sch.* 1986; **18**: 177–8.
2. Stilwell B. Patients' attitudes to a highly developed extended role: the nurse practitioner. *Recent Adv Nurs.* 1988; **21**: 82–100.
3. Department of Health. *Advanced Level Nursing: a position statement.* London: Department of Health; 2010.
4. Nursing and Midwifery Council. *The Proposed Framework for the Standard for Post-Registration Nursing – February.* London: Nursing and Midwifery Council; 2005.
5. Council for Healthcare Regulatory Excellence. *Advanced Practice: Report to the Four UK Health Departments.* London: Council for Healthcare Regulatory Excellence; 2009.
6. Department of Health. *Enabling Excellence.* London: Department of Health; 2011.
7. Carnwell R, Daly W. Advanced nursing practitioners in primary care settings: an exploration of the developing roles. *J Clin Nurs.* 2003; **12**(5): 630–42.
8. Newhouse RP, Stanik-Hutt J, White KM, *et al.* Advanced practice nurse outcomes 1990–2008: a systematic review. *Nurs Econ.* 2011; **29**(5): 1–21.

CHAPTER 2

Setting up a minor illness clinic

Minor illnesses are common and are generally defined as illnesses of short duration.[1] The frequency of consultations for common problems places a huge burden on general practice and it is estimated that, every year, 50 million visits to the GP are made for minor ailments such as coughs and colds, mild eczema, and athlete's foot.[2] In recent years the role of practice nurses has expanded greatly and many are now taking on advanced roles with greater autonomy and responsibility.

Our surgery set up a minor illness clinic in 2007 to be run by an ANP educated to Master's level in advanced clinical practice supported by four GP partners and two part-time salaried doctors.

SETTING UP THE SERVICE

Doctors, receptionists and the practice manager were involved in the initial discussions and planning of the service. The first task was to decide what conditions would be included. A patient leaflet was then devised which was handed out to all new patients registering with the practice and leaflets were left on the reception desk and in the rack in reception for patients to pick up if they wished to do so.

It was decided that the leaflet would incorporate the information shown in Table 2.1.

TABLE 2.1 Leaflet information

Minor illness clinic	Minor illnesses	Exclusions
Did you know that the practice has a minor illness clinic which is run by our advanced nurse practitioner? She has received advanced training and can offer advice and prescribe treatment for the following conditions.	• Coughs and colds • Sore throats • Chest infections • Diarrhoea and sickness • Earache • Hay fever • Head lice • Ingrowing toenail • Insect bites • Skin problems (for example, skin infections, minor rashes and eczema) • Conjunctivitis • Urine infections (females only) • Vaginal infections • Heartburn • Untreated haemorrhoids • Verrucas • Warts • Worms • Constipation • Asthma problems • COPD problems	This clinic may not be suitable for you if your problem is a long-standing one and you are under the care of a consultant (with the exception of asthma and chronic obstructive pulmonary disease (COPD)).

EXCLUSION CRITERIA

Patients deemed unsuitable were babies and young children under the age of three, patients with multiple complex problems and those who have seen a GP several times for a recurring problem.

RECEPTIONIST TRAINING

Reception staff received training from the reception manager. When patients ask for a same-day appointment they are asked, 'Is this something which may be suitable for the minor illness clinic?' If the patient is unsure, the receptionist can quickly cover the conditions included, giving the patient the opportunity to decide whether the service is suitable or not.

Once the problem has been established as potentially suitable for the clinic the following questions are asked:

Has the patient been treated by a doctor for the same problem in the past week?

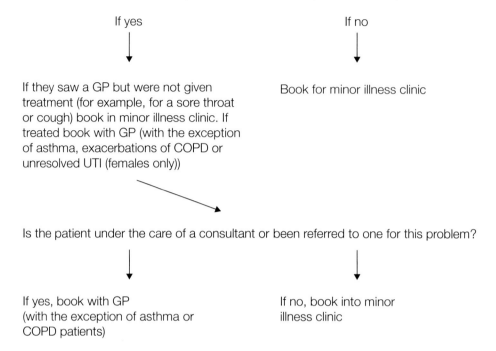

If yes

If no

If they saw a GP but were not given treatment (for example, for a sore throat or cough) book in minor illness clinic. If treated book with GP (with the exception of asthma, exacerbations of COPD or unresolved UTI (females only))

Book for minor illness clinic

Is the patient under the care of a consultant or been referred to one for this problem?

If yes, book with GP (with the exception of asthma or COPD patients)

If no, book into minor illness clinic

AVOIDING PROBLEMS

GP support is available during all sessions.

- Telephone appointment slots are inserted into each clinic (two per session) for the advanced nurse practitioner to speak to the patient if reception staff are unsure whether the problem is suitable. This has also been useful for patients who are reluctant to tell the receptionist their symptoms because the problem is personal, but also where the receptionist is unsure of the suitability.
- Weekly tutorials are held with a senior GP and the content of these may be patient based, or disease based.
- Mistakes do happen in terms of inappropriate bookings, but I avoid calling a GP in to see the patient unless the problem is urgent.
- Advice can be sought by telephoning the on-call GP if this is needed.
- If the booking is inappropriate for the clinic, one of the GPs will see the patient on arrival either as an extra or sooner if the problem is more urgent.

PATIENT SATISFACTION

The service is now established and well used. When audited, the findings mimicked those found elsewhere. One study reported that 90% of their patients accepted an appointment with the nurse, and a few patients who had seen the nurse subsequently requested consultations with her.[3] Secondly, the fact that almost 80% of patients did not return for a further consultation about that episode of illness suggests that the treatment and advice offered were effective. Our findings were similar, and now that the service has been established for nearly six years there are quite a few patients who select the minor illness clinic as their first choice rather than wait for a GP appointment.

FUTURE EXPANSION

It is anticipated that with further training more conditions can be added to those currently seen, which will allow further professional development and will also hopefully enhance the service offered to patients.

REFERENCES

1. Jones R, White P, Armstrong D, *et al. Managing Acute Illness.* The King's Fund. 2010. Available at: www.kingsfund.org.uk/sites/files/kf/field/field_document/managing-acute-illness-gp-inquiry-research-paper-mar11.pdf (accessed 3 February 2013).
2. NHS Choices. *Treating Common Conditions.* Available at: www.nhs.uk/Livewell/Pharmacy/Pages/Commonconditions.aspx (accessed 3 February 2013).
3. Marsh GN, Dawes ML. Establishing a minor illness nurse in a busy general practice. *BMJ.* 1995; **310**: 778.

CHAPTER 3

History taking: general aspects

Taking a thorough and comprehensive history is a vital component of the patient consultation and provides an initial introduction to the problem. From the information provided, the clinician should gain sufficient information to allow them to consider a provisional diagnosis, and decide on further investigations and treatment if these are required. The consultation should be conducted in a professional manner using a systematic structured approach, giving the patient the opportunity to contribute and hence feel confident in the clinician's assessment of their problem. Adequate time should be allowed so that the patient does not feel they have been rushed, with opportunity for the patient to ask questions if they have not understood or need clarification on any aspect of the discussion. The patient should be encouraged to talk, describing their symptoms in their own words. Open questions are invaluable in encouraging the patient to describe the problem in detail. Language used during the consultation should be appropriate and easy to understand, avoiding medical terms and technical terminology.

SETTING THE SCENE
- Use a comfortable but private room.
- Greet the patient, explaining who you are if you have not met them before.
- Try to put the patient at ease and establish a rapport so that he/she will feel comfortable talking to you.
- Give the patient full attention, maintaining eye contact.
- Interruptions should be avoided if at all possible.
- Allow the patient to talk.
- When the patient is giving several symptoms, attempt to determine which of these is bothering them most.
- During the interview use a combination of open and closed questions. Closed questions generate a yes or no answer; open questions give the patient an opportunity to give a lot more information about a particular symptom.
- It is often useful to summarise what the patient has said so that they can offer any additional information or add something they have forgotten to include.

The initial questioning should incorporate the following and is applicable whatever the nature of the patient's problem. *See* Table 3.1.

TABLE 3.1 Initial questioning

History	Additional points
Presenting complaint	How can I help today?
History of the presenting complaint	When did the symptoms start?
	Have symptoms worsened?
	Has patient had anything like this before and if so when?
Specific questions	These will focus on further questions relating to the problem/ diagnosis and the system you are dealing with and are covered in the history-taking section of each chapter under each system.
Past medical history	Anything in the history which may be relevant? Is this a recurrence of a previous problem?
Current medication and past medications including products purchased over the counter (OTC)	Current medications if any?
	Has patient tried to self-treat with OTC products? If so with what?
	Could the problem be a side-effect of medication?
Allergies to any medications	Previous allergic reaction to any medications?
Social and family history	Current employment?
	Anything of importance in the family history?
	Could symptoms be related to patient's employment?
Alcohol and smoking	Both may be important.
Employment history	May identify contact with hazardous substances.
Recent travel abroad	If travelled abroad, were injections required or malaria prophylaxis and did patient take these?
Functional enquiry	Appetite?
	Weight loss?
	Fever?
	Nausea or vomiting?
	Night sweats?
	Fatigue?
	Lumps?
	Itching?

ASSESSMENT OF PAIN

If the presenting problem involves pain, there are several models which can be used to gain information.

One example is the OPQRST model shown in Table 3.2.

TABLE 3.2 OPQRST model of pain assessment

O	Onset	When did the pain start? Was the pain sudden or did it start more gradually?
P	Provocation and palliation	Does anything make the pain worse or anything make it better?
Q	Quality	Can patient describe the pain? Is it a dull ache, throbbing, sharp, and burning or a crushing pain?
R	Radiation	Determine the exact site of the pain and whether it travels or radiates anywhere else.
S	Severity	Is the pain interfering with daily activities, or disturbing patient's sleep?
T	Timing	Is the pain intermittent or is it there all the time?

SYSTEMS ENQUIRY

Once the information relating to the presenting complaint has been gathered, a review of the body's main systems is useful. It can provide an opportunity for the patient to mention any symptoms or concerns that he or she may have failed to mention earlier in the history-taking process. Usually, the questions surrounding the presenting complaint will have provided sufficient information so that once all the information has been gathered it is useful to clarify key points, which ensures nothing has been missed, and gives the patient the opportunity to add anything further. Questions relating to each system are discussed within the following chapters.

Further investigations and treatment if needed can then be commenced and again these are discussed within each chapter in relation to each body system.

FURTHER READING

Bickley LS. *Bates' Guide to Physical Examination and History Taking*. 11th ed. London: Wolters Kluwer Health/Lippincott Williams and Wilkins; 2009.

Epstein O, Perkins D, Cookson J, *et al. Clinical Examination*. 4th ed. London: Mosby; 2008.

CHAPTER 4

Respiratory

INTRODUCTION

Respiratory diseases have a major impact on health and are the most common reason for general practice consultations and emergency medical admission to hospital.[1] Many respiratory diseases have shared or similar signs and symptoms, and to complicate matters some of these symptoms are also shared with some cardiac conditions. A careful and thorough history is therefore essential to raise suspicion of a suspected cause and this together with appropriate investigations will help confirm the diagnosis so that appropriate treatment can be commenced.

CONDITIONS COVERED IN THE CHAPTER

- Upper respiratory tract infection (URTI)
- Influenza
- Acute and chronic cough
- Exacerbation of asthma
- Exacerbation of COPD
- Pneumonia
- Tuberculosis (TB).

COMMON PRESENTING SYMPTOMS

May present with one or several of the following.
- Cough
- Sputum
- Breathlessness
- Wheezing
- Haemoptysis
- Chest pain.

TAKING THE RESPIRATORY HISTORY

Initial history is as described in Chapter 3, followed by a focused enquiry relating to the respiratory system.

Table 4.1 shows symptoms enquiry and further questioning for specific symptoms.

TABLE 4.1 Symptoms enquiry and further questioning for specific symptoms

Symptom	Further questioning
Cough	Productive or non-productive?
	Worse during the day or at night or both?
	Are there additional symptoms as below?
Sputum	Sputum colour, thickness?
	How much? (measures such as a teaspoon or tablespoon may help patient give an estimate)
	Yellow or green?
	Rusty coloured?
	Frothy or blood streaked? (*see* haemoptysis below)
Haemoptysis	If patient mentions blood in the sputum, is it frank bleeding or blood-stained sputum? Is this a new event or has it occurred over a more prolonged period of time?
	Amount?
	Fresh blood or dark in colour?
	Did the episode follow a coughing bout?
Breathlessness	Recent onset or noticed by patient for some time?
	Breathless on exertion, at rest or both?
	Is breathlessness associated with particular activities, e.g. climbing stairs or can it occur when walking on the flat?
	Is the patient breathless when lying flat or do they wake in the night gasping for breath?
	Is it limiting daily living activities?
Wheezing	Present on exertion or at rest or both?
	Associated with tight chest/breathlessness?
	Occurs during the day or at night or both?
	Are there any trigger factors such as exercise?
Chest pain	Use OPQRST (*see* Chapter 3) to get more information.

Table 4.2 shows a summary of presenting signs and symptoms and the diseases they may suggest. Each symptom will then be discussed in more detail in the context of each disease.

TABLE 4.2 Presenting signs and symptoms

	Breathlessness	Cough	Sputum	Wheeze	Chest pain	Haemoptysis
URTI (common cold)	No	Yes	No	No	No	No
Influenza	No	Yes	No	No	No	No
Exacerbation of asthma	Yes	Yes	Possible	Yes	Tight chest	No
Exacerbation of COPD	Yes	Yes	Yes	Yes	Tight chest	No
Pneumonia	Yes	Yes	Yes	Possible	No	Possible (blood streaked sputum)
TB	Yes	Yes	Yes	Possible	No	Possible

FURTHER INVESTIGATIONS

Investigations should be chosen on the basis of the history, signs and symptoms, including the duration of symptoms and the overall clinical picture.

Other investigations selected on the basis of history symptoms and clinical findings

- Peak flow
- Spirometry
- Bloods including full blood count (FBC) and erythrocyte sedimentation rate (ESR)
- Sputum culture
- Oxygen saturation levels (O_2 sats)
- Chest X-ray.

Consultant-initiated investigations

- Bronchoscopy
- Biopsy
- Computerised tomography (CT scan).

Urgent referral to respiratory physician required

- Smokers and ex-smokers over 40 years of age with cough, haemoptysis and weight loss
- Suspicious symptoms even if X-ray is normal
- Chest X-ray suggesting pleural effusion or consolidation
- Finger clubbing
- History of asbestos exposure and recent onset of chest pain, together with shortness of breath and/or any unexplained systemic symptoms.

URTI (COMMON COLD) AND INFLUENZA

The common cold and influenza are often confused by patients, and it is not uncommon for a patient to present saying that they think they may have influenza. Both conditions are highly contagious and although both are unpleasant for the sufferer the common cold is usually short lived and unlikely to result in serious complications; influenza on the other hand can lead to more serious outcomes and in severe cases can potentially result in death. Both are easily spread and are transmitted through coughing, sneezing and close personal contact. Current statistics suggest that there are an estimated 3000–4000 deaths from influenza each year with the majority of these occurring in people over the age of 65.[2] A history and examination of the patient will quickly enable the clinician to identify the correct diagnosis.

As well as the features listed in Table 4.2 there are several other clues to suggest which of the two conditions the patient is suffering from (*see* Table 4.3).

TABLE 4.3 Clues to aid the diagnosis

Common cold	Influenza
Gradual onset	Rapid onset
Slight temperature after first 24 hours	Raised temperature in first 24 hours lasting approximately 3–4 days
Normal appetite	Loss of appetite
Slight headache	Severe headache
Blocked or runny nose with sneezing	Sneezing less common
Sore throat and sometimes earache	Muscular aches and pains
Feeling of lethargy	Feeling of complete exhaustion

Pathophysiology
Common cold

The cause is viral, of which there are many, but some of the commonest are rhinoviruses, adenoviruses and sometimes coxsackie viruses.[3] Once the virus gains entry the immune system is activated in an attempt to fight off the infection. Hairs lining the nose filter and trap some pathogens, and mucus coating much of the upper respiratory tract plays a part in trapping any invading organisms. The anatomy and position of the posterior nose to the pharynx allows large particles to settle on the back of the throat while lower down the respiratory tract the cilia trap any invading pathogens and attempt to transport them up towards the pharynx. This process activates the release of inflammatory mediators including histamines, interleukins and prostaglandins, which then activate sneeze and cough reflexes. This promotes the dilation of blood vessels, which in turn leads to increased production of mucus and this further supports the defence mechanism by trapping any invading organisms.

Influenza

There are potentially three viruses which can cause influenza, type A, B or C. Type A is considered to be more pathogenic and is frequently the cause of major epidemics affecting large numbers of people.[4] If the virus is able to invade the respiratory tract, replication rapidly takes place, leading to the release of inflammatory mediators and the subsequent development of influenza symptoms.

Differential diagnosis

⚠ BEWARE!

As well as the common cold and influenza there are other conditions with shared and/or similar symptoms:
- bronchitis: inflammation of the lining of the bronchial tubes can often follow a cold, and although there are shared symptoms with other respiratory conditions the cough can persist for several weeks
- pneumonia: pp. 25–9
- pharyngitis: pp. 128–31
- exacerbation of COPD: pp. 22–5.

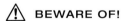

Antibiotics are not recommended for use where viral infection is suspected. Symptoms of the common cold generally resolve without any treatment often by a maximum of approximately 2 weeks. Influenza symptoms usually settle in approximately 5–7 days, but unfortunately symptoms such as tiredness, malaise, and aches and pains may persist for a longer period. Self-help measures can provide some relief, including rest, analgesia, steam inhalations to ease nasal congestion and gargling for the sore throat. Some patients may choose to purchase over-the-counter cough linctuses or cold and flu remedies, but these are thought to be of limited benefit.

Complications

⚠ BEWARE OF!

- Worsening of comorbid conditions such as asthma, COPD, or heart failure (HF).
- Onset of pneumonia.
- Onset of ear infection or sinusitis.

TABLE 4.4 Clinical alerts!

Productive cough with purulent green sputum
Increased breathlessness
Prolonged fever
Worsening symptoms
Dehydration in the presence of severe loss of appetite
Weight loss
Prolonged or atypical symptoms

Key reminders

- Patients often confuse the common cold with influenza.
- Neither condition requires antibiotics unless complications develop.
- Symptoms of common cold are generally milder than those of influenza.
- Both should resolve without specific medical treatment.

ACUTE AND CHRONIC COUGH

One-third of the UK population visit their GP each year with a respiratory condition, with cough the commonest reason for attendance.[5] Coughs are categorised as acute (lasting less than 3 weeks), sub-acute (lasting 3–8 weeks) or chronic (lasting more than 8 weeks).[6] The commonest cause of acute cough is upper respiratory tract infection of viral origin which usually resolves spontaneously. Chronic cough, however, has a number of potential causes both respiratory and non-respiratory (*see* Tables 4.5 and 4.6). Both acute and chronic cough can cause distress and can be particularly upsetting when the cough causes sleep deprivation.

TABLE 4.5 Common respiratory diseases causing chronic cough

Asthma
COPD
Bronchiectasis
Pulmonary fibrosis
Lung cancer
Infection – postviral TB

There are several instances where cough is not respiratory in origin (*see* Table 4.6).

TABLE 4.6 Non-respiratory causes of cough

Gastro-oesophageal reflux (GORD)
Postnasal drip
Foreign body
Medication induced, e.g. ramipril
Pulmonary oedema
Anxiety
Smoking

CLINICAL ALERT!

- Smoking is reported to be one of the commonest causes of persistent cough which appears to be dose related.[7]
- Either singly or in combination, postnasal drip, asthma, and GORD are three of the most common causes of chronic cough.[8]
- Asthma, infection, or HF can cause coughing which potentially wakes patients at night.[7]

Pathophysiology

Cough is an essential part of the body's defence mechanism and its purpose is to assist in clearing respiratory pathogens and noxious substances from the bronchial tree. A cough is thought to develop following inhalation of an irritant substance, which then activates receptors in the respiratory system. Once an irritant substance is inhaled there is an increased sensitivity of the cough receptors, with stimulation of the sensory nerves in the epithelium. High intra-thoracic pressures are needed for the cough to effectively expel foreign bodies or mucus from the airways, and it is thought that this contributes to the discomfort experienced during repeated bouts of coughing.[6] An acute cough in an otherwise healthy person is usually self-limiting and will resolve without intervention. However, those with chronic cough often complain of other symptoms such as disturbed sleep, hoarse voice and chest discomfort.

Treatment

- Acute cough often resolves with no treatment.
- Chronic cough may require treatment, but this will depend on the underlying cause and will be discussed in the relevant chapters.

Complications

⚠ BEWARE OF!

- Spontaneous pneumothorax
- Cough syncope: fainting caused by decreased blood flow to the brain during prolonged or forceful bouts of coughing
- Musculoskeletal pain: costochondritis
- Hernias caused by the degree of raised intra abdominal pressure when coughing
- Loss of faeces or stress incontinence.

CLINICAL ALERT!

Urgent chest X-ray needed for cough with alarm symptoms:
- haemoptysis
- cough persisting for more than 3 weeks with history and symptoms suggestive of lung cancer
- unexplained weight loss
- chest pain
- increased breathlessness
- finger clubbing
- cervical or supraclavicular lymphadenopathy
- assessment in secondary care setting for patients with suspected pneumothorax or pleural effusion with breathlessness.

See p. 13 for recommended referral to a consultant for urgent assessment.

Key reminders

- The majority of coughs are viral.
- They require careful history taking to determine possibility of underlying cause.
- Beware the possibility of undiagnosed asthma in patients with variable symptoms and COPD in current or ex-smokers.
- Be alert to non-respiratory causes such as acid reflux.

EXACERBATION OF ASTHMA

Exacerbations of asthma continue to occur despite improvements in available treatment options, and their occurrence is associated with diminished quality of life, which impacts on both the patient and their family. The exact definition of an exacerbation remains controversial, but it is generally accepted to refer to an increase in symptoms which warrant medical advice and treatment. Exacerbations may be triggered by a number of causes, often as a result of atmospheric or environmental factors encountered either in the home, in schools or in the workplace. A common trigger is a URTI of viral cause, often associated with rhinovirus infection.

TABLE 4.7 Clues to aid the diagnosis

Increased shortness of breath
Cough
Wheeze
Chest tightness
Worsening symptoms despite use of reliever inhaler

Asthma exacerbations can be classified as mild, moderate, severe, or at worst can be life threatening. Assessment of severity is based on symptoms and findings on examination. Although no single parameter has been identified to assess exacerbation severity, lung function is a useful method of assessment. A peak flow (PEF) of 40% or less of predicted function is indicative of a severe attack in patients five years or older.[9]

⚠ BEWARE!

- In children too young to accurately perform peak flow measurements, use of accessory muscles of respiration, chest wall retractions, tachypnoea greater than 60 breaths per minute, cyanosis, and the presence of inspiratory and expiratory wheezing are markers of a severe attack.[10]
- Pulse oximetry on room air with an oxygen saturation of less than 92%–94% 1 hour after beginning standard treatment is a strong predictor of the need for hospitalisation.[9]
- During severe exacerbations the patient will be breathless at rest and have difficulty completing whole sentences.
- During severe exacerbations PEF will be less that 40% predicted or 40% of personal best, and life-threatening exacerbations will present with a patient who is too breathless to speak with a PEF less than 25% predicted or 25% of personal best.[11]

Pathophysiology

The process underpinning the onset of an exacerbation is extremely complex. Once an allergen invades the respiratory tract, a sequence of events follows with inflammation of the airways, airflow obstruction and increased airway responsiveness all important components of the process. Some of the principal cells identified in airway inflammation include mast cells, eosinophils, epithelial cells, macrophages, and activated T lymphocytes.[12] Immunoglobulin E (IgE) also plays a major part in the allergic response, binding to allergens and triggering the release of substances from mast cells which cause inflammation. Once the process of inflammation is under way, it is thought that excess mucus production further clogs the airways, and is followed by the release of prostaglandins, leukotrienes and histamine, further adding to the whole sequence of events. Chronic inflammation over time may lead to structural changes in the airways, including sub-epithelial fibrosis, airway smooth muscle hypertrophy/hyperplasia, and mucus hyperplasia.[3] When inflammation becomes chronic this results in airflow limitation that is only partly reversible, a process which arises as a result of changes to the airways and airway remodelling.

Differential diagnosis

 BEWARE!

There are a number of possible alternative causes of the patient's symptoms. *See* Table 4.8.

TABLE 4.8 Differential diagnoses

Condition	Additional pointers	When to consider
Exacerbation of COPD	pp. 22–5.	pp. 22–5.
Pulmonary embolism (PE)	Do not usually wheeze but will experience chest pain; onset of breathlessness is sudden.	Patient has a history of immobility/ surgery, and there are additional symptoms of productive cough with blood-streaked sputum.
Foreign body	Localised wheeze at the sight of the obstruction.	There is no improvement post bronchodilation.
Pneumothorax	Similar symptoms.	Consider if there is sudden onset of breathlessness with chest pain.
HF	Some shared symptoms such as breathless and cough (pp. 54–60).	Consider if there is peripheral oedema, and inability to lie flat in bed at night.
Anaphylaxis	Usually more stridor than wheeze on auscultation.	Consider if onset of symptoms followed contact with particular substance or product.

Treatment

In most cases inhaled beta-2 agonists given in high doses act quickly to relieve bronchospasm with few side-effects.[14] In acute asthma without life-threatening features, beta-2 agonists can be administered by repeated activations of a metered dose inhaler (MDI) via a large volume spacer, which is as effective as when administered by the nebulised route.[11] Recommended dose is up to 10 puffs of salbutamol 100 mcg, each puff inhaled separately via a spacer and repeated at 10–20-minute intervals or as necessary.[15]

Initial treatment is followed by a short course of oral steroids.

- Adult suggested dose is 40 mg daily for at least 5 days or until recovery.[16]
- Children should be prescribed 2 mg per kilogram of body weight to a maximum of 40 mg daily.[17]

Prescribing tips

- Prednisolone should be taken with food to avoid gastrointestinal symptoms such as dyspepsia.
- If patient is having frequent exacerbations, asthma management needs assessment.
- Drug is present in breast milk but at usual dose is not associated with any effects on the baby.
- Can cross the placenta in pregnancy but is not thought to increase the risk of congenital defects in the baby.

Complications

⚠ BEWARE OF!

- Poor or delayed response to treatment
- Pneumonia
- Pneumothorax
- Respiratory failure.

CLINICAL ALERTS!

⚠ BEWARE OF!

- Cyanosis: signifies hypoxia
- Silent chest: due to severely reduced air entry
- Rapid pulse: due to overuse of ventolin
- Chest pain: may indicate other pathology such as PE, pleurisy or pneumothorax
- Beware of difficulty completing sentences, altered mental status, and use of accessory muscles which may signify impending respiratory failure.

CLINICAL ALERT!

Asthma deaths still occur.
   Risk of death increased in:

- patients who have had a previous severe asthma attack and recent hospital admission
- recent increase in shortness of breath, night waking to use reliever and overuse of reliever at other times

- two or more admissions due to asthma or three or more visits to an accident and emergency department in the past 12 months
- use of two or more reliever inhalers per month
- history of a near-fatal asthma event in the past
- prior severe asthma exacerbation requiring admission to an intensive care unit and intubation.

Key reminders
- Review inhaler technique and if poor review device.
- Review treatment level and step up if needed.
- Review compliance with treatment regime.
- Provide asthma management plan.

EXACERBATION OF COPD

Exacerbations of COPD are a significant cause of distress for both the patient and their family and are a cause for concern because of their association with increased risk of morbidity and mortality. There remains no clear definition, but they are generally accepted as referring to acute episodes of worsening of symptoms that differ from the day-to-day variations, and may require alterations in therapy.[18] As the disease progresses the frequency of exacerbations becomes more frequent, and patients experiencing frequent exacerbations have been found to suffer a more rapid decline in lung function, worse quality of life and decreased exercise tolerance.[19] Once the exacerbation has been treated it may take several months for the patient to recover fully and return to their previous level of health and activity levels. Severe exacerbations of COPD have an impact on prognosis with mortality increasing with the frequency of these exacerbations, and those requiring hospitalisation have been found to have a four or more times greater risk of death than those patients treated at home.[20]

TABLE 4.9 Clues to aid the diagnosis

Symptom	Additional features	Additional information
Increased breathlessness	Often on exertion	Can also be at rest in severe exacerbations
Cough	May be productive or non-productive	Pseudomonas, haemophilus, and pneumococcal species may produce green sputum
Increased sputum production	May be an increase in quantity and/or purulence	Green purulent sputum suggests bacterial infection[21]
Impaired gas exchange	Reduced oxygen levels Raised carbon dioxide levels	Low oxygen saturation levels

COPD is a systemic disorder affecting a number of organs and functions potentially leading to:

- skeletal muscle dysfunction
- muscle wasting
- end organ damage
- pulmonary hypertension
- increased cardiovascular risk
- increased osteoporosis risk.

Pathophysiology

The process underpinning an exacerbation is extremely complex. Bacterial infections are generally considered to be the most common causes of COPD exacerbations and it is estimated that more than 40% of all exacerbations are bacterial in origin,[22] although respiratory viruses can also be a cause. Commonly isolated organisms include *Haemophilus influenza*, *Streptococcus pneumoniae*, *Moraxella catarrhalis*, *Haemophilus parainfluenzae* and *Pseudomonas aeruginosa*.[23] In smokers and ex-smokers there is damage to the cilia, resulting in reduced effectiveness of the body's defence mechanism which allows pathogens to successfully gain entry and colonise the airways. During exacerbations, inflammation becomes marked, with an increased number of neutrophils and eosinophils and increased CD4 lymphocytes within the bronchial tree. Current smokers have been found to have an increase in macrophages and T lymphocytes in the walls of the airways, and increased numbers of leucocytes in the bronchial tree, but during exacerbations neutrophils become the major component of the inflammatory response,[24] leading researchers to believe that an increase in airway inflammation is central to the pathogenesis of episodes. Once airway inflammation commences in response to a stimulus there is an increase in oedema of the bronchial walls, and an increase in mucus production. This manifests itself as an increase in sputum production, which is often present during exacerbations, and if the sputum is viscous leads to difficulty clearing the airways, plugging of the smaller airways and increased breathlessness.

Differential diagnosis

TABLE 4.10 Differential diagnoses: beware

Condition	Additional pointers	When to consider
Pneumonia	*See* p. 25 for clues to aid the diagnosis	pp. 25–9
Pneumothorax	Similar symptoms	p. 20
HF/pulmonary oedema	*See* p. 54 for clues to aid the diagnosis	pp. 54–7
PE	p. 20	p. 20

(continued)

Condition	Additional pointers	When to consider
Lung cancer	May have chronic cough, weight loss, increasing shortness of breath and haemoptysis; finger clubbing may be evident	Consider in smokers and ex-smokers with appetite loss and unexplained weight loss
Pleural effusion	May be asymptomatic	Patient may complain of breathlessness and pleuritic chest pain
Bronchiectasis	Often evidence of finger clubbing	Chronic persistent cough productive of copious amounts of sputum

Treatment

- Increase dose and frequency of short-acting bronchodilators and add spacer device if using metered dose inhalers to aid lung deposition.
- If significant breathlessness and wheeze, prescribe short course of oral steroids (30 mg daily in one dose for 7 days with food).[16]
- Course of antibiotics if sputum is purulent (local guidelines may suggest choices).
- Guidance suggests penicillin, e.g. amoxicillin, a macrolide (e.g. erythromycin or clarithromycin or a tetracycline (e.g. oxytetracycline).[25]

Prescribing tips

- If exacerbations are frequent, consider addition of bone protection and addition of proton pump inhibitor (PPI) to provide gastric protection.
- Longer courses of antibiotics (10–14 days) recommended if the patient has bronchiectasis.
- p. 21: information relating to prescribing oral steroids.

CLINICAL ALERT!

In the event of a severe exacerbation the patient may require admission to hospital. Decision to treat at home should be based on assessment of the following:

- degree of breathlessness
- severity of symptoms
- level of consciousness
- presence of cyanosis
- presence of peripheral oedema
- presence of comorbidities (possible deterioration of these during an exacerbation)
- available support and ability to cope at home.

Complications
- Hypercapnia
- Hypoxaemia
- Cor pulmonale
- Pulmonary hypertension.

⚠ **BEWARE OF!**

Increased risk of mortality in patients with:
- low body mass index
- hypercapnia
- hypoxia
- pulmonary hypertension
- low FEV1
- presence of co-morbidities.

Key reminders
- Progressive disease
- Associated with reduced quality of life
- More rapid deterioration in those who continue to smoke
- Significant cause of morbidity and mortality.

PNEUMONIA: COMMUNITY ACQUIRED

Pneumonia is a serious disease that remains a leading cause of death in both adults and children, and among children the disease is the single largest cause of death, accounting for 18% of all deaths of children in the under-5 age group, yearly around the world.[26] The mortality rate for pneumococcal pneumonia has been estimated to be approximately 10–20 in every 100 people,[27] with mortality rates for older patients in hospital-based studies of community-acquired pneumonia reported to be as high as 30%, increasing to 57% among cases acquired in the nursing home setting.[28] However, many pneumococcal infections may not be investigated so it is possible that both the number of people affected and death rates may be inaccurate.

Clues to aid the diagnosis

Signs and symptoms of pneumonia vary depending on the causative organism and may also be different in different age groups. When the illness is viral, symptoms tend to be milder with the exception of the elderly and those who are immuno-suppressed who are at risk of developing a more severe viral pneumonia with higher morbidity and mortality rates.

Table 4.11 presents viral and bacterial symptoms in children.

TABLE 4.11 Viral and bacterial symptoms in children: clues to aid diagnosis

Viral	Bacterial
Fever (often only mild)	High fever (often above 38.5 degrees)
Lethargy	Rapid breathing rate
Muscle aches and pains	Chest recession
Loss of appetite	Breathing difficulties
Tiredness	Tiredness
May expectorate small amounts of sputum	Sputum

CLINICAL ALERT!

Children with pneumonia may also present with abdominal pain and/or vomiting and may complain of headache.[29]

Table 4.12 presents viral and bacterial symptoms in adults.

TABLE 4.12 Viral and bacterial symptoms in adults: clues to aid diagnosis

Viral	Bacterial
Cough (often non-productive)	Sudden onset
Headaches	Chest pain
Fatigue	Breathlessness
Muscle aches and pains	Haemoptysis
Lethargy	Fever
Fever	Productive cough
Breathlessness	Rapid shallow breathing

Causative organisms

Streptococcus pneumoniae is the most frequently identified pathogen in community GP samples, although other commonly reported organisms include *Mycoplasma pneumoniae, Staphylococcus aureus, Haemophilus influenzae* and influenza viruses.[25] Pneumonia caused by *Legionella* is a rare but serious condition and is a leading cause of community-acquired pneumonia with a high risk of complications among hospitalised patients.[30]

CLINICAL ALERT!

Sputum colour may help in determining the causative organism in suspected bacterial pneumonia: *Streptococcus pneumoniae* is associated with a cough productive of rust-coloured sputum:

● pseudomonas, haemophilus, and pneumococcal species may produce green sputum

- *Klebsiella* species pneumonia is associated with a cough productive of red currant-jelly sputum
- anaerobic infections often produce foul-smelling or bad-tasting sputum.[31]

Pathophysiology

The pathophysiology of pneumonia is again extremely complex. When an organism invades the respiratory tract the defence mechanism includes the cough reflex and mucociliary clearance system, which work in conjunction with an influx of macrophages and neutrophils to produce an antibody response to the invading organism. Effective mucociliary clearance is dependent on efficient functioning of the ciliary system and the production of mucus, which in health work together to trap any invading organisms and propel them via the beating of the cilia towards the mouth for expulsion. Protection offered by the mucus-covered ciliated epithelium, which extends from the larynx to the terminal bronchioles, is impaired in many situations such as chronic cigarette smoking, viral respiratory infections, exposure to hot/cold air or harmful gases and old age.[32] Once bacteria have gained entry to the upper airways they move to the lung parenchyma and, during pulmonary infection, acute inflammation results in the migration of neutrophils out of capillaries and into the air spaces, forming a pool of neutrophils that is ready to respond when needed.[31] The whole process has clearly failed when pneumonia develops and a number of factors are associated with increased risk, including the health of the individual and efficiency of their immune system and also the potency and virulence of the invading organism.

Differential diagnosis

 BEWARE OF!

Table 4.13 shows some possible differential diagnoses in adults. Table 4.14 presents differentiation between bronchitis and pneumonia.

TABLE 4.13 Differential diagnoses in adults

Condition	Additional pointers	When to consider
Acute bronchitis	Very difficult to differentiate from other infections.	*See* Table 4.14 for suggested guidance on differentiating bronchitis from pneumonia.
Pulmonary fibrosis	Many patients present with worsening breathlessness and dry cough and possible weight loss.	Consider when history suggests exposure to toxic substances (either fumes, gases or vapours). Also consider in those who have had contact with asbestos silicon or coal and those who have had frequent contact with birds.
PE	p. 20.	p. 20.
Sarcoidosis	Often asymptomatic and found incidentally.	Consider if there is a dry cough with breathlessness.

(continued)

Condition	Additional pointers	When to consider
Drug-induced pulmonary disease	Often considered only after more common conditions have been excluded. Symptoms may include rash, cough and breathlessness.	Consider in patients taking amiodarone, penicillamine, methotrexate gold, and bleomycin. Also consider in heroin or crack cocaine users.
Lung cancer	p. 24.	p. 24.

TABLE 4.14 Differentiating between bronchitis and pneumonia

Bronchitis (acute)	Pneumonia
May have breathlessness, sputum and/or wheeze, but not always present.	Patient will often have one or more symptoms of sputum production, wheezing, breathlessness, and/or chest pain.
The primary symptom is an acute cough, which is usually productive and lasts for less than 3 weeks in 50% of patients, but for more than 1 month in 25% of patients.[33]	There is usually a cough with purulent sputum, fever, pleuritic chest pain, breathlessness on exertion and anorexia.[3]
Patient may complain of generalised muscle aches and pains with a fever.	Elevated temperature of above 38 degrees with additional symptoms including sweating, and generalised muscle aches and pains.

Treatment

Viral pneumonia

ANTIBIOTICS WILL NOT HELP!

Self-help measures include rest, adequate fluids, analgesia to relieve aches and pains and if not eating well, small meals and often.

Bacterial pneumonia

ADULTS

Amoxicillin 500 mg given three times daily (erythromycin 500 mg four times daily or clarithromycin 500 mg twice daily if allergic to penicillin)[16] usually prescribed for 7 days, but longer courses may be needed in some cases.

CHILDREN

Amoxicillin is first line for all ages, but for poorly children a broader spectrum antibiotic such as co-amoxiclav may be needed.[17]

COMPLICATIONS

Potential complications of bacterial pneumonia include the following:

- destruction and fibrosis of the lung parenchyma which may cause scar tissue to form
- empyema
- pulmonary abscess
- respiratory failure

- acute respiratory distress syndrome
- death
- viral pneumonia may progress to bacterial.

CLINICAL ALERT!

Emergency admission to hospital may be needed if the person develops severe chest pains, extreme shortness of breath (either on exertion and/or at rest), dehydration, haemoptysis or severe vomiting.

⚠ BEWARE!

Mortality risk is higher in the presence of:
- rapid respiratory rate
- hypoxia
- anaemia
- pneumonia affecting multiple lobes
- hypotension
- multiple comorbidities.

Key reminders
- If unrecognised and untreated potentially fatal
- Common cause of death in the young and the elderly
- Numerous causative organisms
- Worldwide problem
- Vaccination available.

TUBERCULOSIS (TB)

TB continues to be a problem around the world and is the second biggest killer worldwide due to a single infectious agent, with only HIV/Aids causing more deaths.[35] The disease affects all age groups and statistics indicate that over 95% of deaths occur in low and middle-income countries, with over a million deaths recorded in 2012.[35] In the UK alone there are approximately 9000 new cases of TB each year, the majority occurring in the major cities with a high prevalence rate in London.[36] Although death rates have reduced in recent years the disease continues to be a problem.

TABLE 4.15 Clues to aid the diagnosis of active TB

Symptom	Additional information
Cough	Often have a productive cough with purulent sputum, associated with increasing breathlessness. Tissue damage leads to destruction of pulmonary capillary and the leakage of blood vessels is believed to cause the patient to cough.[37]
Haemoptysis	Haemoptysis common but volume often small.[16]
Fever	Fever is present and patients will complain of night sweats.
Breathlessness	As lung damage progresses, gas exchange may be impaired, leading to hypoxia which manifests itself as dyspnoea.

Pathophysiology

Once inhaled, infectious droplets settle throughout the airways, but the majority of the invading organisms are trapped in the mucus of the upper airways, and at the same time the cilia which line the airways attempt to beat the infectious droplets upwards for expulsion. Any bacteria that manage to bypass the mucociliary system reach the alveoli where they are quickly surrounded and engulfed by alveolar macrophages in a further attempt by the body to ward off any potential infection. Macrophages then attempt to ingest and surround the tubercle bacilli so that a granuloma is formed, which keeps the bacilli contained. For those who are fit and well with healthy immune systems, the granuloma undergo fibrosis and calcification so that the infection is restrained and subsequently remains but is in a dormant state. Once made inactive, the bacteria remain in the body as latent TB, and any patient with latent TB cannot spread the disease.[38] For those whose immune system is impaired, granuloma formation is initiated but fails to prevent spread of the bacilli. The necrotic tissue undergoes liquefaction, and the fibrous wall loses structural integrity so that the semi-liquid necrotic material can then drain into a bronchus or nearby blood vessel, leaving an air-filled cavity at the original site.[39] In those infected with mycoplasma TB, coughing up of droplets enables the spread of infection to others, and if discharge of any necrotic fluid into a blood vessel occurs, the likelihood of the development of TB at other sites is greatly increased. When this occurs the disease has the ability to spread to a variety of extrapulmonary sites by invading lymph nodes and then settling in the bone marrow, liver, spleen, kidneys, bones, or the brain. The most common sites of extrapulmonary disease are mediastinal, retroperitoneal, and cervical lymph nodes, the vertebral bodies, adrenal glands, the meninges, and the gastrointestinal (GI) tract with the pathology underpinning this process similar to that seen in the lungs.[38]

Persons with latent TB have no signs or symptoms of the disease and do not feel unwell.

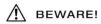 **BEWARE!**

Reactivation of the infection can occur in the presence of:
- impaired immunity (particularly HIV infection)
- use of certain immunosuppressant drugs (e.g. corticosteroids)
- silicosis
- malignancy
- renal insufficiency
- diabetes
- adolescence or advanced age.

TABLE 4.16 Clues to aid the diagnosis of TB at extrapulmonary sites

Site of TB infection	Signs and symptoms
Lymph nodes	Persistent, painless swelling of the lymph nodes, which usually affects nodes in the neck, but can occur in nodes at other sites throughout your body.[40]
Spine	In the active stage, patients present with malaise, loss of weight, loss of appetite, night sweats and evening rise of temperature and the spine is stiff and painful on movement, with localised kyphotic deformity.[41]
Bone and joints	The most common initial symptom of bone TB is pain and there may also be curving of the affected bone or joint, as well as loss of movement and weakening in the affected bone or joint with an increased risk of fracture.[40]
Adrenal glands	Can destroy the adrenal glands, producing symptoms of Addison's disease (muscle weakness, fatigue, loss of appetite and weight loss).[42]
Gastrointestinal tract (GI tract)	The clinical presentation of abdominal tuberculosis can be acute, or chronic with most patients having symptoms of fever, pain, diarrhoea or constipation, or alternating constipation and diarrhoea, weight loss, anorexia and malaise.[43]
Genitourinary tract (GU tract)	Many patients present with lower urinary symptoms typical of bacterial cystitis, and there may also be symptoms of back, flank, and suprapubic pain, haematuria, frequency of micturition and nocturia further suggesting that the problem may be a urinary tract infection.[44]
Central nervous system (CNS)	Greatest prevalence among the immunocompromised and may affect the meninges, brain, or spinal cord.[45]

Diagnosis
- Chest X-ray.
- Minimum of three early morning sputum samples for TB microscopy.
- Treatment should be initiated without confirmation from results if signs and symptoms are highly suspicious of a TB diagnosis.[16]

Differential diagnosis

⚠ BEWARE OF!

- Lung cancer: p. 24
- Community-acquired pneumonia: p. 25
- Fungal lung infections
- Sarcoidosis: p. 27.

CLINICAL ALERT!

- Lung cancer and TB may exist together.
- Community-acquired pneumonia has similar symptoms; sputum analysis will confirm presence of bacteria.
- Fungal lung infections are normally associated with travel to countries where these infections are prevalent (parts of Africa and the US and parts of Mexico).
- Sarcoidosis has similar symptoms and also involves formation of granulomas. Granulomas in sarcoidosis are non-caseating (non-necrotising).

Treatment

NICE Guidance suggests:
- Six months of isoniazid and rifampicin (supplemented in the first 2 months with pyrazinamide and ethambutol) for treatment of active respiratory TB in adults and children.[46]

Prescribing tips
- Risk of side-effects with isoniazid is more likely to occur where the infected patient is also suffering from other comorbid illnesses such as HIV, diabetes or renal failure.
- Several possible side-effects with rifampicin, which have a high incidence.
- Both drugs require monitoring of liver function as both can potentially cause abnormalities.
- Pyrazinamide similarly requires monitoring of liver function.
- Main side-effect of ethambutol is visual disturbances.

Risk of treatment failure
Risk of treatment failure is increased in:
- homeless people (failure to take and/or complete treatment)
- those with HIV infection[47]
- immigrants who have come from parts of the world where drug-resistant strains are common.

Complications
- Spread of TB to other organs

- Pneumothorax
- Coughing up large amounts of blood
- Bronchiectasis.

⚠ **BEWARE!**

The number of drug-resistant cases of TB continues to rise, with a 26% increase in cases between 2010 and 2011.[48] Drug-resistant strains now account for around 10% of deaths from TB.[49]

Key reminders
- Can affect any age
- Worldwide problem
- Greater risk of treatment failure among certain groups
- Drug-resistant strains are increasing
- Continues to cause death, although death rates are reported to be decreasing.

REFERENCES
1. Royal College of General Practitioners. *Respiratory Problems*. RCGP; 2007. Available at: www.rcgp.org.uk/gp-training-and-exams/gp-curriculum-overview/~/media/Files/GP-training-and-exams/Curriculum%20previous%20versions%20as%20at%20July%202012/RCGP-Curriculum-15-8-Respiratory-Problems-2009.ashx (accessed 29 June 2012).
2. Donaldson GC, Keatinge WR. Excess winter mortality: influenza or cold stress? Observational study. *BMJ*. 2002; **324**(7329): 89–90.
3. Simon S, Everitt H, van Dorp F. *Oxford Handbook of General Practice*. Oxford: Oxford University Press; 2010.
4. Derlet RW, Sandrock CE, Nguyen HH, *et al*. *Influenza*. Available at: http://emedicine.medscape.com/article/219557-print (accessed 16 June 2012).
5. Everitt H. Assessing adults who are coughing in primary care. *InnovAiT*. 2008; **1**(3): 216–21.
6. Irwin RS, Boulet LP, Cloutier MM, *et al*. Managing cough as a defence mechanism and as a symptom: a consensus panel report of the American College of Chest Physicians. *Chest*. 1998; **114**(2 Suppl. Managing): S133–81.
7. Morice AH, McGarvey L, Pavord I. On behalf of the British Thoracic Society Cough Guideline Group: recommendations for the management of cough in adults. *Thorax*. 2006; **61**(Suppl. I): i1–24.
8. D'Urzo A, Jugovic P. Chronic cough. Three most common causes. *Can Fam Physician*. 2002; **48**(8): 1311–16.
9. National Heart, Lung, and Blood Institute. *National Asthma Education and Prevention Program. Expert Panel Report 3: guidelines for the diagnosis and management of asthma*. 2007. Available at: www.nhlbi.nih.gov/guidelines/asthma/asthgdln.htm (accessed 19 July 2012).
10. Camargo CA, Rachelefsky G, Schatz M. Managing asthma exacerbations in the emergency department: summary of the national asthma education and prevention program

expert panel report: guidelines for the management of asthma exacerbations. *J Allergy Clin Immunol.* 2009; **124**(2 Suppl.): S5–14.

11. Pollart SM, Comptom RM, Elward KS. Management of acute asthma exacerbations. *Am Fam Physician.* 2011; **84**(1): 40–7.
12. Morris MJ. Asthma. Available at: http://emedicine.medscape.com/article/296301-overview#aw2aab6b2b4 (accessed 10 June 2013).
13. Barnes P. Pathophysiology of asthma. *Eur Respir Mon.* 2003; **23**: 84–113.
14. British Thoracic Society/Scottish Intercollegiate Guidelines Network. *British Guideline on the Management of Asthma: A National Clinical Guideline.* BTS/SIGN guideline 101. BTS/SIGN; 2008. Revised 2012. Available at: www.sign.ac.uk/pdf/qrg101.pdf
15. British National Formulary. 2013. Available at: www.bnf.org/bnf/index.htm
16. Chapman S, Robinson G, Stradling J, *et al. Oxford Handbook of Respiratory Medicine.* 2nd ed. Oxford: Oxford University Press; 2006.
17. Hull J, Forton J, Thomson A. *Paediatric Respiratory Medicine.* 2nd ed. Oxford: Oxford University Press; 2009.
18. Celli BR, Vestbo J. The EXACT-Pro: measuring exacerbations of COPD. *Am J Resp Crit Care Med.* 2011; **183**(3): 287–8.
19. Donaldson GC, Seemungal TAR, Bhowmik A, *et al.* Relationship between exacerbation frequency and lung function decline in chronic obstructive pulmonary disease. *Thorax.* 2002; **57**: 847–52.
20. Soler-Cataluna JJ, Martinez-Garcia MA, Roman Sanchez P, *et al.* Severe acute exacerbations and mortality in patients with chronic obstructive pulmonary disease. *Thorax.* 2005; **60**: 925–31.
21. Stockley RA, O'Brien C, Pye A, *et al.* Relationship of sputum colour to nature and outpatient management of acute exacerbations of COPD. *Chest.* 2000; **117**: 1638–45.
22. White AJ, Gompertz S, Stockley RA. Chronic obstructive pulmonary disease: the aetiology of exacerbations of chronic obstructive pulmonary disease. *Thorax.* 2003; **58**(1): 73–80.
23. Soler N, Torres A, Ewig S, *et al.* Bronchial microbial patterns in severe exacerbations of chronic obstructive pulmonary disease (COPD) requiring mechanical ventilation. *Am J Respir Crit Care Med.* 1998; **157**: 1498–1505.
24. Saetta M, Turato G, Maestrelli P, *et al.* Cellular and structural bases of chronic obstructive pulmonary disease. *Am J Respir Crit Care Med.* 2001; **163**: 1304–9.
25. Scottish Intercollegiate Guidelines Network. *Community Management of Lower Respiratory Tract Infection in Adults.* SIGN guideline 59. Edinburgh: SIGN; 2002. Available at: www.sign.ac.uk/guidelines/fulltext/59/references.html#55
26. World Health Organization. *Pneumonia. Fact sheet 331.* Available at: www.who.int/mediacentre/factsheets/fs331/en/ (accessed 20 June 2012).
27. Cartwright K. Pneumococcal disease in Western Europe: burden of disease, antibiotic resistance and management. *Eur J Pediatr.* 2002; **16**: 188–95.
28. El-Solh AA, Sikka P, Ramadan F, *et al.* Etiology of severe pneumonia in the very elderly. *Am J Respir Crit Care Med.* 2001; **163**: 645–51.
29. British Thoracic Society. Guidelines for the management of community acquired pneumonia in children: update 2011. *Thorax.* 2011; **66**(Suppl. 2): ii1–23.
30. File TM. Community-acquired pneumonia. *Lancet.* 2003; **362**: 1991–2001.
31. Kamangar N. *Bacterial Pneumonia.* Available at: http://emedicine.medscape.com/article/300157-overview#a0104 (accessed 7 June 2012).
32. Singh YD. *Pathophysiology of Community Acquired Pneumonia.* Available at: www.japi.org/january_special_2012/03_pathophysiology_of_community.pdf (accessed 2 July 2012).
33. Worrall G. Acute bronchitis. *Can Fam Physician.* 2008; **54**(2): 238–9.

34. Karnath B, Boyars MC. *Pulmonary Auscultation*. Available at: www.turner-white.com/pdf/hp_jan02_pulmonary.pdf (accessed 5 July 2013).

35. World Health Organization. *Tuberculosis. Factsheet No 4*. Available at: www.who.int/mediacentre/factsheets/fs104/en/ (accessed 7 June 2013).

36. Health Protection Agency. *Tuberculosis*. Available at: www.hpa.org.uk/Topics/InfectiousDiseases/InfectionsAZ/Tuberculosis/ (accessed 10 June 2013).

37. Virtual Medicine. *Pathophysiology behind Classical Symptoms of Pulmonary TB (Pathology)*. Available at: http://virtualmedic.wordpress.com/2011/07/17/pathophysiology-behind-classical-symptoms-of-pulmonary-tuberculosis-pathology/ (accessed 25 April 2013).

38. Herchline T. *Tuberculosis*. Available at: http://emedicine.medscape.com/article/230802-overview (accessed 8 June 2012).

39. Knechel NA. Tuberculosis: pathophysiology, clinical features and diagnosis. *Crit Care Nurse.* 2009; **29**(2). Available at: www.aacn.org/WD/CETests/Media/C0923.pdf (accessed 24 April 2013).

40. NHS Choices. *Tuberculosis (TB) Symptoms*. Available at: www.nhs.uk/Conditions/Tuberculosis/Pages/Symptoms.aspx

41. Agrawal V, Patgaonkar PR, Nagariya SP. Tuberculosis of spine. *J Craniovertebr Junction Spine.* 2010; **1**(2): 74–85.

42. National Institute of Diabetes Digestive and Kidney Diseases. *Adrenal Insufficiency and Addison's Disease*. Available at: http://endocrine.niddk.nih.gov/pubs/addison/addison.aspx (accessed 27 April 2013).

43. Sharma MP, Bhatia V. Abdominal tuberculosis. *Indian J Med Res.* 2004; **120**: 305–15.

44. Eastwood JB, Corbishley CM, Grange JM. Tuberculosis and the kidney. *JASN.* 2001; **12**(6): 1307–14.

45. Joshua Burrill J, Williams CJ, Gillian Bain G, *et al.* Tuberculosis: a radiologic review. *RadioGraphics.* 2007; **27**: 1255–73.

46. National Institute for Health and Clinical Excellence. *Tuberculosis: NICE guideline 117*. London: NIHCE; 2011. Available at: http://guidance.nice.org.uk/CG117/NICEGuidance/pdf/English

47. Khan FA, Minion J, Pai M, *et al.* Treatment of active tuberculosis in HIV-coinfected patients: a systematic review and meta-analysis. *Clin Infect Dis.* 2010; **50**(9): 1288–99.

48. Health Protection Agency. *Drug-resistant TB*. Available at: www.hpa.org.uk/webw/HPAweb&HPAwebStandard/HPAweb_C/1317134905749?p=1317132140479 (accessed 12 June 2012).

49. Houses of Parliament. *Drug-resistant TB*. Parliamentary Office of Science and Technology. Available at: www.parliament.uk/briefing-papers/POST-PN-416 (accessed 8 June 2012).

CHAPTER 5

Cardiology

INTRODUCTION

Cardiovascular disease (CVD) is a major problem, is prevalent around the world and is estimated to account for nearly half of all deaths in Europe (48%).[1] Becoming increasingly prevalent in developing countries, recent statistics indicate CVD now contributes to approximately 80% of deaths in low and middle-income countries.[2] Risk factors have been extensively researched and many are known to be modifiable, yet despite this the prevalence of CVD continues to rise and it is estimated that by 2030 more than 23 million people will be dying from these diseases annually around the world.[3]

CONDITIONS COVERED IN THE CHAPTER
- Atrial fibrillation (AF)
- Hypertension
- Angina
- Heart failure (HF).

COMMON PRESENTING SYMPTOMS

May present with one or several of the following:
- chest pain
- breathlessness
- ankle swelling
- palpitations
- dizziness.

TAKING THE CARDIAC HISTORY

Initial history is as described in Chapter 3, followed by a focused enquiry relating to the cardiac system.

TABLE 5.1 Symptoms enquiry and further questioning for specific symptoms

Symptom	Further questioning
Chest pain	Use OPQRST (see Chapter 3) to get more information.
Breathlessness	Breathless on exertion, at rest or both?
	Waking at night gasping for breath?
	Sleeping with several pillows as unable to lie flat?
	Are there other symptoms (coughing or wheezing) in addition to breathlessness?
Ankle swelling	Are both ankles swollen?
	Are they only swollen at the end of the day?
	On examination can a dent be left in the ankle when pressure is applied?
Palpitations	How fast is the heart beating?
	Is the heart rate regular or irregular?
	Can patient associate the onset with anything in particular?
	Are there any other symptoms when palpitations occur such as feeling dizzy or faint?
	What does patient do during attacks?

Table 5.2 shows a summary of presenting signs and symptoms and the diseases they may suggest. Each symptom will then be discussed in more detail in the context of each disease.

TABLE 5.2 Presenting signs and symptoms

	Chest pain	Breathlessness	Ankle swelling	Palpitations
AF	Possible	Possible	No	Yes
Hypertension	No	No	No	No
HF	No	Yes	Possible	Possible
Angina	Yes	Yes	No	Possible (see clinical alert below)

CLINICAL ALERT!

Palpitations associated with angina may indicate myocardial ischaemia precipitated by increased oxygen demand, which can occur secondary to a rapid heart rate.[4]

ADDITIONAL INFORMATION

- Does the patient look unwell?
- Are they breathless?
- Examine the hands to assess for finger clubbing and cyanosis, staining of the fingers from smoking.
- Are the ankles or feet oedematous?
- Record pulse rate, blood pressure and respiratory rate.

FURTHER INVESTIGATIONS

Investigations should be chosen on the basis of the history and symptoms, including the duration of symptoms and the overall clinical picture.

Other investigations

Other investigations selected on the basis of history, symptoms and clinical findings:
- electrocardiograph (ECG)
- 24-hour blood pressure monitoring
- chest X-ray
- bloods.

REFERRAL TO A CARDIOLOGIST REQUIRED

- Worsening symptoms
- Unstable angina
- Uncontrolled hypertension
- Abnormal heart rhythms
- Treatment failure
- Any patient requiring emergency intervention, e.g. cardioversion for unstable AF.

ATRIAL FIBRILLATION (AF)

AF is reported to be the commonest cardiac arrhythmia, with prevalence rates roughly doubling with each advancing decade of age,[5] affecting as many as 18% of people aged 85 or older.[6] Despite advances in treatment and management, the condition remains a significant cause of morbidity and mortality.

Clues to aid the diagnosis

The condition can be asymptomatic and the presence of an irregular pulse is frequently an incidental finding detected on clinical examination.

The commonest symptoms reported are:
- a feeling of chest discomfort
- dizziness

- breathlessness
- palpitations
- malaise
- reduced exercise tolerance.

Diagnosis and investigations

ECG is needed in both symptomatic and asymptomatic patients. Further testing should include:
- chest X-ray
- ECG
- FBC
- urea and electrolytes (U&Es)
- thyroid function tests (TFTs)
- liver function tests (LFTs).

Types of AF

Table 5.3 shows the classification of AF.

TABLE 5.3 Classification of AF

Type	Additional information
Paroxysmal AF	May return to normal rhythm but problem may recur. Symptoms usually resolve within 7 days, but often the time to recovery is less than this.[7] Paroxysmal AF can change to become persistent of permanent AF (*see* information below).
Persistent AF	AF is regarded as persistent when an episode of AF lasts longer than 7 days and becomes long-standing when symptoms last for 1 year or more.[8]
Permanent AF	AF is regarded as permanent when it is not possible to get the rhythm to revert to sinus rhythm. When episodes of paroxysmal AF last for 2 days or less, conversion to permanent AF occurs in 31% of patients, increasing to 46% when episodes persist for 2 days or more.[9]
Lone AF	Lone AF has been used to describe AF in younger patients where there is no association with comorbidities or obvious cardiac disease.[10]

CLINICAL ALERT!

 BEWARE!

Patients with a first presentation of AF and comorbidities are at higher risk for rapid progression to permanent AF, with older age, diabetes and HF also regarded as independent predictors of risk.[11]

Pathophysiology

AF is associated with a number of conditions: diabetes, hypertension, coronary heart disease (CHD), HF and valvular heart problems,[5] although the mechanism by which these conditions increase the risk is poorly understood. In the healthy heart the sinoatrial node sends electrical impulses at regular intervals, which spread through the atria, causing them to contract at regular intervals. The electrical impulse then reaches the atrioventricular node which carries the impulse to the ventricles, stimulating them to contract and forcing blood out into the major blood vessels for passage around the body. In AF this mechanism goes wrong and impulses are fired in an erratic fashion, resulting in rapid irregular contraction of the atria with a similar effect on the ventricles.

Differential diagnosis

Table 5.4 presents differential diagnoses for AF.

TABLE 5.4 Differential diagnoses: beware of!

Condition	Additional pointers	When to consider
Paroxysmal supraventricular tachycardia	More common in women, but can occur in men and it is the most common arrhythmia in children.[12]	If there are symptoms of chest discomfort or pressure: dyspnoea, fatigue, light-headedness or dizziness, and palpitations.[13]
Atrial flutter	Signs and symptoms may include palpitations, rapid heart rate, chest pain, shortness of breath, light-headedness, fatigue, and low blood pressure; may also be asymptomatic.[14] Detected on ECG.	Prevalence increases with age so consider in older adults; also occurs more frequently in those with known heart disease or comorbidities.[15]
Atrial tachycardia	Very rapid heart rate, which may exceed 100 beats per minute. Detected on ECG.	Consider in patients with palpitations, dizziness, shortness of breath and chest pain (similar symptoms to supraventricular tachycardia).[12]
Wolff–Parkinson–White syndrome	Condition involves an extra (accessory) electrical pathway between the atria and the ventricles present at birth, but the arrhythmias it causes usually become apparent during the teens or early twenties, but can occur at any age.[16] Detected on ECG.	If asymptomatic will complain of feeling light-headed, having palpitations and possible syncope, but may be asymptomatic.[17]

Treatment aims

Treatment depends on the type of AF. There are two aims: rate control or rhythm control. Treatment to control heart rate can be initiated in primary care, but treatment to control heart rhythm requires specialist intervention.

Guidance suggests urgent referral to cardiologist required for any patient with any of the following complications:[18]

- a very rapid pulse
- associated symptoms of chest pain and/or breathlessness
- altered level of consciousness
- suspicion of underlying abnormality requiring specialist intervention (e.g. Wolff–Parkinson–White syndrome)
- presence of comorbidities, such as transient ischaemic attacks (TIAs), HF.

Non-urgent referral

Non-urgent referral is required for:[19]

- younger patients
- suspected paroxysmal AF
- contraindication to prescribed drugs for rate control
- failure to control heart rate with treatment prescribed
- continued symptoms despite treatment implemented in primary care.

Treatment

There are a number of guidelines for the suggested treatment and management of AF, but the underlying aim across all of them is that of reducing symptoms, improving quality of life, and preventing complications, some of which are potentially life threatening. Prevention of complications relies on antithrombotic therapy, control of heart rate and additional optimal treatment of any additional cardiac diseases,[18] which can be commenced in primary care. There are several guidelines relating to the use of rate control or rhythm control, but the decision to use either strategy is generally based on multiple factors including AF type, severity of symptoms, comorbidities and patient preference. Rate control is often more suitable for asymptomatic, older patients with CHD and contraindications to antiarrhythmic drugs,[20] while rhythm control may be more appropriate for patients whose symptoms are severe or persistent[21] and this can be attempted with cardioversion, drug treatment or ablation, but all of the latter options are instigated in secondary care. If patient is suitable for treatment in primary care, assessment of stroke risk and commencement of anticoagulation therapy are key, as implementing this treatment has been shown to reduce mortality rates.[8]

CLINICAL ALERT!

The urgency for antithrombotic treatment is based on the concerns that AF is a major risk factor for stroke, making a person five times more likely to have a stroke.[21]

Assessment of stroke risk

There are now tools available to help clinicians in their assessment of stroke risk and the CHA2DS2-VASc Calculator (*see* Table 5.5) is an updated version of the earlier CHADS2 risk calculator which has been found to significantly increase the percentage of patients indicated for anticoagulation.[22]

TABLE 5.5 CHA2DS2-VASc Calculator[23] Reprinted with kind permission

Criteria	Yes	No
Congestive heart failure	+1	0
Hypertension	+1	0
Age 75 years or older	+2	0
Diabetes	+1	0
Stroke or transient ischaemic attacks (TIA)	+2	0
History of vascular disease	+1	0
Age 65–74	+1	0
Sex (female gender carries higher risk)	+1	0

Those with a CHA2DS2-VASc score of 2 or more are at a high risk of stroke and should receive oral anticoagulation, whereas those with a CHA2DS2-VASc score of 1 are at moderate risk.[24]

Anticoagulation therapy

Patients at low risk of stroke may be treated with aspirin while an increasing stroke risk favours treatment with the more effective warfarin.[25] Clopidogrel is an alternative for patients who are intolerant to or unsuitable for aspirin. Dabigatran is a new treatment recently approved for use and is recommended for patients with a history of stroke, TIA or embolism in the past, heart failure, aged 75 or older or 65 and over with comorbidities, e.g. hypertension, CHD or diabetes.[26]

Drug treatment for rate control commenced in primary care

Table 5.6 shows suggested drug treatments.

TABLE 5.6 Suggested drug treatments

Drug class	Additional information	Prescribing tips
Beta-blockers, e.g. bisoprolol	May cause fatigue, coldness of the extremities and sometimes nightmares.[27]	Useful for patients with ischaemic heart disease (IHD) but unsuitable for patients with asthma or severe unstable HF failure.[28]
Calcium channel blockers (CCBs) (e.g. verapamil and diltiazem)	May also improve exercise tolerance.[29]	Unsuitable for patients with left ventricular dysfunction (LV) and bradycardia.[30]
Digoxin	For elderly less active patients digoxin may be sufficient as monotherapy or it may be added to either a beta-blocker or a CCB as a second-line therapy.[19]	Digoxin can cause toxicity if dose is too high, with symptoms of nausea, vomiting, diarrhoea, abdominal pain, confusion, dizziness, agitation, arrhythmias, heart block and various visual symptoms.[31] Toxicity is confirmed by high drug levels on blood testing.

CLINICAL ALERT!

Beta and rate-limiting calcium antagonists (e.g. diltiazem or verapamil) are often effective as initial monotherapy for rate control, but a combination of drugs is often necessary to achieve adequate rate control.[29]

Target heart rate

Guidance from the Royal College of Physicians has suggested a target heart rate of below 90 bpm at rest and below 80 bpm during exercise in patients with atrial fibrillation.[32]

Where rate control fails or symptoms persist, referral to secondary care for further assessment is recommended.

Complications
- HF: rapid ventricular rate leads to poor filling of the ventricles and subsequent reduced cardiac output leading to LVF.
- Cardiomyopathy: caused by the rapid rate at which the ventricles contract.
- Stroke: this is the most frequent complication of AF.

Key reminders
- Increases in prevalence with increased age
- Erratic heart rate may be an incidental finding
- May be asymptomatic
- Major risk factor for stroke.

HYPERTENSION

Hypertension or high blood pressure is usually asymptomatic, but it is linked to the development of a number of conditions, some of which have potentially fatal outcomes. The incidence increases with age and current estimates suggest that approximately 40% of adults in England have the condition,[33] but more worryingly there may be as many as five million adults with undiagnosed hypertension.[34] Hypertension is the single most important modifiable risk factor for ischaemic stroke,[35] but risk appears to increase further when combined with other risk factors and there is now evidence to suggest that approximately 60%–80% of all ischaemic strokes can be attributed to increasing blood pressure, in combination with elevated blood cholesterol levels, cigarette smoking, carotid stenosis, and diabetes mellitus.[36]

Target blood pressure
- Healthy adult with none of the problems below: 140/90.
- Diabetic: insulin-dependent BP 130/80 or below.[37]
- Diabetic: non-insulin dependent BP 130/80 or below.[38]
- CKD non-diabetic: 140/90 or below.[39]
- CKD diabetic: either insulin or non-insulin dependent target 130/80 or below.[39]

Clues to aid the diagnosis
Hypertension is frequently asymptomatic, which is reflected in the number of patients who are undiagnosed and untreated.

Confirming the diagnosis
Current guidance now advocates that hypertension is diagnosed following 24-hour ambulatory blood pressure (ABPM) recording rather than on measurements recorded in the clinic.[40] This should be offered to all patients with first and second BP measurements taken during consultations, which are both recorded at higher than 140/90 mmHg.

Antihypertensive treatment
Antihypertensive treatment should then be offered to:
- patients in whom initial clinic systolic BP exceeds 160 mmHg and/or diastolic BP exceeds 100 mmHg and subsequent ABPM daytime average or HBPM average is 150/95 mmHg or higher[41]
- patients with initial clinic BP of 140/90 mmHg or higher and subsequent ABPM daytime average or HBPM average of 135/85 mmHg or higher who also have established CVD, target organ damage, renal disease, diabetes or a 10-year CVD risk equal to or greater than 20% also require treatment.[41]

Additional assessment

As part of the initial assessment it is recommended that the following tests are also undertaken to determine the presence of conditions not yet diagnosed and also to assess for the presence of target organ damage.

- Urine dipstick testing for blood and protein
- U&Es
- Blood glucose levels
- Lipids and triglyceride levels
- 12-lead ECG.

CLINICAL ALERT!

- When reviewing the above it is important to remember that proteinuria, microscopic haematuria, and reduced eGFR are frequently asymptomatic but are key indicators of kidney damage.[42]
- High BP and hyperlipidaemia often exist together and are associated with increased cardiovascular risk.[43]

Pathophysiology

The mechanism underpinning hypertension is highly complex and is still not fully understood, but in some cases there may be an underlying or contributing cause (*see* Table 5.7).

BP readings are reported as two numbers: the top is the systolic and the bottom the diastolic. Systolic measurements indicate the pressure in the arteries when the heart muscle contracts; the diastolic figure measures pressure in the arteries when the heart muscle is resting and refilling. Where a cause cannot be identified the condition is labelled 'essential hypertension'. Normal BP levels are achieved with the help of a number of physiological mechanisms and it is thought that essential hypertension develops when these mechanisms go wrong. Maintenance of a normal BP is dependent on the balance between the cardiac output and peripheral vascular resistance. In younger hypertensives, the cardiac output is often elevated, while in older patients there is increased systemic vascular resistance.[44] The autonomic nervous system also plays an important role in the control of BP and in hypertensive patients, both increased release of, and enhanced peripheral sensitivity to norepinephrine can be found and there is also an increased responsiveness to stressful stimuli.[44]

TABLE 5.7 Other causes of hypertension

Possible cause	Additional information
Abnormal excretion of sodium	Abnormality in the excretion of sodium, leading to sodium retention.
Excess dietary intake of salt	A diet high in salt is thought to induce raised blood pressure by increasing fluid volume which then increases cardiac output.
Chronic mental stress	Negative influences that may manifest as depression, anxiety, anger, or hostility, have been associated with the development of hypertension.[45]
Obesity	Hypertension is more common among obese people and its prevalence increases with increased body mass index (BMI), level of upper body obesity and fasting insulin levels.
Insulin resistance	Insulin resistance frequently occurs in obese people but can also occasionally occur in non-obese individuals.
Baroreceptor dysfunction	When activated by a rise in BP, baroreceptors normally reduce heart rate and BP by inhibition of the sympathetic nervous system and vagal stimulation.[46] Dysfunction of this mechanism is therefore thought to lead to perpetuation of hypertension.

Treatment of hypertension
Lifestyle modification
WEIGHT REDUCTION
Weight loss has been studied extensively for its effect on reducing blood pressure. One study reported that a weight loss of 8 kg in moderately obese individuals led to significant decreases in BP.[47]

REDUCED SALT INTAKE
Reduced sodium intake has been shown to be effective in lowering BP measurements but may also play a role in preventing the condition. One clinical trial reported that subjects who continued sodium reduction 10–15 years after the trial ended experienced a 25%–30% lower risk of cardiovascular outcomes.[48]

SMOKING CESSATION
Smoking cessation has been found to reduce systolic BP and heart rate during the daytime, when patients typically smoke, a process thought to occur as a result of reduced sympathetic nervous system activity.[49]

REDUCED ALCOHOL
There is a suspected dose–response relationship between mean percentage of alcohol reduction and mean BP reduction, with the effects of intervention more marked in those with higher baseline BP readings,[50] suggesting that alcohol reduction should form an important component of lifestyle modification for the prevention and treatment of hypertension among those whose alcohol intake is above the recommended levels.

HEALTHY DIET

The effects of three healthy diets were compared, each with reduced saturated fat intake, for their effect on blood pressure and serum lipids. The most successful outcomes were found among those participants whose diet involved partial substitution of carbohydrates with either protein or monounsaturated fat, which resulted in lower BP readings, improved lipid levels, and reduced estimated CVD risk.[51]

Pharmacological treatment

ACE INHIBITORS

ACE inhibitors are now recommended as first line to those under 55 years of age and are particularly beneficial for treating hypertension in diabetic patients, especially those with type 1 diabetes and/or diabetic nephropathy, because they reduce proteinuria and slow the rate of deterioration in renal function.[52]

ANGIOTENSIN RECEPTOR BLOCKERS (ARBS)

Offer an alternative to ACE inhibitors for those patients intolerant of ACE inhibitors, although ACE inhibitors remain the drugs of choice for patients with HF, LV dysfunction after MI, and diabetic nephropathy.[53]

CCBS

Drugs of this class are recommended for patients over 55 or those of black African Caribbean ethnicity and have been shown to be effective in treating hypertension in patients of black African Caribbean ethnicity and also in those aged 55 or older.[54] They may also be an alternative for those patients who develop side-effects from ACE inhibitors or in those who have contraindications to their use.

COMBINATION TREATMENT

Patients often require more than one medication to achieve optimal BP and current guidance indicates a combination of an ace inhibitor (or ARB if ACE not tolerated) in addition to a CCB, or substitution of a thiazide diuretic can be tried if either ACE or CCB is not tolerated or is contraindicated.[41]

DIURETICS

When BP continues to be inadequately controlled with two agents the addition of a diuretic may be needed (e.g. indapamide). The addition of a diuretic is generally offered after the above two steps have been taken, although there is the option to offer one of these drugs earlier if a CCB is inappropriate (either because of intolerance, oedema or risk of HF).[55]

FURTHER TREATMENT

If BP continues to be above target, suggested options are to add in a low dose of spironolactone, or increase dose of the diuretic, but if these options are poorly tolerated or contraindicated an alpha blocker (e.g. doxazosin) or beta-blocker (e.g. atenolol) may be used.[41]

TABLE 5.8 Prescribing tips

Drug	Additional information
ACE inhibitors	Can cause hypotension with the first dose and are therefore best given at night initially. A dry, tickly cough is the most common adverse effect of ACE inhibitors, and studies have indicated that cough may develop in around 10% of those treated with ACE inhibitors.[56]
ARBs	Should be used in caution in patients with renal artery stenosis, and they may not benefit patients of African Caribbean origin, particularly those with LVF.[30]
CCBs	Associated with peripheral oedema which is thought to be both compound-specific and dose-dependent, with more potent CCBs like amlodipine associated with higher rates of oedema than a lower-potency CCB like diltiazem.[57]
Diuretics	Can cause alterations in glucose and lipid profiles and hypokalemia and can also increase the incidence of new-onset diabetes, especially when combined with beta-blockers; therefore, caution is advised in using these drugs in patients at high risk for developing diabetes.[58]
Aldosterone antagonists (e.g. spironolactone)	Can be used if serum potassium is below 4.5 mmol/L but used with caution if eGFR is low, and monitoring of U&Es is needed as may cause hyperkalaemia.[55]
Alpha blockers (e.g. doxazosin)	Useful for patients with benign prostatic hypertrophy, but should be used with caution in patients with a history of postural hypotension or HF and are contraindicated in patients with urinary incontinence.[59]
Beta-blockers	p. 43

Monitoring renal function

 BEWARE!

Certain classes of antihypertensive medications can interfere with U&E levels and may cause a fall in glomerular filtration rate and a rise in serum creatinine levels.[60]

Baseline measurement of renal function is therefore needed before treatment is commenced to assess for any previously unknown problems and also to allow any change to be monitored.

Table 5.9 shows drug classes and suggested frequency of monitoring.

TABLE 5.9 Drug classes and suggested frequency of monitoring

Drug	Suggested monitoring
ACE inhibitors	Baseline measurement, then repeat 2 weeks after increasing the dose and at each subsequent dose increase.[61]
ARBs	As above.
Thiazide diuretics (e.g. indapamide) and loop diuretics (e.g. frusemide)	At baseline then 4–6 weeks after starting treatment with further testing if patient's condition changes or additional potentially interacting drugs are added.[62]
Aldosterone antagonists (e.g. spironolactone)	At baseline then every 5–7 days until optimal dose and potassium values are stable then 6–12 monthly for low-risk patients, more frequently if elderly or there is renal or cardiac dysfunction.[63]

CLINICAL ALERT!

Once patient is stable and antihypertensive treatment is established, monitoring of U&Es should continue to be undertaken every 6–12 months or earlier if any problems arise.

Complications

Undetected and untreated, hypertension has serious consequences and has been described as a silent killer. Even in those with mild to moderate hypertension there is a risk of developing atherosclerosis in approximately 30% of sufferers and 50% will develop end organ damage within 8–10 years of onset.[64] The number of organs which can potentially be affected is numerous with effects ranging from reduced quality of life to a fatal outcome.

Table 5.10 shows organs which may be affected.

TABLE 5.10 Organs which may be affected

Organ/vessels affected	Likely	Additional information
Arteries	Atherosclerosis Angina MI Aneurism	Consistently raised BP has several effects, including thickening of the arteries and the risk of plaque or fatty deposits forming within the blood vessels leading to atherosclerosis. When the coronary arteries are affected the patient may develop angina, irregular heart rhythm or suffer an MI. The constant pressure of blood flowing through an already weakened artery may lead to enlargement and bulging of the vessel resulting in a potentially life-threatening aneurysm, and if the vessel ruptures may cause massive internal bleeding.

(continued)

Organ/vessels affected	Likely	Additional information
Heart	LVF HF	In patients with hypertension, the risk of HF is increased twofold in men and threefold in women.[64] Over time increased BP causes the heart to pump harder to send blood around the body, which results in weakening of the heart muscle. The left ventricle becomes enlarged with thickening of the muscle, increasing the risk of HF.
Brain	TIA Stroke	Hypertension is the single most important risk factor for stroke, thought to cause about 50% of ischaemic strokes.[65] As well as causing blockage to arteries supplying the brain, high BP can also cause rupture or leakage of vessels resulting in haemorrhagic stroke.
	Cognitive impairment	Hypertension is associated with an increased risk of cognitive decline though the mechanism underpinning this is unclear.[66]
Kidneys	Nephropathy Renal failure	Damage can occur to the arteries and the glomeruli, resulting in poor filtration of waste products and impaired excretion with fluid retention. A consistently raised BP is one of the leading causes of kidney failure.[67]
Eyes	Retinopathy	Hypertension has a range of effects on the eye, including retinopathy, which is predictive of stroke, HF and cardiovascular mortality.[68]
	Damaged optic nerve	Blockage to blood flow can cause damage to the optic nerve, resulting in poor vision or loss of vision.
	Fluid behind the retina	Leakage of fluid may cause fluid to collect behind the retina, leading to impaired vision.

CLINICAL ALERT!

 BEWARE!

Death from IHD or stroke increases progressively as BP increases, with the mortality rate for both IHD and stroke doubling for every 20 mmHg systolic or 10 mmHg diastolic increase in BP above 115/75 mmHg.[69]

Key reminders
- Asymptomatic
- Large numbers of affected adults undetected and untreated
- Associated with numerous complications
- High risk of IHD, renal damage, stroke and LVF if untreated.

ANGINA

Studies carried out across the UK have reported various prevalence rates for angina in the UK, but the condition is considered to be relatively common, affecting approximately 9.2% of men aged 55–64, and 16.2% of men aged 65–74, with rates of 4% and 6.8% reported in women in the same age groups.[70] When the condition is poorly treated, symptoms can have an impact on the patient's ability to carry out daily living activities, therefore reducing quality of life, and it can potentially have a fatal outcome. People of South Asian origin in the UK have an increased risk of IHD, while people of black Caribbean ethnicity have a lower risk compared to that of the overall UK population, with higher rates found among both men and women in lower socio-economic groups.[71]

Clues to aid the diagnosis

The patient frequently reports episodes of chest discomfort, typically associated with exertion, although symptoms may occur at rest. Patients will use different terminology to describe the pain and may report radiation to shoulders, neck, arms or to the jaw and may also complain of breathlessness during attacks.

CLINICAL ALERT!

- Dementia may mean the patient has difficulty in reporting their symptoms.
- Angina can also exist in a pain-free form where the patient presents complaining of nausea, shortness of breath and/or abdominal pain.[72]

Pathophysiology

Angina develops when the flow of blood through the coronary arteries is reduced, a problem frequently caused by a build-up of plaque in damaged arteries, which may lead to either partial blockage of vessels and resulting angina pain, or total blockage leading to a subsequent heart attack. The process underlying the development of plaque is highly complex.

Differential diagnosis

Table 5.11 presents differential diagnoses.

TABLE 5.11 Differential diagnoses: beware of!

Condition	Additional pointers	When to consider
Aortic stenosis	Similar symptoms to angina with chest pain on exertion, dizziness and reduced exercise tolerance.	Patient reports a gradual onset of their symptoms with breathlessness on exertion one of the symptoms noticed first.
GORD	May have a chronic cough and associated symptoms of a burning sensation spreading from the stomach up to the chest.	Consider if symptoms are not associated with exercise.
Aortic dissection	Abrupt onset of severe pain in the chest, back or abdomen, but patient may also experience shortness of breath, pain in the arms or legs, weakness, or loss of consciousness.[73]	Consider if onset is sudden, patient is over age 50 and is hypertensive as 70% of those affected are hypertensive.[74]
Pneumothorax	p. 20.	p. 20.
Anxiety and panic attacks	Anxious, nervous patients. Pain not related to activity.	Patient is having palpitations alongside their chest pain.
Mitral valve problems	Chest pain if experienced is less severe, but there are shared symptoms of shortness of breath, with exertion or when lying flat.	Consider when symptoms include fatigue, dizziness, palpitations and sometimes cough.[75]
Pericarditis	Pain described as stabbing and may worsen during coughing, taking a deep breath and sometimes when swallowing.	Consider when patient reports that pain improves with leaning forward or sitting upright.
PE	p. 20.	p. 20.

Treatment

CLINICAL ALERT!

 BEWARE!

- Risk factors for CHD, including hypertension, diabetes mellitus, obesity, and hyperlipidaemia, should be treated.
- Smoking cessation where needed should be a key component of management as this has been shown to result in a significant reduction in acute adverse effects and may reverse, or at least slow, atherosclerosis.[76]

Stable angina

First-line treatment is to commence a short-acting nitrate, e.g. glycerol trinitrate (GTN).[71]

- Patient should be advised to use before any activity which may bring on symptoms.
- Dose can be repeated after 5 minutes if symptoms are not resolved, but patient should be advised to seek medical advice if pain persists after the second dose.
- GTN may cause throbbing headaches and dizziness.[30]

Additional treatment

Before prescribing further treatment it is important to take into consideration comorbidities and contraindications to ensure an appropriate treatment is prescribed. Current guidance suggests further addition of either a beta-blocker or CCB, both of which are effective in reducing symptoms, which they achieve by reducing myocardial demand for oxygen.[77]

- A beta-blocker and CCB can be prescribed together if symptoms remain uncontrolled on one of these drugs.
- If the above cannot be prescribed in combination either because of adverse effects or contraindications, a long-acting nitrate (such as nicorandil) can be considered. However, while long-acting nitrates are effective anti-anginal drugs during initial treatment, their effectiveness is compromised by the rapid development of tolerance during sustained therapy, which means that their clinical efficacy is decreased during long-term use.[78]

CLINICAL ALERT!

Beta-blockers, CCBs and nitrates are all effective in reducing angina symptoms, i.e. prolonging the duration of exercise before the onset of angina and reducing the frequency of angina, but none has been shown to prevent MI or death in people being treated for chronic stable angina.[79]

Additional therapy for secondary prevention

- Aspirin 75 mg daily
- Clopidogrel is an alternative to aspirin if it is contraindicated or poorly tolerated
- Statin if lipids are elevated.

CLINICAL ALERT!

May need addition of gastric protection (omeprazole) for prevention of GI symptoms if aspirin is initiated.

Complications

The most important complication is MI and risk of death.

Key reminders

- Increased prevalence in older age
- Can become unstable angina where chest pain occurs at rest
- Uncontrolled angina reduces quality of life.

HEART FAILURE (HF)

The number of people affected by HF increases with age, and with longer life expectancy the numbers of people affected is likely to increase substantially in the years to come. There are around 900 000 known cases of HF at present in the UK,[80] although this is likely to be an underestimate as it is thought there are people with the condition whose symptoms are not troublesome enough for them to see their GP and have therefore not yet received a diagnosis. The condition worsens progressively over time, and when symptoms become severe enough to interfere with daily living activities, it can potentially significantly affect quality of life.

CLINICAL ALERT!

- IHD is the dominant cause of HF and is often associated with acute or prior MI.[81]
- Other causes include non-ischaemic cardiomyopathy, which may have an identifiable cause such as hypertension, thyroid disease, valvular disease, alcohol excess or myocarditis, or the cause may be unknown.[82]

Clues to aid the diagnosis

Patient may complain of:
- breathlessness on exertion
- fatigue
- loss of appetite
- nocturia
- ankle oedema.

Examination may reveal:
- tachycardia
- distended neck veins
- weak, rapid pulse
- possible wheeze
- ascites.

CLINICAL ALERT!

 BEWARE!

Orthopnoea, paroxysmal nocturnal dyspnoea and oedema have a high specificity and if present suggest HF is almost certainly the correct diagnosis.[83]

Diagnosis

Table 5.12 shows tests which are usually requested with additional information.

TABLE 5.12 Tests usually requested and additional information

Test	Additional information
FBC	Anaemia is more common in HF and is associated with a more advanced clinical severity, a more rapid deterioration, and an increased mortality risk.[84]
U&Es	U&E levels may be abnormal because of impaired renal function in the elderly.
LFTs	Aspartate transaminase (AST) and alanine transaminase (ALT) are elevated, and marked elevations in these enzymes have been linked to a poor prognosis.[85] Albumin synthesis may also be impaired, leading to low albumin levels, which leads to a greater accumulation of fluid.[85]
TFTs and lipids	Abnormal thyroid function and hyperlipidaemia are frequently found together and hypothyroidism is associated with an increased risk of CHF among older adults,[86] while hyperlipidaemia is a known risk factor for CHD which potentially leads to HF.[87]
Glucose	In both diabetic and non-diabetic patients with symptomatic HF, elevated glucose levels and elevated HbA1C is an independent progressive risk factor for CV death, hospitalisation for HF, and increased mortality risk.[88]
ECG	ECG may suggest abnormal heart rhythms, or a prior MI as the cause.
Chest X-ray	May report cardiomegaly.
Serum natriuretic peptides	Low levels make HF diagnosis unlikely; very high levels indicate a poor prognosis.[89]
Echocardiograph	Can help determine whether the ventricles are functioning normally or abnormally and will also identify any abnormal heart rhythms or detect previous MI which may now be the cause of HF.

Classification

The New York Heart Association (NYHA) classification system categorises HF on a scale of I to IV according to symptoms and impact on activity levels.[90]

- Class I: No limitation of physical activity. No symptoms at all on activity.
- Class II: Slight limitation of physical activity. No symptoms at rest but may experience breathlessness and fatigue with exertion.
- Class III: Marked limitation of physical activity. Symptoms on any activity but may be fine when at rest.
- Class IV: Symptoms occur even at rest; discomfort with any physical activity.

Pathophysiology

The underlying pathophysiology involves several processes. The impairment in normal functioning of the left ventricle leads to reduced cardiac output, which leads to the initiation of a number of mechanisms that are the body's attempt at compensating for any reduced efficiency. The sympathetic nervous system is activated in an attempt to keep up an adequate cardiac output. Heart rate increases and there is peripheral vasoconstriction and an increase in the contractility of the myocardium, which leads to an increase in blood volume and subsequent retention of salt and water.

Differential diagnosis

 BEWARE!

There are a number of differential diagnoses. Table 5.13 shows the commonest conditions with additional information.

TABLE 5.13 Differential diagnoses

Condition	Additional pointers	When to consider
COPD	pp. 22–5	pp. 22–5
Pneumonia	pp. 25–9	pp. 25–9
PE	p. 20	p. 20
Pulmonary fibrosis	p. 27	p. 27
Acute renal failure	Similar symptoms of breathlessness, fluid retention causing swollen ankles feet and legs, nausea	May be detected on bloods with abnormal urea and electrolyte levels detected

Treatment

Both non-pharmacological and pharmacological interventions are important in the management of HF.

Table 5.14 shows non-pharmacological advice with supporting evidence and Table 5.15 shows pharmacological treatments.

TABLE 5.14 Non-pharmacological advice with supporting evidence

Non-pharmacological treatment	Supporting evidence
Exercise	Patients may be reluctant to increase exercise levels for fear of causing breathlessness, but exercise performed under medical supervision may be beneficial. Resistance training is useful for HF patients, since it strengthens muscles, while daily handgrip exercises can improve blood flow through the arteries.[91] Exercise may not be appropriate for all patients with the condition.
Smoking cessation	Quitting smoking appears to have a substantial and early effect (within 2 years) on decreasing morbidity and mortality in patients with LVF dysfunction.[92]
Healthy diet	There is limited information on diet and nutritional advice for HF. However, there is some evidence to suggest that weight reduction achieved by healthy eating has been shown to be associated with improvements in both diastolic and systolic ventricular function.[93]
Reduced salt intake	In patients with known HF, a high salt intake aggravates the retention of salt and water, exacerbating HF symptoms and progression of the disease.[94] Daily salt intake should be restricted and should not exceed 6 g maximum per day.[82]

Non-pharmacological treatment	Supporting evidence
Fluid restriction	Patients, especially those with renal dysfunction or hyponatraemia, should be advised to restrict fluid intake to 1.5–2 L per day.[95]
Reduced alcohol intake	Alcohol consumption should be restricted to moderate levels, because alcohol has direct toxic effect on the myocardium and also predisposes to arrhythmias (especially AF) and hypertension and may lead to alterations in fluid balance.[95]
Vaccinations	Influenza and pneumococcal vaccinations recommended.
Compliance with advice and treatment	Non-compliance with non-pharmacological and pharmacological treatment is obviously detrimental and can potentially result in worsening HF symptoms, which may result in hospital admission and fatal outcomes.

⚠ **BEWARE!**

- Chronic HF can be exacerbated by lung infections, therefore the need for influenza and pneumonia vaccinations is particularly important for these patients.
- Worsening HF, increased rates of hospital admissions and increased mortality are associated with continued smoking when compared to non-smokers and ex-smokers.[92]
- Patients should be advised against using low-salt products as these have high potassium content.

Pharmacological treatment options and benefits

TABLE 5.15 Pharmacological treatment options

Drug	Evidence	Additional information	Prescribing tips
ACE inhibitors	ACE inhibitors have consistently shown beneficial effects on mortality, morbidity, and quality of life and are indicated in all stages of symptomatic HF resulting from impaired left ventricular systolic function.[96]	First-line treatment for HF.[89]	pp. 47–9.
ARBs	Alternative for patients intolerant to ACE inhibitors.	A study of patients intolerant to ACE inhibitors found that treatment with candesartan led to a risk reduction of 23% in cardiovascular deaths and hospitalisation for CHF.[97]	pp. 47–9.
Beta-blockers	There is consistent evidence for positive benefits from beta-blockers in patients with HF, with risk of mortality from cardiovascular causes reduced by 29%, mortality due to pump failure reduced by 36% and all cause mortality reduced by 23%.[98]	Commencing a beta-blocker can worsen HF symptoms initially and should therefore be introduced at a low dose and titrated upwards.[99] Should be used with caution in those with low initial BP.[82]	p. 43.
Aldosterone antagonists (e.g. spironolactone)	An ACE inhibitor in addition to spironolactone has been shown to reduce all-cause mortality by 30% and mortality from cardiac causes by 31%.[100]	Used in patients with Class 111-1V HF in addition to ACE inhibitors and beta-blockers.	p. 48.
Loop diuretic/ diuretics	Loop diuretics such as furosemide are commonly prescribed and are effective in reducing symptoms of dyspnoea and oedema but effect on reducing mortality is unclear.[101]	Absorption rates vary and may be affected by several factors. As the glomerular filtration rate (eGFR) decreases, a higher dose of diuretic is necessary to achieve effect.[101]	Require monitoring of urea and electrolytes at baseline, then 1–2 weekly after each dose increase and then 3–6 monthly in higher risk patients or annually in lower risk patients.[62] May cause hyponatraemia and hypokalaemia.

Drug	Evidence	Additional information	Prescribing tips
Digoxin	Digoxin can lead to a small increase in cardiac output, improvement in HF symptoms, and decreased rate of HF hospitalisations.[102]	In patients with HF and sinus rhythm, digoxin may reduce symptoms and hospital admission for worsening HF, although its use is usually reserved for patients with severe HF who have not responded to other treatments.[103]	p. 43.
Statins	Frequently prescribed, although evidence for their direct benefit in HF is not conclusive.	Evidence suggests that statins are often commenced in primary care prior to HF diagnosis and appear to benefit patients probably through their effect on cardiovascular comorbidities.[104]	Current guidance suggests simvastatin as first-line following fasting cholesterol triglycerides and TFTs prior to commencing with monitoring of LFTs at 3 months and then 12-monthly.[105] Alternative statins are available if needed.
Aspirin/ warfarin	In patients with AF as well as HF warfarin is needed because of increased stroke risk.	Both aspirin and warfarin have been shown to reduce the incidence of further coronary events in patients with CVD.[82]	Warfarin is monitored in secondary care, but patients on aspirin may need addition of PPI for gastro protection.
Hydralazine and isosorbide	Considered in patients unsuitable for ACE inhibitors and ARBs.	Can be used in addition to ACE inhibitor and a beta-blocker in symptomatic patients, or as an alternative if ACE or ARB is contraindicated.[30]	This combination has been found particularly beneficial for black patients with HF taking standard therapy and has been shown to increase survival rates.[106]

Complications

- AF is present in approximately one third of patients with chronic HF and can be either a cause or a consequence of HF.[107]
- Stroke and thromboembolism: HF increases the risk of stroke and thromboembolism, with an overall estimated annual incidence of approximately 2%.[107]
- There are a number of respiratory problems associated with HF which include airflow obstruction, hypoxaemia, air trapping and sleep apnoea, which are associated with a worse prognosis.[108]
- In advanced disease, patients often have reduced exercise tolerance and therefore reduced activity levels with subsequent muscle wasting.
- As HF progresses and physical activity levels decrease, there can be substantial salt and water retention, leading to oedema with many patients eventually dying from progressive pump dysfunction, which includes hypotension, low cardiac output, and multi-organ dysfunction.[109]

Key reminders

- Progressive condition
- Prevalence increases with increasing age
- Associated with serious complications
- Advancing disease has a substantial effect on patients' quality of life.

REFERENCES

1. British Heart Foundation. *European Cardiovascular Disease Statistics 2008*. Available at: www.bhf.org.uk/publications/view-publication.aspx?ps=1001443 (accessed 13 December 2012).
2. World Health Organization. *Preventing Chronic Diseases: a vital investment*. Available at: www.who.int/chp/chronic_disease_report/contents/en/index.html (accessed 14 December 2012).
3. World Health Organization. *Cardiovascular Disease: global atlas on cardiovascular disease prevention and control*. Available at: www.who.int/cardiovascular_diseases/en/ (accessed 12 December 2012).
4. Yalamanachi M, Khurana A, Smaha L. Evaluation of palpitations: aetiology and diagnostic methods. *Hospital Physician*. 2003. Available at: www.turner-white.com
5. Kannel WB, Wolf PA, Benjamin EJ, *et al*. Prevalence, incidence, prognosis, and predisposing conditions for atrial fibrillation: population-based estimates. *Am J Cardiol*. 1998; **82**(8A): 2N–9N.
6. Lafuente-Lafuente C, Mahe I Extramiana F. Management of atrial fibrillation. *BMJ*. 2009; **23**(339): b5216.
7. Rosenthal L. *Atrial Fibrillation*. Available at: http://emedicine.medscape.com/article/151066-overview (accessed 17 December 2012).
8. Camm AJ, Lip GY, Caterina R, *et al*. 2012 focused update of the ESC guidelines for the management of atrial fibrillation: an update of the 2010 ESC guidelines for the management of atrial fibrillation. *Eur Heart J*. 2012; **33**(21): 2719–47.
9. Lip GYH, Saw Hee LI. Paroxysmal atrial fibrillation. *QJ Med*. 2001; **94**: 665–78.

10. Sankaranarayanan R, Kirkwood G, Dibb K, *et al.* Comparison of atrial fibrillation in the young versus that in the elderly: a review. *Card Res Pract.* Available at: www.hindawi.com/journals/crp/2013/976976/abs/ (accessed 15 August 2013).

11. Pappone C, Radinovic A, Manguso F, *et al.* Atrial fibrillation progression and management: a 5-year prospective follow-up study. *Heart Rhythm.* 2008; **5**: 1501–7.

12. American Heart Association. *Tachycardia: fast heart rate.* Available at: www.heart.org/HEARTORG/Conditions/Arrhythmia/AboutArrhythmia/Tachycardia_UCM_302018_Article.jsp (accessed 29 June 2013).

13. Colucci RA, Silver MJ, Schubrook J. Common types of supraventricular tachycardia: diagnosis and management. *Am Fam Physician.* 2010; **82**(8): 942–52.

14. Boyer M, Koplan BA. Atrial flutter. *Circulation.* 2005; **112**: e334–6.

15. Rosenthal L. *Atrial Flutter.* Available at: http://emedicine.medscape.com/article/151210-overview (accessed 17 December 2012).

16. Merck Manual. *Wolff-Parkinson White syndrome.* Available at: www.merckmanuals.com/home/heart_and_blood_vessel_disorders/abnormal_heart_rhythms/wolff-parkinson-white_wpw_syndrome.html (accessed 9 September 2013).

17. Ellis CR. *Wolff-Parkinson White syndrome.* Available at: http://emedicine.medscape.com/article/159222-overview (accessed 12 December 2012).

18. World Heart Federation. *Atrial Fibrillation.* Available at: www.world-heart-federation.org/what-we-do/awareness/atrial-fibrillation/

19. National Institute for Health and Clinical Excellence. *Atrial fibrillation: NICE guideline 3.* London: NICE; 2006. www.nice.org.uk/CG36

20. Wyndham CRC. Atrial fibrillation: the most common arrhythmia. *Tex Heart Inst J.* 2000; **27**(3): 257–67.

21. Stroke Association. *Atrial Fibrillation and Stroke.* Available at: www.stroke.org.uk/sites/default/files/Atrial%20fibrillation%20(AF)%20and%20stroke.pdf (accessed 25 June 2012).

22. Lip GYH, Nieuwlaat R, Pisters R, *et al.* Refining clinical risk stratification for predicting stroke and thromboembolism in atrial fibrillation using a novel risk factor-based approach: the Euro heart survey on atrial fibrillation. *Chest.* 2010; **137**(2): 263–72.

23. Giralt-Steinhauer E, Cuadrado-Godia E, Ois A, *et al.* Comparison between CHADS2 and CHA2 DS2-VASc score in a stroke cohort with atrial fibrillation. *Eur J Neurol.* 2013; **20**(4): 623–8.

24. Gorin L, Fauchier L, Nonin E, *et al.* Antithrombotic treatment and the risk of death and stroke in patients with atrial fibrillation and a CHADS2 score = 1. *Thromb Haemost.* 2010; **103**: 683–5.

25. Andersen LV, Vestergaard P, Deichgraeber P, *et al.* Warfarin for the prevention of systemic embolism in patients with non-valvular atrial fibrillation: a meta-analysis. *Heart.* 2008; **94**: 1607–13.

26. National Institute for Health and Clinical Excellence. *Dabigatran etexilate for the prevention of stroke and systemic embolism in atrial fibrillation: NICE guideline 249.* London: NICE; 2012. http://guidance.nice.org.uk/TA249

27. Barber P, Robertson D. *Essentials of Pharmacology for Nurses.* 2nd ed. London: Open University Press; 2012.

28. National Prescribing Centre. Primary care management of atrial fibrillation. *MeReC Bulletin,* 2002; **12**(5): 17–20.

29. Segal JB, McNamara RL, Miller MR, *et al.* The evidence regarding the drugs used for ventricular rate control. *J Fam Pract.* 2000; **59**: 4947–59.

30. British National Formulary. 2013. Available at: www.bnf.org/bnf/index.htm

31. Barclay M, Begg E. The practice of digoxin therapeutic drug monitoring. *New Zeal Med J.*

Available at: http://journal.nzma.org.nz/journal/116-1187/704/content.pdf (accessed 14 July 2012).

32. Boyd KM, Clark DH, Colthart AB, *et al.* Final consensus statement of the Royal College of Physicians of Edinburgh consensus conference on atrial fibrillation in hospital and general practice, 3–4 September 1998. *Br J Haematol.* 1999; **104**(1): 195–6.

33. NHS Evidence. *Hypertension.* Available at: www.evidence.nhs.uk/topic/hypertension (accessed 5 November 2012).

34. British Heart Foundation. *Hypertension.* Available at: www.bhf.org.uk/heart-health/conditions/high-blood-pressure.aspx (accessed 14 June 2012).

35. Sacco RL, Benjamin EJ, Broderick JP, *et al.* Stroke: risk factors. *Stroke.* 1997; **28**: 1507–17.

36. Hankey GJ. Potential new risk factors for ischaemic stroke: what is their potential? *Stroke.* 2006; **37**: 2181–8.

37. National Institute for Clinical Excellence. *Type 1 diabetes. Diagnosis and management of Type 1 diabetes in children, young people and adults. NICE guideline 15.* London: NICE; Updated March 2010. Available at: http://guidance.nice.org.uk/nicemedia/live/10944/29391/29391.pdf

38. National Institute for Health and Clinical Excellence. *Type 2 diabetes. NICE guideline 87.* London: NICE; Updated March 2010. Available at: www.nice.org.uk/nicemedia/pdf/cg66niceguideline.pdf

39. National Institute for Health and Clinical Excellence. *Chronic Kidney Disease. NICE Guideline 73.* London: NICE; 2008. Available at: www.nice.org.uk/cg73

40. Hodgkinson J, Mant J, Martin U, *et al.* Relative effectiveness of clinic and home blood pressure monitoring compared with ambulatory blood pressure monitoring in diagnosis of hypertension: systematic review. *BMJ.* 2011; **342**: d3621.

41. National Institute for Health and Clinical Excellence. *NICE Consults on New Guideline for Diagnosing and Treating High Blood Pressure.* London: NICE; 2011. Available at: www.nice.org.uk/newsroom/pressreleases/NewGuidelineForDiagnosingAndTreatingHighBloodPressure.jsp

42. Chadban SJ, Briganti EM, Kerr PG, *et al.* Prevalence of kidney damage in Australian adults: the Aus Diab Kidney Study. *J Am Soc Nephrol.* 2003; **14**: S131–8.

43. Wierzbicki AS. Lipid lowering: another method of reducing blood pressure? *J Human Hypertension.* 2002; **16**: 753–60.

44. Foex P, Sear JW. Hypertension: pathophysiology and treatment. *Contin Educ Anaesth Crit Care Pain.* 2004; **4**(3): 71–5.

45. Pickering TG. Mental stress as a causal factor in the development of hypertension and cardiovascular disease. *Curr Hypertens Rep.* 2001; **3**(3): 249–54.

46. Vikrant S, Tiwani SJ. Essential hypertension: pathogenesis and pathophysiology. *J Ind Acad Clin Med.* 2001; **2**(3): 140–61.

47. Su H, Sheu WH, Chin HM, *et al.* Effect of weight loss on blood pressure and insulin resistance in normotensive and hypertensive obese individuals. *Am J Hypertens.* 1995; **8**(11): 1067–71.

48. Cook NR, Cutler JA, Obarzanek E, *et al.* Long term effects of dietary sodium reduction on cardiovascular disease outcomes: observational follow-up of the trials of hypertension prevention (TOHP). *BMJ.* 2007; **334**: 885.

49. Oncken CA, White WB, Cooney JL, *et al.* Impact of smoking cessation on ambulatory blood pressure and heart rate in postmenopausal women. *Am J Hypertens.* 2001; **14**(9 Pt 1): 942–9.

50. Xin X, He J, Frontini MC, *et al.* Effects of alcohol reduction on blood pressure: a meta-analysis of randomised controlled trials. *Hypertension.* 2001; **38**: 1112–17.

51. Appel LJ, Sacks FM, Carey VJ, *et al.* Effects of protein, monounsaturated fat and carbohydrate

intake on blood pressure and serum lipids: results of the OmniHeart randomized trial. *JAMA*. 2012; **308**(9): 875–81.

52. Carretero OA, Oparil S. Essential hypertension: Part II treatment. *Circulation*. 2000; **101**: 446–53.

53. Rodgers JE, Patterson JH. Angiotensin II-receptor blockers: clinical relevance and therapeutic role. *Am J Health Syst Pharm*. 2001; **58**(8): 671–83.

54. Samiullah R, Rao Saad R, Khan A, *et al.* Comparison of efficacy of calcium channel blockers with angiotensin converting enzyme inhibitors in the treatment of essential hypertension in elderly men. Available at: www.pafmj.org/showdetails.php?id=386&t=o (accessed 4 July 2013).

55. Mcormack T, Arden C, Begg A, *et al.* Optimizing hypertension treatment. *Brit J Cardiol*. 2013; **20**(Suppl. 1): S1–16.

56. Overlak A. ACE inhibitor-induced cough and bronchospasm: incidence, mechanisms and management. *Drug Saf*. 1996; **5**(1): 72–8.

57. Kubota K, Pearce GL, Inman WH. Vasodilation-related adverse events in diltiazem and dihydropyridine calcium antagonists studied by prescription-event monitoring. *Eur J Clin Pharmacol*. 1995; **48**: 1–7.

58. Salvetti A, Ghiadoni L. Thiazide diuretics in the treatment of hypertension: an update. *JASN*. 2006; **17**(4 Suppl. 2): S25–9.

59. British Hypertension Society. Alpha adrenoceptor blockers (alpha blockers). Available at: www.bhsoc.org/pdfs/therapeutics/Alpha-Adrenoceptor%20Antagonists%20(Alpha-Blockers).pdf (accessed 25 July 2013).

60. Martin U, Coleman JJ. Monitoring renal function in hypertension. *BMJ*. 2006; **333**(7574): 896–9.

61. Ritter JM. Angiotensin converting enzyme inhibitors and angiotensin receptor blockers in hypertension. *BMJ*. 2011; **342**: 1673–80.

62. Martin M. Monitoring renal function in hypertension. *BMJ*. 2006; **333**(7574): 896–9.

63. BPAC. Medical management of angina. *Best Practice J*. Available at: www.bpac.org.nz/BPJ/2011/october/angina.aspx

64. Riaz K. *Hypertension*. Available at: http://emedicine.medscape.com/article/241381-overview#aw2aab6b2b5aa (accessed 20 November 2012).

65. World Heart Federation. *Stroke and Hypertension*. Available at: www.world-heart-federation.org/cardiovascular-health/stroke/stroke-and-hypertension/ (accessed 24 November 2012).

66. Reitz C, Tang M, Manly J, *et al.* Hypertension and the risk of mild cognitive impairment. *Arch Neurol*. 2007; **64**(12): 1734–40.

67. The National Kidney and Urologic Diseases Information Clearinghouse (NKUDIC). *High Blood Pressure and Kidney Disease*. Available at: http://kidney.niddk.nih.gov/kudiseases/pubs/highblood/#how (accessed 17 June 2012).

68. Wong TY, Mitchell P. The eye in hypertension. *Lancet*. 2007; **369**(9559): 425–35.

69. Chobanian AV, Bakris GL, Black HR, *et al.* Seventh report of the joint national committee on prevention, detection, evaluation, and treatment of high blood pressure. *Hypertension*. 2003; **42**(6): 1206–52.

70. Lampe FC, Morris RW, Walker M, *et al.* Trends in rates of different forms of diagnosed coronary heart disease 1978 to 2000: prospective, population based study of British men. *BMJ*. 2005; **330**(7499): 1046.

71. National Institute for Health and Clinical Excellence. *The Management of Stable Angina: NICE guideline 126*. London: NICE; 2007. www.nice.or.uk/guidance/cg126

72. Almeda FQ, Kason TT, Nathan S, *et al.* Silent myocardial ischaemia: concepts and controversies. *Am J Med*. 2004; **116**(2): 112–18.

73. Juang D, Braverman AC, Eagle K. Aortic dissection. *Circulation.* 2008; **118**: e507–10.

74. Khoynezhad A, Plestis KA. Managing emergency hypertension in aortic dissection and aortic aneurysm surgery. *J Card Surg.* 2006; **21**(Suppl. 1): S3–7.

75. Turi ZG. Mitral valve disease. *Circulation.* 2004; **109**: e38–41.

76. Alaeddini J. *Angina Pectoris.* Available at: http://emedicine.medscape.com/article/150215-treatment (accessed 14 February 2013).

77. Sharma V, Henderson R. *Managing Stable Angina in Primary Care.* Available at: www.gponline.com/Clinical/article/1165106/Managing-stable-angina-primary-care/ (accessed 15 July 2013).

78. Kosmicki MA. Long term use of short and long acting nitrates in stable angina pectoris. *Curr Clin Pharmacol.* 2009; **4**(2): 132–41.

79. Abrams J. Chronic stable angina. *N Engl J Med.* 2005; **352**(24): 2524–33.

80. Cowie MR, Wood DA, Coats AJ, *et al.* Incidence and aetiology of heart failure; a population-based study. *Eur Heart J.* 1999; **20**(6): 421–8.

81. Armstrong PW. Left ventricular dysfunction: causes, natural history, and hopes for reversal. *Heart.* 2000; **84**(Suppl. I): i15–17.

82. Scottish Intercollegiate Guidelines Network. *Management of Chronic Heart Failure: a national clinical guideline. SIGN guideline 95.* Edinburgh: SIGN; 2007. www.sign.ac.uk/pdf/sign95.pdf

83. Skinner JS, Adams PC, Blades S, *et al. Diagnosis and Management of Heart Failure due to Left Ventricular Systolic Dysfunction.* Available at: www.gp-training.net/protocol/cardiovascular/lvsd.htm (accessed 15 February 2013).

84. Coats AJS. Anaemia and heart failure. *Heart.* 2004; **90**(9): 977–9.

85. Alvarez AM, Mukherjee D. Liver abnormalities in cardiac diseases and heart failure. *Int J Angiol.* 2011; **20**(3): 135–42.

86. Rodondi N, Newman AB, Vittinghoff E, *et al.* Subclinical hypothyroidism and the risk of heart failure, other cardiovascular events, and death. *Arch Intern Med.* 2005; **165**(21): 2460–6.

87. Mayo Foundation for Medical Education and Research (MFMER). *Heart Disease. Complications.* Available at: www.mayoclinic.com/health/heart-disease/DS01120/DSECTION=complications (accessed 12 July 2013).

88. Gerstein HC, Swedburg K, Carlsson J, *et al.* The Haemoglobin A1c level as a progressive risk factor for cardiovascular death, hospitalisation for heart failure, or death in patients with chronic heart failure: an analysis of the Candesartan in Heart failure: Assessment of Reduction in Mortality and Morbidity (CHARM). *Arch Intern Med.* 2008; **168**(15): 1699–1704.

89. National Institute for Health and Clinical Excellence. *Chronic Heart Failure: management of chronic heart failure in adults in primary and secondary care. NICE guideline 108.* London: NICE; 2010. www.nice.org.uk/CG108

90. American Heart Association. AHA medical/scientific statement: 1994 revisions classification of functional capacity and objective assessment of patients with diseases of the heart. *Circulation.* 1994; **90**(1): 644–5.

91. University of Maryland Medical Centre. *Exercise Effects on the Heart.* Available at: www.umm.edu/patiented/articles/what_effects_of_exercise_on_heart_circulation_000029_3.htm (accessed 24 February 2013).

92. Suskin NS, Sheth T, Negassa A, Yusuf S. Relationship of current and past smoking to mortality and morbidity in patients with left ventricular dysfunction. *J Am Coll Cardiol.* 2001; **37**(6): 1677–82.

93. Lavie CJ, Milani RV. Obesity and cardiovascular disease: the Hippocrates paradox? *J Am Coll Cardiol.* 2003; **42**: 677–9.

94. He FJ, Burnier M, Macgregor GA. Nutrition in cardiovascular disease: salt in hypertension and heart failure. *Eur Heart J.* 2011; **32**(24): 3073–80.

95. Gibbs CR, Jackson G, Lip GYH. ABC heart failure: non-drug management. *BMJ.* 2000; **320**(7231): 366–9.

96. Davies MK, Gibbs CR, Lip GYH. Management: diuretics, ACE inhibitors, and nitrates. *BMJ.* 2000; **320**(7232): 428–31.

97. Granger CB, McMurray JJ, Yusuf S, *et al.* Effects of candesartan in patients with chronic heart failure and reduced left-ventricular systolic function intolerant to angiotensin converting-enzyme inhibitors: the CHARM-Alternative trial. *Lancet.* 2003; **362**(9386): 772–6.

98. Domanski MJ, Krause-Steinrauf H, Massie BM, *et al.* A comparative analysis of the results from 4 trials of beta-blocker therapy for heart failure: BeST, CIBIS-II, MeRIT-HF, and COpeRNICUS. *J Cardiac Fail.* 2003; **9**(5): 354–63.

99. Fletcher P. Using beta blockers in heart failure. *Aust Prescr.* 2000; **23**: 120–3.

100. Pitt B, Zannad F, Remme WJ, *et al.* The effect of spironolactone on morbidity and mortality in patients with severe heart failure. Randomised aldactone evaluation study investigators. *N Engl J Med.* 1999; **341**(10): 709–17.

101. Friedman EA. *Diuretics and Heart Failure.* Available at: http://emedicine.medscape.com/article/2145340-overview#aw2aab6b2b2 (accessed 25 April 2013).

102. Dumitru I. *Heart Failure.* Available at: http://emedicine.medscape.com/article/163062-overview (accessed 23 February 2013).

103. Hood WJ, Dans A, Guyatt G, *et al.* Digitalis for treatment of congestive heart failure in patients in sinus rhythm: a systematic review and meta-analysis. *J Card Failure.* 2004; **10**(2): 155–64.

104. Ryan RP, McManus RJ, Mant J, *et al.* Statins in heart failure: retrospective cohort study using routine primary care data. *Ann Med.* 2009; **41**(7): 490–6.

105. National Institute for Health and Clinical Excellence. *Lipid Modification: NICE Guideline 67.* London: NICE; 2008. Updated 2010. Available at: www.nice.org.uk/nicemedia/live/11982/40675/40675.pdf

106. Taylor AL, Ziesche S, Yancy C, *et al.* Combination of isosorbide dinitrate and hydralazine in blacks with heart failure. *N Engl J Med.* 2004; **351**(20): 2049–57.

107. Watson RDS, Gibbs CR, Lip GYH. ABC of heart failure: clinical features and complications. *BMJ.* 2000; **320**(7229): 236–9.

108. Gehlback BK, Geppert E. The pulmonary manifestations of left heart failure. *Chest.* 2004; **125**(2): 669–82.

109. Francis GS, Wilson Tang WH. Pathophysiology of congestive heart failure. *Rev Cardiovasc Med.* 2003; **4**(Suppl. 2): S14–20.

CHAPTER 6

Gastrointestinal

INTRODUCTION

Gastrointestinal conditions cover a wide spectrum of diseases, with an extensive range of signs and symptoms. Their severity ranges from mild to more severe (often regarded as chronic), while others may be potentially life threatening. Gastrointestinal disease is the third most common cause of death, after circulatory and respiratory disease, and is the most common cause of admission to hospital for both the total number of people admitted and the total number of episodes of care.[1]

CONDITIONS COVERED IN THE CHAPTER

- Gastroenteritis
- Diverticulitis
- Cholecystitis
- Constipation
- Haemorrhoids
- Irritable bowel syndrome (IBS)
- Dyspepsia.

COMMONLY PRESENTING SYMPTOMS

May present with one or several of the following:

- nausea
- vomiting
- diarrhoea
- constipation
- indigestion
- heartburn.

TAKING THE GASTROINTESTINAL HISTORY

Initial history is as described in Chapter 3, followed by a focused enquiry relating to the gastrointestinal system.

TABLE 6.1 Symptoms enquiry and further questioning for specific symptoms

Symptom	Further questioning
Nausea	Productive or non-productive?
	Worse during the day or at night or both?
	Are there additional symptoms as shown below?
Vomiting	Does vomiting occur after meals or at any time?
	Is the vomit bloodstained?
	Are there other associated features such as abdominal pain?
	Does the vomit contain undigested food?
	Does it have the appearance of ground coffee?
Diarrhoea	How often would patient normally open their bowels?
	How many stools are they passing daily?
	Needing to open the bowels during the night and if so how many times?
	Is stool watery, blood streaked or contains mucus?
	Additional symptoms? Nausea, vomiting or abdominal pain?
	Any contact with anyone with similar symptoms?
	Any foreign travel?
	Recent antibiotics?
Constipation	How often would patient normally open their bowels?
	Is it difficult to pass stools?
	Is there any alteration to bowel habit? Does the problem alternate with diarrhoea?
	Are there additional symptoms, abdominal pain, nausea or vomiting?
Heartburn	Is the problem worse after meals?
	A problem when lying down?
	Can the patient identify specific foods which cause symptoms?

Table 6.2 shows a summary of presenting signs and symptoms and the diseases they may suggest. Each symptom will then be discussed in more detail in the context of each disease.

TABLE 6.2 Presenting signs and symptoms and diseases they suggest

	Nausea	Vomiting	Diarrhoea	Constipation	Indigestion
Gastroenteritis	Yes	Yes	Yes	No	No
Diverticulitis	Yes	Yes	Yes	Yes	No
Cholecystitis	Yes	Yes	No	No	No
Constipation	Possible	No	No	Yes	No
Haemorrhoids	No	No	No	No	No
IBS	Possible	No	Yes	Yes	No
Dyspepsia	Yes	Possible	No	No	Yes

FURTHER INVESTIGATIONS

Investigations should be chosen on the basis of the history and symptoms, including the duration of symptoms and the overall clinical picture.

Other investigations selected on the basis of history symptoms and clinical findings
● Abdominal ultrasound
● Endoscopy
● Abdominal X-ray
● Barium enema
● Barium swallow.

URGENT REFERRAL TO A GASTROENTEROLOGIST REQUIRED
● Dysphagia
● Mass found on examination
● Any suspicion of malignancy
● Unexplained symptoms.

GASTROENTERITIS

Gastroenteritis is a common condition affecting people of any age with varying degrees of severity. The condition may be caused by a variety of organisms that may be viral or bacterial, with symptoms and severity varying according to the causative organism. Acute gastroenteritis is a common cause of morbidity and mortality and is ranked as one of the five leading causes of deaths worldwide, the majority of these occurring in young children in poorer under-developed countries.[2] In the UK there are approximately one in five people affected each year, and in England and Wales alone there are an estimated 190 deaths each year, the majority of these occurring in those over the age of 65.[3]

TABLE 6.3 Clues to aid diagnosis

Viral	Bacterial	Additional information
Mild fever	High fever	High fever more likely with certain causative organisms.
Vomiting	Vomiting	Not present with all causes of gastroenteritis.
Watery diarrhoea, non-bloody	Bloody diarrhoea	Diarrhoea a prominent feature.
Self-limiting	Severe abdominal pains	Cramping abdominal pain accompanies the majority of causes of bacterial gastroenteritis.

TABLE 6.4 Possible causative organisms

Type of organism	Causative organism	Usual duration of symptoms	Source of infection
Viral	Norovirus	Usually resolves within 2–3 days	Contaminated food or water and from contaminated surfaces and from other infected individuals.
Viral	Rotavirus	3–8 days	As above.
Viral	Adenovirus	Approximately 7 days or slightly longer	From other infected individuals, contaminated surfaces.
Bacterial	*Salmonella*	4–7 days	Contaminated meat, eggs, poultry and milk, and can be spread from person to person.
Bacterial	*Escherichia coli* (E. coli)	1–2 weeks	Contaminated food (meat of various types, dairy products such as cheese, milk or yoghurt, contaminated water). Contaminated surfaces and from other infected persons.
Bacterial	*Shigella*	Usually 5–7 days	Contaminated food and water and from other infected individuals.
Bacterial	*Campylobacter*	May persist beyond 7 days	Raw meat, or undercooked meat, chicken and poultry.
Parasitic	*Giardia intestinalis*	Often persists for more than 10 days and can persist for 6 weeks or longer	Contaminated food, water, soil, and from contaminated surfaces or passed from other infected persons.
Parasitic	*Cryptosporidium parvum*	Up to 1 month	Found in food, soil and water.

Pathophysiology

Viral gastroenteritis

A source contaminated by a virus capable of causing gastroenteritis may be acquired by the faecal–oral route or in some cases may be airborne. Although most viruses are spread by the faecal–oral route, some are airborne (e.g. norovirus), but in either case the mechanism by which diarrhoea subsequently develops is poorly understood. Rotavirus has received a lot of attention and it is thought that the organism causes poor digestion of carbohydrates, and malabsorption of nutrients together with inhibition of water reabsorption.[2]

Bacterial gastroenteritis

The pathophysiology underpinning bacterial gastroenteritis varies according to the causative organism. Some bacteria are able to enter the gastrointestinal tract and attach to the intestinal mucosa where they begin to secrete toxins. The absorption of nutrients is then impeded, causing cells to secrete electrolytes and water. Other bacteria are capable of invading the mucosal cells, leading to ulceration and bleeding, which causes an inflammatory diarrhoea associated with significant abdominal pain.[4]

Differential diagnosis

TABLE 6.5 Differential diagnoses: beware of!

Condition	Additional pointers	When to consider
Appendicitis	pp. 86–7.	pp. 86–7.
Large bowel obstruction	May be caused by a growth or a stricture.	There are symptoms of abdominal distension, nausea, vomiting, and colicky abdominal pain.[5]
Clostridium difficile (C. Diff)	pp. 297–8.	pp. 297–8.
Inflammatory bowel disease (IBD)	Symptoms vary according to the portion of bowel affected.	There may be symptoms of weight loss, fever, malaise, and a low-grade fever with additional feature of IBS such as cramping, irregular bowel habits, diarrhoea with mucus and blood.[6]

Treatment

Viral gastroenteritis is usually self-limiting and rehydration and adequate fluids is usually all that is required. Many bacterial causes are also self-limiting, but there may be cases where antibiotics are needed.

TABLE 6.6 Suggested treatment of bacterial causes requiring antibiotics

Bacterial causes	Treatment
Salmonella	Ciprofloxacin
Shigella	Ciprofloxacin
Giardia intestinalis	Metronidazole

CLINICAL ALERT!

- There is no specific treatment for cryptosporidium.[7]
- Although usually asymptomatic, treatment with antibiotics may be needed in severe cases and the infection is usually susceptible to fluoroquinolones (e.g. ciprofloxacin).[8]

Prescribing tips
- Antimotility drugs are not recommended for acute diarrhoea for children under the age of 12.[9]
- Loperamide should be avoided in bloody or suspected inflammatory diarrhoea where fever is present.[10]
- Loperamide is not recommended for use in pregnancy but is not known to have adverse effects in breastfeeding women.

Complications

⚠ BEWARE OF!

- Dehydration.
- Electrolyte imbalance occurs when there is excessive loss of water and salts through diarrhoea and/or vomiting.
- Dehydration is the most common complication.[4] Severe dehydration and excess fluid loss can lead to low BP.
- In cases of severe diarrhoea and vomiting reduced blood flow to vital organs can potentially lead to renal failure if left untreated.
- Lactose intolerance can follow damage to lining of the stomach.
- Very rarely gastroenteritis caused by *Salmonella* can spread to other sites (e.g. the meninges or the joints), causing infection.
- IBS has been reported to occur rarely following gastroenteritis.
- When diarrhoea is severe, absorption of regular medication may be impaired, which will result in reduced effectiveness.

CLINICAL ALERT!

Urgent treatment and admission to hospital in the event of the following:
- clinically unwell with worsening symptoms
- altered level of consciousness

- severe dehydration with signs of sunken eyes, low urine output, and thirst
- tachypnoea.

Key reminders
- Many causes, infections are very common
- Viral gastroenteritis usually self-limiting
- Variable duration according to causative organism
- No available treatment for some causative organisms
- Complications are rare, but are more likely in the elderly or the very young.

DIVERTICULITIS

Diverticula are small protrusions through the muscular wall of the colon that can become inflamed and infected, leading to diverticulitis. The condition is extremely common, particularly among the elderly, and in the developed world diverticular disease of the colon is present in more than 65% of those over the age of 65,[11] and although many with the condition will remain asymptomatic, an estimated 25% of sufferers will develop some symptoms and 75% of these will have at least one episode of diverticulitis at some point in time.[12]

Clues to aid the diagnosis

Once diverticula are inflamed and infected the patient will present with:
- fever
- feeling generally unwell
- lethargy and malaise
- lower abdominal pain
- feeling of bloatedness
- rarely there may be rectal bleeding.

CLINICAL ALERT!

⚠ BEWARE!

- Regular rectal bleeds require further investigation to exclude other causes.
- Raised white cell count (WCC), raised ESR and raised C-reactive protein (CRP) levels are suggestive of infection.
- May present with acute constant abdominal pain, most often occurring in the left lower quadrant with fever, nausea and vomiting, and constipation or diarrhoea may also be present.
- More severe diverticulitis may present with severe pain, nausea, vomiting and loss of appetite and a change in bowel habit, patient may also complain of dysuria, frequency and urgency caused by bladder irritation from the adjacent inflamed colon.[13]

Pathophysiology

The colon is a common site for diverticula to occur (usually the sigmoid colon), but they can develop anywhere along the GI tract. The initial development of diverticula without inflammation and infection is referred to as diverticulosis. Although the cause is not conclusive, it appears to be associated with poor diet, particularly low fibre diets, obesity and constipation.[14] The process by which infection occurs is also not clear, but it is thought that undigested food particles and faecal matter collect in the diverticula, causing obstruction, a process which leads to an overgrowth of normal bacteria in the colon along with excess mucus production.

Differential diagnosis

 BEWARE OF!

The number of differential diagnoses is extensive because of the number of organs and structures in close proximity to the colon.

TABLE 6.7 Differential diagnoses

Condition	Additional pointers	When to consider
Colorectal cancer	Absence of fever with rectal bleeding or blood in the stool.	Symptoms persist for more than 3 weeks and are accompanied by unintentional weight loss.
Pelvic inflammatory disease (PID)	pp. 108–10.	pp. 108–10.
Crohn's disease	Stools may be loose, watery and frequent.	Consider if there are additional symptoms of cramping abdominal pain with rectal bleeding, fever and loss of appetite when patient is symptomatic.
Appendicitis	pp. 86–7.	pp. 86–7.
Ulcerative colitis	Diarrhoea is watery with blood.	Consider if the patient complains of cramping abdominal pains and the need to open the bowels urgently.
Pancreatic disease	Pain from pancreatic disease may be cramping but can radiate to the back.	Consider if there are additional symptoms of low back pain, nausea and vomiting.
IBS	pp. 88–91.	pp. 88–91.

Treatment

Patients with mild symptoms can be managed at home. Table 6.8 suggests pharmacological and non-pharmacological interventions.

TABLE 6.8 Pharmacological and non-pharmacological interventions

Intervention	Additional information
Analgesia	Simple analgesia for pain relief.
Antibiotics	Suggested treatment is amoxicillin plus co-amoxiclav plus trimethoprim for 7–14 days or a quinolone (e.g. ciprofloxacin) plus metronidazole for 7–10 days.[15]
Fluids	Avoidance of food until symptoms begin to improve. Light diet can be reintroduced when symptoms are improving.

Prescribing tips

See Chapter 16 for further information relating to antibiotics.

CLINICAL ALERT!

 BEWARE!

Admission is required in the following circumstances:

- frail elderly, and patients with comorbidities which may worsen or compromise recovery
- worsening symptoms or persistent symptoms despite treatment
- patients not able to tolerate prescribed antibiotics, requiring treatment in secondary care
- any patient who has developed complications as shown below.

Complications

Complications are shown in Table 6.9.

TABLE 6.9 Complications

Complication	Common or rare	Treatment
Abscess	Commonest	Small abscesses may be treated with antibiotics. Larger abscesses require drainage.
Fistula	Common	May require surgery to remove the portion of bowel affected.
Peritonitis	Rare	Potentially life threatening. Requires urgent treatment with antibiotics but may also require surgery to drain the pus.
Rectal bleeding	Rare	Cautery may be attempted to stop the bleeding or if this is unsuccessful, surgery will be needed to remove the affected part of the colon.
Intestinal obstruction	Rare	Partial or total blockage can occur as a result of scarring. Surgery will be required, and may be urgent or non-urgent, depending on the severity of the blockage.

Key reminders
- Common condition, particularly among the elderly
- Many patients with the condition are asymptomatic
- In some cases a high-fibre diet may be all that is necessary
- Early treatment of signs of infection will reduce the risk of complications.

CHOLECYSTITIS

The incidence of acute cholecystitis is approximately the same in Western Europe as in the United States, but the exact incidence worldwide is not known. However, in the UK 16 884 cases of cholecystitis were reported in the 1-year period between 2009 and 2010, with approximately two thirds of these occurring in females.[16] In England alone more than 49 000 operations are performed each year,[17] and in the US an estimated 10%–20% of the population have gallstones, and as many as one third of these people develop acute cholecystitis, which results in approximately 500 000 operations being performed annually.[18]

Clues to aid the diagnosis
- Patient frequently presents with sudden onset of acute severe pain, centred in the right upper quadrant.
- There may be nausea and vomiting.
- Anorexia may be present.
- Abdominal pain on examination.
- Low-grade fever.

CLINICAL ALERT!

⚠ BEWARE!
- In elderly patients, localised tenderness may be the only presenting sign; right upper quadrant pain has been reported to be absent in 27% of elderly patients in one study and fever was absent in 45% of subjects.[18]
- Jaundice is unusual in the early stages of acute cholecystitis and may be found in fewer than 20% of patients.[19]
- Patient may complain that the pain radiates up towards the right shoulder.

Pathophysiology

Ninety per cent of cases are caused by gallstones, which have caused blockage to either the cystic duct or the neck of the gallbladder with resulting inflammation and distension.[18] The remaining 10% are therefore acalculous (without stones). This type is thought to occur as a result of bile stasis, resulting in a change in bile composition, sepsis and ischaemia,[20] and occurs more commonly in elderly patients with chronic debilitating disease, or patients with critical illness, typically trauma, or in association with major burns.[21] Risk factors for each of the two types differ (*see* Table 6.10).

TABLE 6.10 Risk factors for cholecystitis with or without gallstones

Cholecystitis associated with gallstones	Acalculous cholecystitis
Older age	Debilitation
Obesity	Prolonged periods of fasting
History of CVD	Sickle cell
Past CVA	Severe burns
Diabetes	More common in critically ill patients

Differential diagnosis

The differential diagnosis is extensive and there are a number of possible alternative causes of the symptoms experienced (*see* Table 6.11).

TABLE 6.11 Differential diagnoses

Condition	Additional pointers	When to consider
Appendicitis	pp. 86–7.	pp. 86–7.
Gallbladder cancer	Often detected at a late stage as symptoms mimic those of benign gallbladder diseases.	Consider in those presenting with abdominal pain predominantly in the epigastric and right upper quadrant. Jaundice, nausea, vomiting, anorexia and weight loss are present in 50% of cases.[22]
Gastritis	Symptoms include indigestion and pain in the upper abdomen that may become either worse or better with eating.[23]	Consider if there are additional symptoms of nausea, vomiting and a feeling of fullness.[23] May occur in association with prolonged use of nonsteroidal anti-inflammatory drugs (NSAIDs) or with high alcohol intake.
Gastric ulcers	Epigastric pain is a common symptom and occurs with both gastric and duodenal ulcers.	Consider if there is gnawing or burning sensation which often occurs after meals, classically, shortly after meals with gastric ulcer and 2–3 hours afterwards with duodenal ulcer.[24]
Liver disease	Numerous symptoms depending on the underlying cause, but there will be abdominal pain in the right upper quadrant if the cause is a liver tumour.[5]	Consider if there are additional symptoms, feeling generally unwell or tired, having poor appetite, weight loss, a tender abdomen, feeling itchy or vomiting.[25] Possible history of high alcohol intake.
IBS	pp. 88–91.	pp. 88–91.

- Uncomplicated cholecystitis has a low mortality rate and is usually associated with a positive prognosis.
- However, approximately 25%–30% of patients either require surgery or develop a complication.[18]
- The development of complications significantly worsens prognosis and in patients with acalculous cholecystitis, mortality rates of 10%–50% have been estimated compared to 1% for calculous cholecystitis.[21]

Treatment

Admission to hospital is usually required and initial treatment of acute cholecystitis is often conservative, comprising of bed-rest, analgesia, anti-emetics, fluids and intravenous antibiotics. If symptoms settle sufficiently, most patients will be discharged home until surgery can be arranged. Routine referral to hospital may be appropriate for patients who are reasonably well with mild symptoms that are intermittent.

For some patients surgery may be inappropriate. In the frail elderly, conservative treatment and management may be the safest option.

Complications

There are a number of complications some of which can have fatal consequences.

 BEWARE!

The following are potentially life threatening.
- Septicaemia, in which patient presents with fever, tachycardia, tachypnoea and mental confusion.
- Perforated gallbladder, most commonly seen in patients who delay seeking treatment or in those who have not responded to treatment; occurs in an estimated 10% of cases.[26] Once perforation occurs pain is drastically reduced, confusing the clinical picture. Peritonitis develops shortly afterwards with potentially fatal consequences.
- Gallbladder gangrene can be a complication in up to 20% of cases of cholecystitis and usually occurs in diabetics, the elderly or immunocompromised persons.[19]
- Empyema (pus in the gallbladder), which is potentially life threatening if septicaemia develops.
- A fistula can develop between the gallbladder and nearby organs such as the small intestine.
- Infection of the bile duct requires urgent antibiotics to avoid risk of spread of infection and resulting septicaemia.

- Pancreatitis can develop when stones obstruct the pancreatic duct, leading to inflammation of the pancreas.
- Abscesses are possible in the presence of severe cholecystitis.
- Gallstones can become lodged in the intestine, a problem more frequent in patients over age 65, and can sometimes be fatal.[26]

Key reminders

- More common in females
- Increased prevalence with increasing age
- Majority of cases caused by gallstones
- Cholecystectomy is one of the commonest surgical procedures performed
- Complications are rare.

CONSTIPATION

Constipation is a common problem which can affect adults and children alike. Within the UK it is estimated that three million GP consultations relating to constipation take place each year,[27] with the condition affecting approximately 3% of adults with a significantly greater prevalence among women and among those from less privileged backgrounds.[28] Among children around 5%–30% are affected, with the problem becoming chronic in more than one third of patients.[29] True prevalence rates are difficult to determine because of variations in diagnostic criteria and also patient preference to self-treat rather than seek help from healthcare professionals.

Clues to aid the diagnosis

Diagnosis is made on the patients' description of their bowel habits.

The ROME criteria[30] (cited with kind permission) indicates that there is constipation if patients who do not take laxatives report at least two of the following in any 12-week period during the previous 12 months:

- fewer than three bowel movements per week
- hard stool in more than 25% of bowel movements
- a sense of incomplete evacuation in more than 25% of bowel movements
- excessive straining in more than 25% of bowel movements
- a need for digital manipulation to facilitate evacuation.

Consultation may be made more difficult because of patient perception of what they believe to be constipation.

Pathophysiology

Constipation can involve problems relating to actual passing of stools where the patient may describe infrequent opening of the bowels, straining or difficulty in expelling the stool, or there may be concerns relating to the consistency of the stools passed where the patient may describe hard or pellet-like stools, which then similarly cause difficulties in passing the stool. Although hard stools frequently result in problems with passing, soft bulky stools may also be associated with constipation, particularly in elderly patients with anatomic abnormalities and in patients with impaired colorectal motility.[31] Causes of constipation may originate from problems with the bowel itself or occur as a result of external factors (*see* Table 6.12).

TABLE 6.12 Causes of constipation

Bowel conditions causing constipation	Other possible factors
Obstruction of the colon caused by neoplasm	Poor diet low in fibre
Diverticular disease (pp. 72–4).	Medications known to cause constipation (e.g. analgesia containing codeine)
Reduced motility of the bowel	Pregnancy or old age
Hirschsprung disease	Dehydration
	Hypothyroidism

CLINICAL ALERT!

Constipation in children usually is functional and the result of stool retention.[32]

Differential diagnosis

 BEWARE!

There are many differential diagnoses. Table 6.13 shows some of the commonest in both adults and children.

TABLE 6.13 Differential diagnoses: adults and children

Differential diagnosis in adults	Differential diagnosis in children
Colonic obstruction	Hirschsprung disease (disease of the large intestine, which causes constipation)
Cancer of the colon	Neurofibromatosis: this is a genetic disease frequently associated with constipation, although the underlying pathology and reason for its association with the condition is poorly understood
Crohn's disease	Hypothyroidism
Diverticular disease	Hypokalaemia
Hypothyroidism	Hypercalcaemia
IBS	Imperforate anus

Treatment

Lifestyle advice should be offered and should include the following.
- Dietary advice relating to increasing fibre intake.
- Ensure patient has an adequate fluid intake.

- Exercise should be encouraged.
- Review medications where patient is taking treatment that may aggravate the problem (analgesia, antacids, certain antihypertensives, iron supplements, diuretics, antispasmodics and antidepressants are known to potentially cause constipation).

Table 6.14 shows treatment options for constipation in adults.

TABLE 6.14 Treatment options for constipation in adults

Laxative type	Examples	Dose	Additional information
Bulk forming laxatives	Ispaghula husk (e.g. fybogel)	Prescribed as sachets. Contents of sachets are dissolved in water, which can be taken twice daily if needed.	They act by causing retention of fluid and an increase in faecal mass but may cause flatulence and distension.[29]
Stimulant laxatives	Bisacodyl	Prescribed as tablets and dose can range from one tablet at night up to four tablets if needed.	Stimulant laxatives achieve their effects through alteration of electrolyte transport by the intestinal mucosa[33] and generally work within several hours. Patients may complain of abdominal discomfort and cramping after use.[34]
	Senna	Two tablets at night.	
Osmotic laxatives	Lactulose	15 mL twice daily which can be adjusted once effect achieved.	Achieve its effect by retaining fluid and are safe and effective but are also associated with bloating and flatulence.[35]
Stool softeners	Docusate	Given in divided doses, maximum is 500 mg daily.	Work by softening the faeces and have been shown to produce a modest improvement; other forms of treatment may be more effective.[36]

Treatment of constipation in children

- Movicol plain is the recommended first-line treatment.[29] Children aged 1–6 should be prescribed one sachet daily, two sachets daily for those aged 6–12, titrated up to four sachets daily for both age groups if needed.[9]
- If problem persists a stimulant laxative (e.g. bisacodyl) may be added or if the above is not tolerated substitution with a stimulant laxative may be tried; these are generally well tolerated, but may induce abdominal pain.[37]
- If needed bisacodyl can be prescribed for children aged 4–18 at a dose of 5–10 mg in children over 10, and 5 mg for children aged 4–10 years of age, given at bedtime.[38]
- Lactulose can also be prescribed either singly if the above is not tolerated or in combination with a stimulant laxative if needed at a dose of 2.5 mL twice daily if under 1 year of age, 5 mL twice daily for ages 1–5, 10 mL for ages 5–10 and 15 mL for 10–18 years of age.[9]

Prescribing tips

ADULTS

- Bulk-forming laxatives may take several days for full effect to develop and need to be taken with plenty of water to avoid causing obstruction.[39]
- Stimulant laxatives exert their effect within hours and are therefore best given at night.
- Use of lactulose can cause diarrhoea if the patient has difficulty titrating the dose once symptoms ease.

CHILDREN

- In children maintenance therapy may need to continue for several weeks, bearing in mind the above recommendations.
- If problem persists despite treatment, advice from a paediatrician may be needed.
- Doses should be tapered over a period of months and never stopped abruptly.
- Some children may require longer term treatment.

Complications

⚠ **BEWARE OF!**

- Anal fissures
- Faecal impaction
- Rectal prolapse.

Key reminders

- Very common in adults and children alike
- Easily treatable
- Lifestyle interventions such as adjustment to diet often effective
- Several treatment options available
- Complications are rare.

HAEMORRHOIDS

Worldwide, the prevalence of symptomatic haemorrhoids is estimated at around 4% in the general population, prevalence increasing with age, with a peak in persons aged 45–65 years.[40] However, it is thought that the true prevalence is not accurate because many sufferers may be too embarrassed to seek advice and treatment.

Clues to aid the diagnosis

Haemorrhoids can be internal or external. The commonest reported symptom is fresh blood either on the stool itself, or on the toilet paper or in the bowl after a bowel movement.

Internal haemorrhoids are usually not painful unless they prolapse, when they can cause pain or discomfort and itching around the anal area. Once prolapsed, external haemorrhoids can become thrombosed, which produces a hard painful palpable lump. This can become painful and lead to further bleeding, and discomfort. Many sufferers will give a history of constipation and difficulty opening the bowels, and in older people weakening of the support structures increases the risk of haemorrhoids becoming prolapsed.[41]

Pathophysiology

Haemorrhoids are caused by swellings in the anal or rectal veins, but they may also be caused by weakening of the connective tissue in the rectum and anus that occurs with age.[42] In pregnancy, veins in the rectum and anus can become distended because of increased pressure in the abdomen, although the problem generally resolves once the baby is born. During defecation, contraction of the sphincter muscle normally returns any residual faecal matter from the anal canal back to the rectum. Although the exact cause of haemorrhoids is not known, a number of factors are thought to contribute. Straining to pass stools is believed to cause congestion and this in combination with inadequate fibre intake, prolonged sitting on the toilet, constipation or diarrhoea, and conditions such as pregnancy, ageing and hereditary tendencies are believed to contribute to the development of the problem.[42] Haemorrhoids can be external or internal. The former develop from ectoderm and are covered by squamous epithelium, whereas the latter are derived from embryonic endoderm and lined with the columnar epithelium of the anal mucosa.[40] Nerve supply is important as external haemorrhoids are innervated by cutaneous nerves that supply the perianal area and hence can be painful, while internal haemorrhoids are not supplied by somatic sensory nerves and therefore do not cause pain.

Differential diagnosis

Table 6.15 presents differential diagnoses.

TABLE 6.15 Differential diagnoses: beware of!

Condition	Additional pointers	When to consider
Proctitis	Rectal or anal pain with a change in bowel habit, passage of mucus.	Consider if there is rectal bleeding and a frequent sensation that bowels need to be opened.
Rectal prolapse	Rectal or anal pain with rectal bleeding.	Consider if patient complains of sensation of something around the anus, and a mass outside the anus is visible on examination.
IBD	p. 70.	p. 70.

⚠ BEWARE!

- Colorectal cancer may also have symptoms of rectal bleeding, perianal pain or painless bleeding but will also be associated with change in bowel habit and unexplained weight loss.[43]
- Anal cancer is associated with rectal bleeding, anal pain, mucus from the back passage and lumps around the anus which may be confused with haemorrhoids.[44]

Treatment

Treatment will depend on the severity of the haemorrhoids at examination. Haemorrhoids are graded according to the degree of severity (*see* Table 6.16).

TABLE 6.16 Haemorrhoids severity grades

Grade of haemorrhoids	Description
Grade one	Not visible on examination and are in the lining of the rectum.
Grade two	May prolapse during defecation but return inside when bowel movement is finished.
Grade three	Prolapsed and palpable outside the anus. There may be one or several. Sometimes possible for them to be pushed back inside the anus.
Grade four	At this stage haemorrhoids are permanently prolapsed. Size may be variable but they may be quite large.

Suggested treatment options for each grade are shown in Table 6.17.

TABLE 6.17 Treatment options for various haemorrhoid grades

Grade	Suggested management	Additional information	Treatment
One	High fibre diet	Adequate fluid intake Increased fruit and vegetables	
	Laxatives if constipated	*See* pages 80–1 for suggested treatment	
	Topical cream or ointment	e.g. Anusol Anusol HC Proctosedyl	Can be applied morning and night and after each bowel movement

Grade	Suggested management	Additional information	Treatment
	Sclerotherapy	Sclerotherapy is suitable for treating small, internal, first or second-degree haemorrhoids	It uses a hardening chemical that scars the inflamed tissue, reducing blood flow and alleviating both the cause of the haemorrhoid and its symptoms. Cheap and easy to perform, but less widely used than banding because of the high failure rate.[45]
	Rubber band ligation	Tying off of haemorrhoids using rubber bands	Haemorrhoids must be large enough for this to be undertaken. Complications such as pain, abscess formation, urinary retention, bleeding, band slippage and sepsis occur in less than 2% of patients undergoing rubber band ligation.[46] Procedure is contraindicated in those who are on anticoagulation treatment.
Two	High fibre diet		As above.
	Laxatives if constipated		As above.
	(see pages 80–1)		As above.
	Topical cream or ointment (see above)		As above.
	Sclerotherapy (see above)		As above.
	Rubber band ligation (see above)		As above.
Three	Haemorrhoidectomy	Surgical excision	Suitable for patients where rubber band ligation has failed, or bleeding is persistent or the haemorrhoid cannot be reduced. Approximately 10% of patients will have bleeding, fissure, fistula, abscess, stenosis, urinary retention, soiling or incontinence.[45]
	Stapled haemorrhoidopexy	Surgical procedure	A stapled haemorrhoidopexy uses a stapling device to return the haemorrhoids to a position inside the rectum. Staples used remain inside the rectum permanently. Carries a higher recurrence rate than haemorrhoidectomy.[47]

Grade	Suggested management	Additional information	Treatment
	Doppler guided haemorrhoidal artery ligation		The Doppler probe is used to identify areas in the bowel where an artery supplies blood to a haemorrhoid. A stitch is then placed in each artery blocking blood supply to the haemorrhoid, causing the haemorrhoid to shrink. Painless procedure with minimal morbidity, and studies have indicated high satisfaction rates with the outcome.[48]
Four	Haemorrhoidectomy	Information as above.	Information as above.
	Stapled haemorrhoidopexy	Information as above.	Information as above.
	Doppler-guided haemorrhoidal artery ligation	Information as above.	Information as above.

Complications

 BEWARE OF!

- Chronic blood loss may lead to anaemia with symptoms of tiredness and fatigue.
- If blood supply to an internal haemorrhoid is cut off, the haemorrhoid can become strangulated, leading to death of the tissue and severe pain.
- Common complications following surgical procedures are rectal bleeding and faecal incontinence.
- Uncommon complications are rectal perforation, recto-vaginal fistula, faecal incontinence, and urgency of defaecation.[49]

CLINICAL ALERT!

Although rare, pelvic sepsis occurring in the postoperative period following stapled haemorrhoidectomy can be potentially life threatening.[50]

Key reminders

- Common condition
- Prevalence increases with age
- Easily treatable
- Surgical and non-surgical treatments available.

APPENDICITIS

Appendicitis is swelling and infection of the appendix and is reported to be the commonest cause of emergency abdominal surgery.[51] The condition is very common and although it can occur at any age it is particularly prevalent among those aged 10–20 years of age and occurs more frequently in males than females.[52]

Clues to aid the diagnosis

The following signs and symptoms signify the condition.
- Central abdominal pain which moves down to settle in the right iliac fossa over the course of a few hours.
- Pain usually worsens with any movement.

Other symptoms

Other symptoms may include:
- fever
- nausea and vomiting
- loss of appetite
- constipation or diarrhoea.

CLINICAL ALERT!

⚠ **BEWARE!**

- Diagnosis of appendicitis in young children is particularly difficult as they often have abdominal pain from other causes and signs and symptoms are often non-specific in this age group.[53]
- In the elderly, diagnosis of appendicitis is often delayed because even with advanced inflammation, pain may be minimal and fever is frequently absent.[54]

Pathophysiology

Appendicitis may occur for several reasons, such as an infection of the appendix, but the most important factor is the obstruction of the appendiceal lumen, which leads to an increase in pressure within the lumen.[55] As a result mucus builds up and stagnates and allows bacteria that normally live inside the appendix to multiply and flourish with the subsequent development of infection.

There are several possible causes of obstruction, which include:
- faeces
- infection of the gastrointestinal tract, which has managed to spread to the appendix
- IBD (e.g. Crohn's disease or ulcerative colitis).

Differential diagnosis

⚠ BEWARE!

Appendicitis shares symptoms with a number of other conditions including:
- constipation: pp. 78–81
- gastroenteritis: pp. 68–71
- diverticulitis: pp. 72–4
- ectopic pregnancy (normal signs of pregnancy but associated symptoms of abdominal or pelvic pain).

Treatment

Appendicectomy remains the only curative treatment for appendicitis, but there may be instances where surgery is not an option. When this is the case nonsurgical treatment with antibiotics and IV fluids and light diet may be the only option.

Complications
- Complications occur in 1%–5% of patients with appendicitis, and postoperative wound infections account for almost one third of the associated morbidity.[55]
- A ruptured appendix results in leakage of infection into the abdominal cavity, resulting in peritonitis.
- Abscess formation can occur when a pocket of pus forms around the appendix.

CLINICAL ALERT!

⚠ BEWARE!

- Perforation of the appendix is more common in young children, who may present with vague signs and symptoms, making diagnosis more difficult. Perforation rates of up to 50% are reported in this age group.[53]
- Both rates of perforation and mortality rates are higher among the elderly where signs and symptoms of the condition may be atypical and the presence of comorbidities complicates the illness further.
- Mortality rates of 4%–10% have been reported,[56] with even higher rates of 25%–32% among those with perforated appendix or over 75 years of age.[57]

Key reminders
- Very common condition, which can affect any age, but is particularly common in young children
- Diagnosis more difficult in the very young and in the elderly
- Perforation and mortality rates highest in the elderly
- Appendicectomy remains the treatment of choice.

IRRITABLE BOWEL SYNDROME (IBS)

IBS is a chronic, relapsing and remitting gastrointestinal problem, with variable symptoms that have the ability to have a significant negative impact on quality of life of those affected. Estimates suggest a prevalence rate of 5%–11% of the population of most countries, peaking in the third and fourth decades, with a female predominance.[58] While the precise prevalence and incidence depends on the criteria used, many studies agree that it is a relatively common condition affecting a substantial number of individuals in the general population and is a frequent cause of GP consultations and referral to secondary care for further investigation. However, the true numbers of people affected may be underestimated as it is thought that a number of people manage their symptoms without seeking medical advice.

Clues to aid the diagnosis

Commonly reported symptoms include:
- abdominal pain or discomfort
- altered bowel habit
- pain relieved when bowels are opened
- lethargy and malaise
- nausea
- backache.

NICE guidance[59] suggests that these symptoms should be accompanied by at least two of the following symptoms and should be present for at least 6 months before a diagnosis is made:
- feeling of abdominal bloating or distension
- passage of stool associated with mucus
- straining or urgency or a feeling of incomplete passage of stool
- symptoms worsen after a meal.

Many sufferers report that either diarrhoea or constipation dominates their symptoms with estimates suggesting that around one third of patients have diarrhoea-predominant IBS, a further one third have constipation-predominant IBS and the remainder have a mixed pattern with alternating constipation and diarrhoea.[60]

CLINICAL ALERT!

⚠ BEWARE!

- Anxiety and depression are common in IBS, and patients frequently report worsening symptoms during times of stress and personal problems.[61]
- In Western countries, women are two to three times more likely to develop IBS than men.[62]

- In 50% of patients, symptoms start before 35 years of age while almost all report onset of symptoms before they are 50 years of age.[62]

⚠ BEWARE OF THE PATIENT WITH:

- unexplained weight loss
- symptoms of altered bowel habit
- presence of a mass on examination
- rectal bleeding
- anaemia
- raised inflammatory markers (ESR and CRP) on blood testing (*see* Chapter 15)
- family history of bowel or ovarian cancer.

All of the above are regarded as 'red flag' symptoms and need further investigation as their presence suggests an alternative cause. Any suspicion of malignancy requires an urgent referral for further investigation.

Pathophysiology

The pathophysiology of IBS is not well understood, but a number of factors are believed to contribute to development of the condition.

- Abnormalities in gut motility: when motility of the colon is slow this may lead to constipation, while rapid motility may lead to diarrhoea.
- Abnormal signals from the brain to the gut, leading to changes in bowel habits and associated pain or discomfort.[63]
- Abnormal production of gas may be a factor.
- Food intolerance: some patients report increased symptoms after eating particular foods.

Differential diagnosis

Differential diagnosis includes consideration for conditions where abdominal pain is a feature and occurs in conjunction with diarrhoea and/or constipation (*see* Table 6.18).

TABLE 6.18 Differential diagnoses

Condition	Additional pointers	When to consider
Constipation	pp. 78–81.	pp. 78–81.
IBD	Two of the main conditions under the umbrella term IBD are Crohn's disease and ulcerative colitis, which share symptoms but affect different sections of the bowel.	Consider if there are symptoms of abdominal pain, bloody diarrhoea, and weight loss occurring intermittently with periods of remission between exacerbations.[64]

(continued)

Condition	Additional pointers	When to consider
Coeliac disease	Genetic condition.	Consider if the patient is anaemic and there are additional complaints of tiredness, bloating and occasional or chronic diarrhoea.[65]
Pancreatitis	Usually the pain is sharp in nature and may radiate to the back.	Consider if there is tenderness on examination with rapid heart rate and rapid respiratory rate.[66]
Peptic ulcer	Similar symptom to those of IBS but there may be nausea and belching.	Food or antacids relieve the pain of duodenal ulcers, but provide minimal relief of gastric ulcer pain.[67]
Gallstones	pp. 75–8.	pp. 75–8.
Diverticular disease	pp. 72–4.	pp. 72–4.

Treatment

Both non-pharmacological and pharmacological treatments are available. *See* Tables 6.19 and 6.20.

TABLE 6.19 Non-pharmacological treatment of IBS with supporting evidence

Non-pharmacological treatment	Supporting evidence
Dietary modification	Some patients may find certain foods aggravate their symptoms. Foods potentially associated with onset of symptoms include smoked and spicy foods, cabbage, onions, peas and beans, coffee and fried foods.[68]
Lifestyle advice	NICE guidance suggests a number of lifestyle changes that may be beneficial, including eating regular meals, with avoidance of long gaps between meals, restricted intake of tea, coffee, alcohol and fizzy drinks.[59]
Fibre intake	Where constipation is a feature an increase in insoluble fibre (e.g. whole grain cereals) and soluble fibre (cereals, fruit and vegetables) may help improve symptoms. Ispaghula husk has been shown to be effective in increasing stool frequency and improving symptoms of constipation-dominant IBS but may cause bloatedness and wind.[69]
Fat intake	Many patients with IBS have been found to experience fat intolerance and high levels of fat in the diet have been shown to increase retention of gas.[70]
Increased exercise	Exercise may be beneficial for patients with IBS as it has been shown to increase colonic motility, transit time, and intestinal gas, although it does not seem to have any impact on symptoms of bloating.[71]

TABLE 6.20 Pharmacological treatment with supporting evidence

Drug	Supporting evidence
Antispasmodics (e.g. mebeverine)	Mebeverine has been found to be useful and can potentially diminish stool frequency in both diarrhoea and constipation-predominant IBS, and it does not incur significant adverse effects.[72]
Antidepressants	Guidance suggests low-dose tricyclic antidepressants are the preferred choice before selective serotonin reuptake inhibitors (SSRIs), which may be effective in reducing pain.[59]
Laxatives	Numerous choices (pp. 80–1).
Antidiarrhoeal agents	When IBS is diarrhoea predominant, loperamide can help reduce symptoms but does little to relieve abdominal pain.

Prescribing tips

- Mebeverine is unsuitable during pregnancy and breastfeeding. The drug has minimal side-effects and can be prescribed in combination with a laxative if constipation is a problem.
- Antidepressants have numerous side-effects, which may affect compliance, and they may take several weeks to take effect.
- Laxatives may be helpful where constipation predominates. Osmotic laxatives have been shown to improve stool frequency but did not have any effect on abdominal pain.[73]
- Loperamide can be taken on a daily basis for chronic diarrhoea in divided doses.

Other treatment options

Cognitive behavioural therapy (CBT) aims to teach problem-solving skills to deal with factors such as stressful situations that aggravate symptoms. One study reported a clinically significant decline in IBS symptoms and improvement in quality of life after treatment, with these improvements substantially maintained at follow-up.[74] Referral for psychological interventions can be considered if patient is unresponsive to pharmacological therapy and symptoms become continuous.[59]

RELAXATION THERAPY

Stress management and relaxation therapy may be beneficial for some patients and may reduce abdominal pain and diarrhoea.[61]

Complications

IBS is not known to be linked to onset of any other disease and is not to be associated with increased mortality. However, the chronic relapsing nature of symptoms which can vary considerably in severity from patient to patient may have a significant impact on the patient's quality of life.

Key reminders
- Relatively common condition
- More common in females than males
- Association with anxiety and depression
- Relapsing and remitting condition with variable symptoms
- Non-pharmacological and pharmacological treatment options available
- Potential impact on quality of life if poorly managed.

DYSPEPSIA

Dyspepsia is a common problem with prevalence rates in the Western world estimated at 23%–41% and approximately 25% of those suffering symptoms seek further advice from their GP, resulting in around 10% of these being referred to secondary care for further investigations.[75] There is often confusion around the terminology used and the relationship between dyspepsia, indigestion and heartburn. Guidelines suggest this confusion can be minimised if clinicians recognise that heartburn and dyspepsia describe symptoms, whereas GORD is a collective term embracing all diseases caused by acid reflux.[76]

Clues to aid the diagnosis
Patient may present with symptoms of:
- abdominal discomfort
- nausea
- worsening symptoms after eating particular foods
- bloatedness
- retrosternal heartburn and acid indigestion will be a feature of GORD.[76]

CLINICAL ALERT!

⚠ BEWARE OF!

The following symptoms are regarded as alarm symptoms suggestive of other underlying pathology and require urgent referral for further investigation.[77]
- Unintentional weight loss
- Difficulty swallowing
- Vomiting
- Gastrointestinal bleeding
- Abdominal mass.

Pathophysiology
The pathophysiology underpinning dyspepsia is highly complex and therefore only a simplified explanation will be provided. Delayed gastric emptying has been shown to be associated with symptoms of early satiety, nausea, vomiting and fullness and has

been reported to occur in 30%–70% of patients with functional dyspepsia (dyspepsia of no known cause).[78] It is also thought that hypersensitivity to gastric distension is associated with the symptoms of postprandial pain, belching and weight loss and is observed in 37% of patients with functional dyspepsia.[79]

Differential diagnosis

CLINICAL ALERT!

 BEWARE!

There are a number of medications which can potentially cause dyspepsia. These include:

- NSAIDs (e.g. ibuprofen)
- steroids (e.g. prednisolone)
- bisphosphonates (e.g. alendronic acid)
- CCBs (e.g. verapamil or diltiazem)
- nitrates (e.g. isosorbide dinitrate).

Differential diagnosis
Differential diagnoses include the following (*see* Table 6.21).

TABLE 6.21 Differential diagnoses

Condition	Additional pointers	When to consider
Peptic ulcer	p. 91.	p. 91.
Pain caused by biliary disease (e.g. gallstones)	pp. 75–8.	pp. 75–8.
Oesophageal cancer	Difficulty swallowing is the most common symptom of oesophageal cancer.[80]	Consider if there are additional symptoms of heartburn, coughing up of blood and unexplained weight loss in association with swallowing difficulties.
Stomach cancer	Similar symptoms to dyspepsia in the early stages.	Consider if there is loss of appetite and unexplained weight loss, nausea, abdominal pain and a feeling of bloatedness.
IBS	pp. 88–91.	pp. 88–91.

Treatment
Treatment options are based on clinical findings and available choices include both non-pharmacological (*see* Table 6.22) and pharmacological (see below).

TABLE 6.22 Non-pharmacological treatment options

Action	Supporting evidence
Avoiding foods which cause symptoms	One study reported that 80% of patients had an improvement in dyspeptic symptoms following a period of avoidance of foods found to aggravate the problem.[81]
Avoidance of smoking and alcohol	Evidence is controversial but smoking, alcohol and also caffeine have been implicated as factors associated with an increase in symptoms.[82]
Stress	Reduction in stress levels may improve symptoms as these are often increased during times of stress, hence the reason for dyspepsia sometimes being referred to as 'nervous indigestion'.[83]

Simple uncomplicated dyspepsia with no alarm features may respond to antacids (e.g. Gaviscon).

Suggested additional management if needed

SIMPLE DYSPEPSIA NOT REQUIRING INVESTIGATION

- Medication review for any causative drugs (e.g. NSAIDs).
- If symptoms persist, trial of a PPI. Found to be effective where there are no symptoms causing concern.[84]
- If symptoms continue to persist, testing for *Helicobacter pylori* (*H. pylori*) may be appropriate.
- If negative for *H. pylori*, trial of addition of a prokinetic drug (e.g. metoclopramide) or ranitidine. Prokinetic drugs may be useful but may need to be taken long term.[85] Ranitidine although not as effective as a PPI[86] may provide benefit if used in addition.

CLINICAL ALERT!

Endoscopy is not recommended where there are no symptoms of concern but should be undertaken for any patient with onset of symptoms over the age of 55 or if any of the warning symptoms above are present.[75]

GORD FOUND ON ENDOSCOPY

Follow treatment as above and review. A high dose of PPI can be trialled before adding in further treatment, although a standard dose has been proved to be equally as effective in reducing the risk of any recurrent bleeding.[87]

PEPTIC OR DUODENAL ULCER FOUND ON ENDOSCOPY

Those with recurrent symptoms or ulcer disease found on endoscopy may benefit from testing for and treating *H. pylori* infection if found. After successful eradication of *H. pylori* with antibiotics, the risk of ulcer recurrence is reduced dramatically to 5%–20% at 1 year.[87]

Prescribing tips

- Recent concerns surrounding long-term use of PPIs has identified a higher risk of community-acquired pneumonia in those using this type of medication long term.[88]
- A meta-analysis of 11 papers found a significant association between PPI use and the development of *C. difficile* infection, with higher risk among those taking higher doses.[89]

CLINICAL ALERT!

For simple dyspepsia not requiring investigation there is no guidance as to whether PPI should be commenced prior to or after testing for *H. pylori*.[77]

H. pylori testing

PPI should be stopped for 2 weeks prior to testing for *H. pylori*. Testing is undertaken with a breath test or a stool antigen test.[90] Table 6.23 presents suggested treatments.

TABLE 6.23 Suggested treatment of *H. pylori*[77]

Option one	Option two
Double dose PPI (e.g. omeprazole 20 mg) twice daily.	Double dose PPI (e.g.20 mg omeprazole) twice daily.
Plus amoxicillin 1 g twice daily.	Plus metronidazole 400 mg twice daily.
Plus clarithromycin 500 mg twice daily.	Clarithromycin 250 mg twice daily.

Two weeks of treatment is preferred as this achieves higher eradication rates, but adverse effects are common and compliance may be poor.[92]

CLINICAL ALERT!

- Routine referral for endoscopy in patients of any age when there are no worrying symptoms is not recommended.
- Urgent referral needed for any patient with worrying signs and symptoms.
- Treatment for *H. pylori* should only be prescribed following a positive test result.
- It is advisable that patient stops taking drugs for 7–14 days prior to testing for *H. pylori*. This is because studies have reported that 33%–50% of patients taking conventional doses of a PPI develop a false-negative test if treatment is continued.[91]

Complications

Complications stem from any untreated underlying disease. Self-medicating with antacids can potentially mask underlying disease, causing a delay in diagnosis of in some cases potentially fatal conditions.

Key reminders
- Common condition
- Numerous underlying causes
- May be medication induced
- Lifestyle factors may also be relevant.

REFERENCES

1. Williams JG, Roberts SE, Ali MF, *et al.* Burden of disease. *Gut.* 2007; **56**: 1–113.
2. Tablang MV. *Viral Gastroenteritis.* Available at: http://emedicine.medscape.com/article/176515-overview (accessed 2 August 2012).
3. NHS Choices. *Gastroenteritis in Adults.* Available at: www.nhs.uk/Conditions/Gastroenteritis/Pages/Introduction.aspx (accessed 10 August 2012).
4. Bonheur JL. *Bacterial Gastroenteritis.* Available at: http://emedicine.medscape.com/article/176400-overview#aw2aab6b2b2aa (accessed 2 August 2012).
5. Longmore M, Wilkinson I, Turmezei T, *et al. Oxford Handbook of Clinical Medicine.* 7th ed. Oxford: Oxford University Press; 2007.
6. Simon S, Everitt H, van Dorp F. *Oxford Handbook of General Practice.* Oxford: Oxford University Press; 2010.
7. Health Protection Agency. *Cryptosporidium.* Available at: www.hpa.org.uk/Topics/InfectiousDiseases/InfectionsAZ/Cryptosporidium/ (accessed 4 August 2012).
8. Glandt M, Adachi JA, Mathewson JJ, *et al.* Enteroaggregative esericha coli as a cause of travellers diarrhoea: clinical response to ciprofloxacin. *Clin Inf Dis.* 1999; **29**(2): 335–8.
9. British National Formulary for Children. 2013. www.bnf.org/bnf/org_450055.htm
10. World Gastroenterology Organisation Practice Guideline. *Acute Diarrhoea.* Available at: www.worldgastroenterology.org/assets/downloads/en/pdf/guidelines/01_acute_diarrhea.pdf (accessed 20 August 2012).
11. West AB. The pathology of diverticulitis. *J Clin Gast.* 2008; **42**(10): 1137–8.
12. Janes SEJ, Meagher A, Frizelle FA. Management of diverticulitis. *BMJ.* 2006; **332**(7536): 271–5.
13. Salzman H, Lillie D. Diverticular disease: diagnosis and treatment. *Am Fam Physician.* 2005; **72**(7): 1229–34.
14. Eastwood M. Diverticular disease of the colon. *BMJ.* 2009; **339**: b4309.
15. World Gastroenterology Guidelines. *Diverticulitis.* Available at: www.worldgastroenterology.org/assets/downloads/en/pdf/guidelines/07_diverticular_disease.pdf (accessed 25 April 2013).
16. British Medical Journal. *Cholecystitis: best practice.* Available at: http://bestpractice.bmj.com/best-practice/monograph/78/basics/epidemiology.html (accessed 4 August 2012).
17. Gossage JA, Forshhaw MJ. Prevalence and outcome of litigation claims in England after laparoscopic cholecystectomy. *Int J Clin Pract.* 2010; **64**(13): 1832–5.
18. Bloom AA. *Cholecystitis: clinical presentation.* Available at: http://emedicine.medscape.com/article/171886-clinical (accessed 21 January 2014).
19. Steele PD. *Cholecystitis and Biliary Colic in Emergency Medicine.* Available at: http://emedicine.medscape.com/article/1950020-overview#aw2aab6b4 (accessed 5 September 2012).

20. Huffman JL, Schenker S. Acute acalculous cholecystitis – a review. *Clin Gastroenterol Hepatol.* 2010; **8**(1): 15–22.

21. Sahebally SM, Burke JP, Niamh Nolan N, *et al.* Synchronous presentation of acute acalculous cholecystitis and appendicitis: a case report. *J Med Case Reports.* 2011; **5**: 551.

22. Tran H, Giang TH, Ngoc TTB, Hassell LA. *Carcinoma Involving the Gallbladder: a retrospective review of 23 cases – pitfalls in diagnosis of gallbladder carcinoma.* Available at: www.diagnosticpathology.org/content/7/1/10 (accessed 14 September 2012).

23. Mayo Foundation for Medical Education and Research (MFMER). *Gastritis Symptoms.* Available at: www.mayoclinic.com/health/gastritis/DS00488/DSECTION=symptoms (accessed 14 September 2012).

24. British Society for Gastroenterology. *Peptic ulcers.* Available at: www.bsg.org.uk/patients/general/peptic-ulcers.html (accessed 11 July 2013).

25. British Liver Trust. *Pioneering Liver Health.* Available at: http://79.170.44.126/britishlivertrust.org.uk/home-2/faq/ (accessed 12 October 2012).

26. University of Maryland. *Gallstones and Gallbladder Disease: prognosis and complications.* Available at: www.umm.edu/patiented/articles/how_serious_gallstones_gallbladder_disease_000010_3.htm (accessed 15 March 2013).

27. Christer R. Constipation: causes and cures. *Nursing Times.* 2003; **99**(25): 26.

28. Ford AC, Talley NJ. Laxatives for chronic constipation in adults. *BMJ.* 2012; **345**: e6168.

29. National Institute for Health and Clinical Excellence. *Constipation in Children and Young People: NICE guideline 99.* London: NICE; 2010.

30. World Gastroenterology Guidelines. *Constipation.* Available at: www.worldgastroenterology.org/assets/.../en/.../05_constipation.pdf (accessed 15 July 2012).

31. Holson D. *Constipation in Emergency Medicine.* Available at: http://emedicine.medscape.com/article/774726-overview (accessed 10 August 2012).

32. Biggs WS, Dery WH. Evaluation and treatment of constipation in infants and children. *Am Fam Physician.* 2006; **73**(3): 469–77.

33. Schiller LR. Review article: the therapy of constipation. *Aliment Pharmacol Ther.* 2001; **15**: 749–63.

34. Klaschik E, Nauck F, Ostgathe C. Constipation: modern laxative therapy. *Support Care Cancer.* 2003; **11**: 679–85.

35. Vasanwala FF. Management of chronic constipation in the elderly. *Sing Fam Physician.* 2009; **35**(3): 84–92.

36. Ramkumar D, Raos SSCR. Efficacy and safety of traditional medical therapies for chronic constipation: systematic review. *Am J Gastroenterology.* 2005; **100**(4): 936–71.

37. Tack J, Muller-Lissner S. Treatment of chronic constipation: current pharmacologic approaches and future directions. *Clin Gastroenterol Hepatol.* 2009; **7**: 502–8.

38. Electronic Medicines Compendium. *Duloclax.* Available at: www.medicines.org.uk/emc/medicine/2344/spc

39. University of Maryland Medical Centre. *Constipation.* Available at: http://umm.edu/health/medical/altmed/condition/constipation (accessed 12 September 2013).

40. Thornton S. *Haemorrhoids.* Available at: http://emedicine.medscape.com/article/775407-overview#aw2aab6b2b2 (accessed 2 June 2012).

41. National Digestive Diseases Clearing House. *Haemorrhoids.* Available at: http://digestive.niddk.nih.gov/ddiseases/pubs/hemorrhoids/#causes (accessed 27 March 2013).

42. American Society of Colon and Rectal Surgeons. *Haemorrhoids.* Available at: www.fascrs.org/patients/conditions/hemorrhoids/ (accessed 20 July 2012).

43. Cancer Research UK. *Bowel Cancer Symptoms.* Available at: www.cancerresearchuk.org/cancer-help/type/bowel-cancer/about/bowel-cancer-symptoms (accessed 29 March 2013).

44. Cancer Research UK. *Symptoms of Anal Cancer*. Available at: www.cancerresearchuk.org/cancer-help/type/anal-cancer/about/symptoms-of-anal-cancer (accessed 29 March 2013).
45. Acheson AG, Scholefield JH. Management of haemorrhoids. *BMJ*. 2008; **336**(7640): 380–3.
46. Holzheimer RG. Haemorrhoidectomy: indications and risks. *Eur J Med Res*. 2004; **9**: 18–36.
47. Jayaraman S, Colquhoun PH, Malthaner RA. Stapled versus conventional surgery for haemorrhoids. *Cochrane Database Syst Rev*. 2006; **4**: CD005393.
48. Scheyer M, Antonietti E, Rollinger G, *et al*. Doppler-guided haemorrhoidal artery ligation. *Am J Surg*. 2006; **191**: 89–93.
49. Pescatori M, Gagliardi G. Postoperative complications after procedure for prolapsed haemorrhoids (PPH) and stapled transanal rectal resection (STARR) procedures. *Tech Coloproctol*. 2008; **12**(1): 7–19.
50. Molloy RG, Kingsmore D. Life threatening pelvic sepsis after stapled haemorrhoidectomy. *Lancet*. 2000; **355**: 810.
51. National Digestive Diseases Information Clearing House. *Appendicitis*. Available at: http://digestive.niddk.nih.gov/ddiseases/pubs/appendicitis/appendicitis_508.pdf (accessed 2 June 2012).
52. Humes DJ, Simpson J. Acute appendicitis. *BMJ*. 2006; **333**(7567): 530–4.
53. Hardin DM. Acute appendicitis: review and update. *Am Fam Physician*. 1999; **60**(7): 2027–34.
54. Saddique M, Iqbal P, Rajput A, *et al*. Atypical presentation of appendicitis. Diagnosis and management. *J Surg Pak (Int)*. 2009; **14**(4): 157–60.
55. Craig S. *Appendicitis*. Available at: http://emedicine.medscape.com/article/773895-overview#aw2aab6b2b4aa (accessed 12 June 2012).
56. Gurleyik G, Gurleyik E. Age related clinical features in older patients with acute appendicitis. *Eur J Emerg Med*. 2003; **10**: 200–3.
57. Frantz MG, Norman J, Fabri PJ. Increased morbidity of appendicitis with advancing age. *Am Surg*. 1995; **61**: 40–4.
58. Spiller R, Aziz Q, Creed F, *et al*. Guidelines on the irritable bowel syndrome: mechanisms and practical management. *Gut*. 2007; **56**: 1770–98.
59. National Institute for Clinical Excellence. *Irritable Bowel Syndrome in Adults: NICE guideline 61*. London: NICE; 2008. Available at: www.nice.org.uk/nicemedia/live/11927/39622/39622.pdf
60. Drossman DA, Morris CB, Hu YM, *et al*. A prospective assessment of bowel habit in irritable bowel syndrome in women: defining an alternator. *Gastroenterology*. 2005; **128**: 580–9.
61. Drossman DA, Camilleri M, Mayer EA, *et al*. AGA technical review on irritable bowel syndrome. *Gastroenterology*. 2002; **123**: 2108–31.
62. Maxwell PR, Mendall MA, Kumar D. Irritable bowel syndrome. *Lancet*. 1997; **350**: 1691–5.
63. National Digestive Diseases Information Clearinghouse. *Irritable bowel syndrome*. Available at: http://digestive.niddk.nih.gov/ddiseases/pubs/ibs/#5 (accessed 28 January 2013).
64. Schoultz M, Atherton I, Hubbard G. *Assessment of causal link between psychological factors and symptom exacerbation in inflammatory bowel disease: a protocol for systematic review of prospective cohort studies*. Available at: www.systematicreviewsjournal.com/content/2/1/8 (accessed 3 January 2013).
65. National Foundation for Coeliac Awareness. *Coeliac Disease*. Available at: www.celiaccentral.org/Celiac-Disease/21/ (accessed 4 January 2013).
66. University of Maryland Medical Centre. *Pancreatitis*. Available at: www.umm.edu/altmed/articles/pancreatitis-000122.htm (accessed 3 January 2013).
67. Anand BS. *Peptic Ulcer Disease*. Available at: http://emedicine.medscape.com/article/181753-overview (accessed 19 January 2013).

68. Simren M, Mansson A, Langkide AM. Food-related gastrointestinal symptoms in the irritable bowel syndrome. *Digestion.* 2001; **63**(2): 108–15.
69. Bijkerk CJ, Muris JW, Knottnerus JA, *et al.* Systematic review: the role of different types of fibre in the treatment of irritable bowel syndrome. *Aliment Pharmacol Ther.* 2004; **19**(3): 245–51.
70. Serra J, Salvioli B, Azpiroz F, *et al.* Lipid-induced intestinal gas retention in irritable bowel syndrome. *Gastroenterology.* 2002; **123**: 700–6.
71. Johnson DA. *Does Exercise Improve Symptoms of IBS?* Available at: www.medscape.com/viewarticle/737389 (accessed 4 January 2013).
72. Darmish Damavandi M, Nikfar S, Abdollahi M. A systematic review of efficacy and tolerability of mebeverine in irritable bowel syndrome. *World J Gastroenterol.* 2010; **16**(5): 547–53.
73. Khoshoo V, Armstead C, Landry L. Effect of a laxative with and without tegaserod in adolescents with constipation predominant irritable bowel syndrome. *Aliment Pharmacol Ther.* 2006; **23**: 191–6.
74. Hunt MG, Moshier S, Milonova M. Brief cognitive behavioural internet therapy for irritable bowel syndrome. *Behav Res Therapy.* 2009; **47**(9): 797–802.
75. British Society for Gastroenterology. *Dyspepsia: management guidelines.* Available at: www.bsg.org.uk/pdf_word_docs/dyspepsia.doc (accessed 5 January 2013).
76. Scottish Intercollegiate Guidelines Network (SIGN). *Dyspepsia Guideline: SIGN guideline 68.* Edinburgh: SIGN; 2003. Available at: www.sign.ac.uk/pdf/sign68.pdf (accessed 21 January 2013).
77. National Institute for Health and Clinical Excellence. *Dyspepsia: managing dyspepsia in adults in primary care. NICE guideline 17.* London: NICE; 2004. Available at: http://guidance.nice.org.uk/CG17
78. Tack J, Bisschops R, Sarnelli G. Pathophysiology and treatment of functional dyspepsia. *Gastroenterology.* 2004; **127**(4): 1239–55.
79. Lee KJ, Kindt S, Tack J. Pathophysiology of functional dyspepsia. *Best Pract Res Clin Gastroenterol.* 2004; **18**(4): 707–16.
80. Cancer Research U.K. *Oesophageal cancer.* Available at: www.cancerresearchuk.org/cancer-help/type/oesophageal-cancer/about/symptoms-of-oesophageal-cancer (accessed 19 January 2013).
81. Mullan A, Kavanagh P, O'Mahony P, *et al.* Food and nutrient intakes and eating patterns in functional and organic dyspepsia. *Eur J Clin Nutr.* 1994; **48**: 97–105.
82. Nandurkar S, Talley NJ, Xia H, *et al.* Dyspepsia in the community is linked to smoking and aspirin use but not to Helicobacter pylori infection. *Arch Intern Med.* 1998; **158**: 1427–33.
83. MD guidelines. *Dyspepsia.* Available at: www.mdguidelines.com/dyspepsia (accessed 15 January 2013).
84. Peura DA, Kovacs TO, Metz D, *et al.* Low-dose lansoprazole: effective for non-ulcer dyspepsia (NUD). *Gastroenterology.* 2000; **118**: A2418.
85. Moayyedi P, Soo S, Deeks J, *et al.* Pharmacological interventions for non-ulcer dyspepsia. *Cochrane Database Syst Rev.* 2006; **4**: CD001960.
86. Veldhuyzen van Zanten SJ, Chiba N, Armstrong D, *et al.* A randomized trial comparing omeprazole, ranitidine, cisapride, or placebo in helicobacter pylori negative, primary care patients with dyspepsia: the CADET-HN Study. *Am J Gastroenterol.* 2005; **100**(7): 1477–88.
87. Andriulli A, Loperfido S, Focareta R, *et al.* High- versus low-dose proton pump inhibitors after endoscopic haemostasis in patients with peptic ulcer bleeding: a multicentre, randomized study. *Am J Gastroenterol.* 2008; **103**(12): 3011–18.
88. Ford AC, Delaney BC, Forman D, *et al.* Eradication therapy in Helicobacter pylori positive

peptic ulcer disease: systematic review and economic analysis. *Am J Gastroenterol.* 2004; **99**: 1833–55.

89. Madenick RD. Proton pump inhibitor side effects and drug interactions: much ado about nothing? *Clev Clin J Med.* 2011; **78**(1): 39–49.

90. Leonard J, Marshall JK, Moayyedi P. Systematic review of the risk of enteric infection in patients taking acid suppression. *Am J Gastroenterol.* 2007; **102**: 2047–56.

91. Chey WD. *Discontinuation of PPI Prior to Urea Breath Test.* Available at: www.medscape.com/viewarticle/465198 (accessed 7 June 2013).

92. British National Formulary. 2013. Available at: www.bnf.org/bnf/index.htm

CHAPTER 7

Gynaecology

Gynaecological problems cover a range of conditions affecting each woman differently and often presenting with varying levels of severity. Some conditions are particularly common in younger women, others more frequent among older women. Pelvic pain, for example, is reported to be particularly common among women of child-bearing age.[1] Abnormal menstrual bleeding patterns, on the other hand, can potentially affect women from the onset of menarche right through to the menopause.

CONDITIONS COVERED IN THIS CHAPTER

- Vaginal infections:
  - bacterial vaginosis (BV)
  - vaginal candida
  - trichomonas
  - chlamydia
  - gonorrhoea
- Pelvic inflammatory disease (PID)
- Dysmenorrhoea
- Menorrhagia.

COMMON PRESENTING SYMPTOMS

May present with one or several of the following:
- vaginal discharge
- itching
- offensive smelling discharge
- abnormal menstrual bleeding
- abdominal pain.

TAKING THE GYNAECOLOGICAL HISTORY

Initial history is as described in Chapter 3, followed by a focused enquiry relating to the gynaecological system.

TABLE 7.1 Symptoms enquiry and further questioning for specific symptoms

Symptom	Further questioning
Vaginal discharge	What colour is the discharge?
	How much is there?
	Is there a smell?
	Can patient describe the consistency?
	Is there itching?
Itching	Is the itching there all the time?
	Is there a discharge? (If so questions as above.)
Abnormal menstrual bleeding	Have the periods always been abnormal or is this a new problem?
	Are the periods regular or irregular?
	How long do they last and how heavy is the blood flow?
	Is there significant pain?
Abdominal pain	Use the OPQRST guidance in Chapter 3.

Table 7.2 shows a summary of presenting signs and symptoms and the diseases they may suggest.

TABLE 7.2 Signs and symptoms and possible diseases

	Vaginal discharge	Itching	Abnormal menstrual bleeding	Abdominal pain
BV	Yes	No	No	No
Vaginal candida	Yes	Yes	No	No
Trichomonas	Yes	Possible but less severe than with candida	No	No
Chlamydia	Possible	No	Possible	Possible
Gonorrhoea	Possible	No	Possible	No
PID	Yes	No	Possible	Yes
Dysmenorrhoea	No	No	Yes	Yes
Menorrhagia	No	No	Yes	Possible if there is an underlying cause

FURTHER INVESTIGATIONS
- Triple swabs (high vaginal, endocervical and chlamydia).
- Cervical smear (if over 25 years of age and test is due or overdue).

Other investigations
Other investigations selected on the basis of history, symptoms and clinical findings may include the following:
- pelvic ultrasound
- transvaginal ultrasonography
- hysteroscopy and biopsy
- dilatation and curettage (D and C)
- endometrial biopsy.

URGENT REFERRAL TO A GYNAECOLOGIST REQUIRED
- Abdominal mass.
- Abnormal smear test result (with HPV detected).
- Menorrhagia with suspected underlying pathology.
- Dysmenorrhoea with suspected underlying pathology.

VAGINAL INFECTIONS
Vaginal infections are common and can have a number of underlying causes. Vaginal discharge is a common symptom of infection and is a frequent reason for consultations in primary care. Statistics indicate that sexually transmitted diseases (STIs) among both males and females are increasing in prevalence, with the latest figures showing a 2% increase between 2010 and 2011 with higher rates of gonorrhoea, syphilis and genital herpes.[2]

There are many pathogens that may cause this problem, each giving rise to specific symptoms, and there are instances when more than one infection may be present, complicating the clinical picture. Of the cases which present in GP surgeries, 95% are accounted for by five causes: BV, candida, cervicitis (caused by gonorrhoea, chlamydia or herpes), trichomonas and excessive normal secretions.[3] Of these, BV is the commonest infection followed by gonorrhoea, which is the second most common bacterial sexually transmitted infection in the UK.[4]

Clues to aid the diagnosis
Symptoms vary according to the underlying pathogen. *See* Table 7.3.

TABLE 7.3 Causative organisms and associated symptoms

Causative organism	Discharge characteristics	Additional features
BV	Grey/whitish discharge with a distinctive fishy-smelling odour	Not usually associated with soreness
Candida	Thick white discharge	Itching and soreness May cause discomfort passing urine
Trichomonas	Yellow/green discharge	Discharge has a frothy appearance and a fishy-smelling odour
Chlamydia	Often asymptomatic but there can be some vaginal discharge	Can present with abnormal vaginal bleeding, dyspareunia or dysuria
Gonorrhoea	Whitish to green-coloured discharge	There may also be pelvic pain, dysuria with cervicitis

CLINICAL ALERT!

The vagina, ectocervix and endocervix are all susceptible to various pathogens, with the type of epithelium present influencing susceptibility to particular infections. The squamous epithelium of the vagina and ectocervix is prone to infection with candida species and *Trichomonas vaginalis*, the columnar epithelium of the endocervix to infection with *Neisseria gonorrhoeae* and *Chlamydia trachomatis*, while the *Herpes simplex* virus may infect both types of epithelium.[5]

Pathophysiology

Pathophysiology for each of the infections differs slightly.

BV

In BV, the vaginal flora becomes altered through known and unknown mechanisms, causing an increase in the vaginal pH that is thought to arise as a result of a reduction in the hydrogen peroxide-producing lactobacilli.[6] In healthy vaginas, lactobacilli serve to maintain an acidic environment that is effective in inhibiting any invading microorganisms. Even though high concentrations of lactobacilli are present, infection with BV substantially reduces the population of these organisms while at the same time other organisms increase in number.

Trichomoniasis

During infection with *T. vaginalis*, epithelial cells are destroyed by direct cell contact and by release of cytotoxic substances.[7] During infection, defence mechanisms are activated, with an increase in the number of leukocytes and an increase in the pH. The active organism divides by binary fission, giving rise to a population of organisms in the lumen and on the mucosal surfaces of the urogenital tract.[8]

Candida

Candida is a yeast whose cells reproduce by a process called budding. The organism is capable of flourishing well in a variety of environments. The first step in the development of a candidal infection is colonisation, which occurs when host defences are impaired and the organism is able to gain access to tissues and to the bloodstream, potentially leading to sepsis.[9]

Chlamydia

The pathophysiology of chlamydia infections is poorly understood. *Chlamydia trachomatis* is a gram-negative pathogen with a life cycle made up of two phases. The infectious form of the organism is referred to as the elementary body (EB), which attaches to and enters the host cell, and once inside host cells the EBs begin their second life cycle as metabolically active reticulate bodies (RBs) using host-derived adenosine triphosphate (ATP) to replicate by binary fission.[10]

Gonorrhoea

The pathology and symptoms of gonorrhoea result from activation of the inflammatory response and the infection is usually characterised by vaginal discharge and sometimes dysuria in women (about 50% of women with cervical infections are asymptomatic), and males may also be asymptomatic or present with urethral discharge, prostatitis or orchitis.[11] The organism has the potential to spread to other sites causing other problems (e.g. PID), and its ability to do this may be influenced by the virulence of the invading organism, any impairment in the immune system of the host and any changes in the vaginal pH.

Differential diagnosis

⚠ **BEWARE OF!**

- Foreign bodies (for example, retained tampons, condoms).
- Malignancies (vulva, vagina, cervix, endometrium).
- Atrophic vaginitis.

Treatment

Table 7.4 shows suggested treatment for each infection.

TABLE 7.4 Suggested treatments

Infection	Suggested treatment	Side-effects
BV	Guidance suggests: Oral metronidazole: 400 mg twice daily for 5–7 days.[12] or	Many side-effects but commonest are nausea and vomiting, anorexia, taste disturbances and furred tongue.
	Vaginal metronidazole gel: applied nightly for 5 days.	May cause vaginal burning or itching.
	Clindamycin gel: applied nightly for 7 days.[12]	Vaginal burning or itching.
Candida	A variety of antifungal treatments are available that include creams, pessaries and tablets, and are for use either intravaginally or to be taken orally. Some preparations require single use only. Canesten pessary is usually used as a one-off dose at night or alternatively fluconazole 150 mg can be used as a one-off oral dose. Recurrent symptoms may require a longer course of 7–14 days of topical therapy or oral fluconazole every third day for a total of three doses.[13]	Rarely local irritation from creams. Oral treatment may cause nausea, abdominal discomfort, diarrhoea and rashes.
Trichomonas	Oral metronidazole: 400 mg twice daily for 5–7 days.[14]	See information for BV as above.
Chlamydia	Doxycycline 100 mg twice daily for 7 days, or azithromycin 1 g immediately.[15]	Commonest include nausea, vomiting and diarrhoea, and possible rashes.
Gonorrhoea	Referral to GU Medicine advised. Cefixime 400 mcg as a single dose, but its use is unlicensed.[16]	Commonest include nausea, vomiting, diarrhoea, abdominal discomfort, rashes and allergic reactions. Headaches.

Prescribing tips
- Metronidazole: no alcohol while taking and for up to 2 days after completing the course and is not recommended for use during menstruation.
- Vaginal creams damage latex condoms and diaphragms.
- For breastfeeding and pregnant women needing treatment for chlamydia, erythromycin is best choice as it is not known to be harmful.

Additional alerts

TABLE 7.5 Alerts: beware!

Infection	Alerts
BV	Be alert to: women with several partners or frequent change of partner (including sex workers), which increases susceptibility to any sexually transmitted infection and HIV.
	In patients with HIV, BV is associated with increased risk of both acquisition and transmission of HIV infection.[17]
	Lesbian women: association between BV and having an increased number of female sexual partners.[18]
Candida	Be alert to: women with several partners or frequent changes of partner. Candida can arise as a result of poorly controlled diabetes or undiagnosed diabetes and also recent antibiotic use.
Trichomoniasis	Be alert to: women with several partners or frequent changes of partner (including sex workers: risk of BV increased among those with several partners in the preceding 30 days).[19]
	Drug addicts: increased risk of BV among those with drug use in the preceding 30 days.[20]
Chlamydia	Be alert to: multiple change of partners or recent new partner (including sex workers).
Gonorrhoea	Be alert to: increased prevalence among those with multiple sexual partners or frequent change of partner (including sex workers).[11] Homosexuality, with reported high rates among homosexual males.[21]

CLINICAL ALERT!

Contact tracing recommended for chlamydia, gonorrhoea and trichomoniasis.

Complications

Complications vary according to the type of infection.

BV

Frequently causes no complications; however, the following should be considered.

- BV can increase susceptibility to HIV infection if exposed to the virus.[22]
- An HIV-infected woman has a greater chance of passing HIV to her partner if infected with BV.[22]
- During pregnancy BV increases the risk for some complications of pregnancy (e.g. preterm delivery).[23]
- Risk of gonorrhoea, and chlamydia is increased in those infected with BV.[19]

Candida

Possibility of:
- recurrent episodes
- treatment failure
- male partner can develop balanitis.

Trichomoniasis

The following are a cause for concern:
- the infection is a risk factor for HIV transmission[24]
- increased risk of post-hysterectomy infections, tubal infertility and cervical cancer in women and increased risk of infection of the prostate and foreskin, and epididymitis, as well as decreased sperm motility in males[25]
- in HIV-positive men infected with trichomonas there is a substantial increase in HIV concentration in the semen[26]
- increased risk of premature birth or low birth weight baby.[24]

Chlamydia

Of particular concern because:
- damage caused is often 'silent'
- chlamydia is a preventable cause of ectopic pregnancy, PID and infertility[27]
- in males complications are rare but can cause pain, fever, sterility and epididymitis; untreated, chlamydia may increase risk of acquiring or transmitting HIV.[28]

Gonorrhoea

Possible concerns are:
- untreated gonorrhoea can increase a person's risk of acquiring or transmitting HIV[29]
- in women there is increased risk of PID, leading to infertility, and in males epididymitis can develop[30]
- if infection spreads it can result in prostatitis, joint pains, salpingitis, prostatitis and septicaemia.[27]

Key reminders
- Relatively common
- Easily spread
- Associated with several problems if left undiagnosed and untreated
- Infections can coexist.

PELVIC INFLAMMATORY DISEASE

PID is an inflammation in the pelvis and is usually caused by an infection that has spread from the vagina and cervix to the uterus, fallopian tubes, ovaries and pelvic area. It is estimated to account for approximately 1 in 60 GP visits in women under the age of 45 each year.[31]

Clues to aid the diagnosis

Presenting signs and symptoms are variable and may be relatively mild or more severe where the woman presents feeling acutely unwell. The commonest presenting features are:

- abnormal vaginal discharge
- lower abdominal pain
- fever
- pain and discomfort on vaginal examination
- the woman may also complain of painful intercourse.

CLINICAL ALERT!

- When PID is suspected, high vaginal and endocervical swabs should be taken as well as testing for chlamydia infection.
- Raised WCC, ESR and raised leucocyte levels help to confirm the diagnosis, although in some patients results will be normal or only mildly elevated. Very raised values can help with the evaluation of disease severity.[32]

Pathophysiology

The first stage is the development of a vaginal or cervical infection, which then transcends to the uterus, fallopian tubes and upper genital tract, although the exact mechanism by which this takes place is not known. However, it is thought that a number of factors may contribute. Hormonal changes during menstruation and ovulation may alter the efficiency of the cervical mucus in providing protection against infection, and antibiotic treatment and the presence of STIs can interfere with the balance of the normal flora, allowing pathogens which are usually non-pathogenic to multiply and ascend.[33]

Differential diagnosis

The differential diagnosis of lower abdominal pain is shown in Table 7.6.

TABLE 7.6 Differential diagnoses: beware!

Condition	Additional pointers	When to consider
Appendicitis	pp. 86–7.	pp. 86–7.
Ectopic pregnancy	p. 87.	p. 87.
Endometriosis	Lower abdominal pain described as cramping in nature.	Consider if pain is associated with menstruation with possible heavy bleeds with clots, and there may also be bleeding between periods.

CLINICAL ALERT!

- Nausea and vomiting are features of appendicitis and PID, but are far more common in appendicitis, occurring in only 50% of women with PID.[34]
- Pain and discomfort on moving the cervix occurs in PID but are found in only 25% of women with appendicitis.[34]

Treatment

Current guidance suggests the following.

Intramuscular ceftriaxone 500 mg stat. followed by:

- oral doxycycline 100 mg twice daily plus metronidazole 400 mg twice daily for 14 days

or

- oral ofloxacin 400 mg twice daily plus oral metronidazole 400 mg twice daily for 14 days.[14]

Guidance recommends partners within the last 6 months should be contacted and offered screening and advice (referral to GU clinic usually required for this). Sexual intercourse should be avoided until treatment is completed.[35]

Prescribing tips

- Women using the oral contraceptive pill (COC) taking a broad-spectrum antibiotic (e.g. doxycycline) should be advised to use additional contraception for the duration of treatment and for 7 days afterwards. This is because drugs of this type interfere with absorption of oestrogen, hence making the pill ineffective.[36]

Complications

⚠ BEWARE!

- Fertility problems can occur if there is scarring and adhesions.
- Up to 10%–15% of women with PID may become infertile, and this is more likely to occur in women who have had multiple infections.[37]
- Damage to fallopian tubes increases risk of ectopic pregnancy by as much as 50%.[33]

Key reminders

- Relatively common, particularly in young women
- Severe episodes require hospitalisation for treatment
- Use of condoms may help reduce risk of infections
- Repeated infections raise the risk of complications.

DYSMENORRHOEA

Dysmenorrhoea literally means painful menstrual cramps originating within the uterus, and it is reported to be one of the commonest gynaecological conditions seen by doctors in the primary care setting. Although the condition is not life threatening, it can be extremely distressing and is a significant cause of time lost from school or work, and at its worst can cause disturbance to the ability to perform activities of daily living, affecting women's ability to function normally. Because some women may choose to self-treat, a percentage of sufferers may never receive a formal diagnosis, which suggests that the condition may be underdiagnosed and undertreated, a factor thought to be attributed to the fact that many women expect some degree of pain during menstruation and are unaware that theirs may be excessive, believing it to be expected.

Classification

Dysmenorrhoea is usually categorised as two distinct types, primary or secondary, based on signs and symptoms and the clinical features. Primary dysmenorrhoea is defined as menstrual pain occurring in the absence of underlying pelvic disease.[38] This type is more frequently found in younger women, with symptoms commencing early after the initial onset of the menarche. Secondary dysmenorrhoea, however, is defined as menstrual pain that occurs with an underlying pathology as its cause and commonly appears in the third and fourth decade of life,[39] often commencing after many years of painless menses.

Table 7.7 presents clues to aid diagnosis and gives differences between primary and secondary dysmenorrhoea. Table 7.8 presents the causes of secondary dysmenorrhoea.

TABLE 7.7 Clues to aid diagnosis and differences between primary and secondary dysmenorrhoea

Primary dysmenorrhoea	Secondary dysmenorrhoea
Onset typically occurs within 6–12 months of the onset of menstruation.	Although onset can occur at any time, much more likely to be seen in women over the age of 30.
There is no pelvic abnormality found on clinical examination.	Abnormality found on pelvic examination.
Pain is usually centred in the lower abdomen and commences with the onset of the menstrual blood flow and may last for up to 72 hours.[40]	Women may report a change in the intensity and timing of pain during each menstrual cycle. Pain may not be solely limited to the onset of menstruation and there may be other symptoms such as back pain, and a feeling of bloatedness.

TABLE 7.8 Causes of secondary dysmenorrhoea

Condition	Brief description
Endometriosis	Tissue similar to that of the endometrium is found outside the uterus and myometrium.
PID	pp. 108–10.
Intrauterine device (IUD)	May cause period pain.
Fibroids	Benign growths that can occur at various sites within the uterus.
Adenomyosis	This condition occurs when endometrial tissue, which normally lines the uterus, exists within and grows into the muscular walls, causing uterine thickening.[41]

Pathophysiology

The pathophysiology of dysmenorrhoea is still not fully understood, but there is evidence to suggest that prolonged uterine contractions and decreased blood flow to the myometrium are instrumental in causing the symptoms.[38] It is thought that prostaglandin release underpins this process, as it is released by the sloughing endometrial cells, a process which leads to contraction of the myometrium, ischaemia and vasoconstriction. In women with severe dysmenorrhoea, prostaglandin levels have been found to be particularly high, especially during the first 2 days of bleeding.[42] In women with primary dysmenorrhoea, ovulatory cycles are normal, and it is now thought that excessive production and release of uterine prostaglandins is the main reason for abnormal uterine activity causing pain. In secondary dysmenorrhoea, elevated prostaglandin levels may also play a part, but in the presence of an underlying medical condition pathophysiology is even more complex.

Differential diagnosis

There are a number of differential diagnoses (*see* Table 7.9).

TABLE 7.9 Differential diagnoses: beware!

Condition	Additional pointers	When to consider
Ovarian cysts	Small cysts may be asymptomatic.	There are additional symptoms of dyspareunia, bowel and/or urinary symptoms.[43]
PID	pp. 108–10.	pp. 108–10.
UTI	Sudden onset of symptoms with frequency of micturition and lower abdominal pain.	Patient complains of burning sensation when passing urine and that urine has an offensive smell.
Ectopic pregnancy	p. 87.	p. 87.
IBS	pp. 88–91.	pp. 88–91.

Treatment

Treatment aims to relieve pain and symptoms. There is a range of options available, with choice of treatment offered depending on the type of dysmenorrhoea, the severity of symptoms and patient choice. Table 7.10 shows some of the more frequently used treatment options.

TABLE 7.10 Treatment options

Treatment	Mode of action	Effectiveness
Simple analgesia, NSAIDs (e.g. ibuprofen) often effective	Achieve their effects by inhibiting the production and release of prostaglandins, effectively reducing painful contractions caused by their release during menstruation. NSAIDs have the additional benefit of reducing blood flow.	A Cochrane review reported that 17%–95% of women achieved effective pain relief.[44] There are several side-effects, including headaches, GI discomfort, nausea and diarrhoea. It is recommended these drugs are taken with food to minimise this.
COC	Effective in suppressing ovulation and reducing the thickness of the lining of the uterus, which in turn reduces prostaglandin levels and the volume of menstrual blood flow.[45]	Limited evidence to support their use.
Levonorgestrel-releasing intrauterine system	Achieves its effects by releasing levonorgestrel into the uterine cavity. Prevents thickening of the lining of the womb and remains in situ for five years.	Studies have shown this method produced spontaneous reduction in dysmenorrhoea with 50% of women amenorrhoeic after 12 months' use.[46]
Depot medroxyprogesterone acetate (Depo Provera)	Suppresses ovulation.	Has been found to induce amenorrhoea in up to 60% of women after 12 months' use and 68% of women after 2 years' use.[47]
Tranexamic acid	An antifibrinolytic agent that competitively inhibits breakdown of fibrin clots by blocking the binding of plasminogen and plasmin to fibrin.[48]	Up to 93% reduction in symptoms.[49]
Danazol	Suppresses the menstrual cycle.	Limited evidence but reserved for women with endometriosis and secondary dysmenorrhoea. Associated with significant side-effects.

(continued)

Treatment	Mode of action	Effectiveness
Uterine ablation (several techniques)	Destroys or removes the lining of the uterus.	One study reported that further surgical treatment was later needed by 38% of women who underwent uterine ablation, but satisfaction rates were high.[50] Failure of the procedure has been found more likely to occur in women younger than 45 years and in women with parity of five or more.[51] Procedure may be unsuitable for women who wish to conceive at a later date as there is a risk of complications in the event of subsequent pregnancy.
Surgical intervention (hysterectomy)	Complete removal of the uterus.	100% effective.
Transcutaneous electrical nerve stimulation (TENS)	This method stimulates the skin, using electrodes which emit various frequencies. It is thought to alter the body's ability to receive and understand pain signals rather than by having a direct effect on the uterine contractions.[52]	A Cochrane review reported that high-frequency TENS may be helpful but that there is not enough evidence to support use of low-frequency TENS.[52]
Acupuncture	Achieves its effects by stimulating receptors and nerve fibres, which then through complex interaction with serotonin and endorphins block pain impulses.[53]	Limited evidence relating to its effectiveness.
Exercise	Improves blood flow and stimulates the production of endorphins, which act as non-specific analgesics.[53]	Inconclusive evidence to support effectiveness.
Topical heat	Thought to reduce the response to a painful stimulus. This analgesic effect may be due to increased levels of endorphins and suppression of cortical pain sensation.[54]	Found to be as effective as ibuprofen, and when used in conjunction with ibuprofen faster pain relief was achieved.[55]
Dietary supplements		
Omega 3–omega 6 fatty acids	Thought to decrease the formation of pro-inflammatory prostaglandins.	Limited evidence obtained from small studies.
Thiamine, magnesium	Possibly reduce prostaglandin synthesis.	Limited evidence for either thiamine or magnesium.
Vitamin E	Interferes with prostaglandin biosynthesis.	Limited evidence.

BEWARE!

The following need urgent referral and further investigation:
- persistent abnormal bleeding
- any abdominal mass found on examination
- abnormal cervix found on examination
- post-coital and inter-menstrual bleeding.

Key reminders
- Dysmenorrhoea can occur at any time in the menstrual years with or without underlying pathology.
- Some women may tolerate symptoms, leaving their condition undiagnosed and untreated.
- Treatment options are numerous, and include both pharmacological and non-pharmacological.

MENORRHAGIA

Menorrhagia is a distressing condition that has a significant impact on many women's lives, as well as workload in primary and secondary care resulting in more than 5% of women aged 30–49 years consulting their GP each year with this complaint.[56] The condition is reported to be one of the commonest problems seen in gynaecology clinics and estimates suggest that approximately 12% of hospital referrals to a gynaecologist are for this condition.[57] In the primary care setting, one in 20 women aged between 30 and 49 years of age consults her GP with heavy menstrual bleeding.[58] In the past, treatment options were limited, but with advances in medical interventions, there are now many more options available. For women who suffer symptoms month after month, the condition can become debilitating, leading to ill health.

Clues to aid the diagnosis
The normal interval between monthly bleeds is 21–35 days, with bleeding expected to last anywhere between 1 and 7 days.[59] The amount of blood lost is regarded as excessive when it exceeds 80 mL.[60] Actually measuring the amount of blood loss is obviously difficult as it relies on the women's description and is therefore subjective. Assessment of blood loss may involve recording how often pads are changed per day and whether this needs to be undertaken during the night as well as during the day.

CLINICAL ALERT!

⚠ BEWARE!

It is important to be clear on the exact nature of the bleeding pattern so that treatment can be selected appropriately.

Other common bleeding patterns are:

• metrorrhagia, which is used to describe heavy or prolonged menstrual bleeding that may occur as a single episode or occur on a chronic basis[61]
• polymenorrhoea, which describes bleeding that occurs at much more frequent intervals than would normally be expected
• menometrorrhagia occurs when bleeding is frequent and when it does occur it is associated with heavy blood loss.

When blood loss is excessive, women may experience other associated symptoms. Table 7.11 shows some of the effects women may experience when bleeding is excessive.

TABLE 7.11 Side-effects of severe blood loss

Fatigue
Breathlessness
Anaemia
Feeling cold
Palpitations

CLINICAL ALERT!

In the presence of symptoms as shown in Table 7.11, an FBC should be requested to assess for anaemia.

Pathophysiology

In healthy women the hypothalamus releases a gonadotrophin-releasing hormone which stimulates the pituitary gland to synthesise the follicle stimulating hormone (FSH) and luteinising hormone (LH). The release of these two hormones then stimulates the ovaries to produce oestrogen and progesterone. The release of oestrogen then stimulates the thickening of the endometrium, a phase described as the proliferative phase. During the second half of the menstrual cycle progesterone takes over, leading to further thickening of the endometrium in preparation for a fertilised embryo. If fertilisation does not take place oestrogen and progesterone levels fall, resulting in menstruation. In women who do not ovulate, the corpus luteum does not develop, which ultimately leads to the release of oestrogen only but no progesterone is released. Oestrogen alone results in the continued proliferation and thickening of the endometrium, until it finally reaches a point where it has outgrown its blood supply and degeneration of the lining begins. In anovulatory women the breakdown of the lining occurs in an erratic manner and this is why anovulatory bleeding is heavier than normal menstrual flow.[62]

- In young women aged 12–18, the most common cause of heavy bleeding is anovulatory cycles, while in older women aged 30–50 fibroids or polyps are more frequently the cause.[62]
- In approximately 40%–60% of women no cause for menorrhagia can be found and in these cases the bleeding is classified as dysfunctional uterine bleeding.[63]
- For the remaining women there are a number of potential causes, which have been broadly classified into ovulatory, anovulatory and anatomic (*see* Table 7.12).

TABLE 7.12 Classification of menorrhagia

Ovulatory	This may occur on a regular monthly basis and be associated with dysmenorrhoea or premenstrual discomfort.
Anovulatory	This type occurs more commonly in adolescents and bleeding is often heavy and irregular.
Anatomic	This type occurs when there is an underlying abnormality such as fibroids or polyps. Bleeding is usually heavy and painful and on clinical examination the uterus may be enlarged.
Caused by medical treatment (iatrogenic)	Iatrogenic causes include chemotherapy, certain drugs such as anticoagulants, treatment with steroid hormones, and use of an IUD.
Systemic conditions	Systemic causes include hypothyroidism and Von Willebrand disease (a genetic bleeding disorder which affects the clotting mechanism).

Differential diagnosis

Other possible causes of menorrhagia are shown in Table 7.13.

TABLE 7.13 Differential diagnoses

Condition	Additional pointers	When to consider
Endometriosis	Pelvic pain is the most common presenting symptom.[64]	Symptoms appear to be strongest before the onset of menstruation, with symptoms of pelvic pain, back pain, dyspareunia and loin pain.[64]
PID	pp. 108–10.	pp. 108–10.
Polycystic ovary disease	Periods may be irregular.	There is also obesity and hirsutism.
Endometrial carcinoma	Usually presents with post-menopausal bleeding but 20%–25% of cases present with abnormalities of the menstrual cycle.[65]	Woman is nulliparous and obese (obesity is associated with a two to threefold increased risk with a similar increased risk in nulliparous women).[66]

CLINICAL ALERT!

⚠ **BEWARE!**

There are a number of symptoms that are a cause for concern and may indicate underlying pathology. Urgent referral is required when there is any suspicion of gynaecological cancer.

Symptoms which may point towards underlying malignancy

These include:

- palpable mass found either on abdominal examination or vulval examination
- vaginal discharge, which has an unpleasant odour
- regular and persistent post-coital bleeding
- inter-menstrual bleeding
- painful intercourse.

Treatment

There are several treatment options available and choice is guided by a combination of factors. Prior to selecting and commencing treatment consideration should be given to the following factors (*see* Table 7.14).

TABLE 7.14 Factors to consider prior to commencing treatment

Factor to consider	Concern
Age of the woman	Some treatments more suitable for specific age groups.
Medical history	Some hormonal treatments are unsuitable for women with a history of embolism or deep vein thrombosis (DVT).
Desire to have children	Some treatment options are unsuitable for women who wish to remain fertile.
Adverse effects	May affect women's willingness to continue treatment.

Treatment options available

Table 7.15 shows the treatment options available, evidence to support their use, common side-effects and possible advantages of the methods discussed below.

TABLE 7.15 Treatment options, side-effects and advantages

Treatment	Side-effects Evidence	Disadvantages Side-effects	Advantages
Levonorgestrel-releasing IUD: **First line**[67]	p. 113 for mode of action.	Irregular bleeding. Breast tenderness.	Provides contraception. Cost-effective. Reduces need for surgery.
Tranexamic acid: **Second line**[67]	p. 113 for mode of action.	Does not provide contraceptive protection. Side-effects include headaches and muscle cramps.	Gives quick relief in reducing blood loss. Only taken for a few days each month. Fertility is not affected.
NSAIDs **Second line**[67]	p. 113 for mode of action. A Cochrane review reported that NSAIDs reduce heavy bleeding when compared with placebo but are less effective than either tranexamic acid, danazol or the levonorgestrel IUD.[68]	May cause gastric irritation.	Available without a prescription so useful for women who have to pay for their prescription. Helps where pain is a problem. Can be used in conjunction with other menorrhagia treatments.
COC **Third line**[67]	p. 113 for mode of action. Little data on the effectiveness of the COC in actually reducing blood loss. However, one study reported that 87% of those allocated to the COC group reported reduced blood loss.[69]	Breast tenderness. Headaches. Loss of libido. Hypertension. Fluid retention. Weight gain.	Provides contraception. Useful if pain is a problem.

(continued)

Treatment	Side-effects Evidence	Disadvantages Side-effects	Advantages
Danazol	p. 113 for mode of action.	Weight gain. Acne. Depression. Raised cholesterol levels. Increase in male characteristics, such as deep voice and increased body hair. Oily skin and hair.	Effective in relieving pain.
Depot medroxyprogesterone acetate (Depo Provera)	p. 113 for mode of action and some effects of treatment.	Side-effects include weight gain. Reduces bone mineral density over time. May cause irregular bleeding patterns or amenorrhoea.	Provides contraceptive cover. Given three monthly, which may be more suitable for some women.
Norethisterone	Less commonly prescribed because of the unpleasant side-effects that may be incurred. A Cochrane review reported that progestogens administered from day 15 or 19 to day 26 of the cycle offered no advantage over danazol, tranexamic acid, NSAIDs or the IUD in women with ovulatory cycles, but when taken for 21 days menstrual blood loss reduced considerably, but treatment was less acceptable than levonorgestrel IUD.[70]	Nausea, vomiting, headaches, mood swings, breast tenderness and abdominal pain.	Provides contraceptive cover. Useful if pain is a problem.

Treatment	Side-effects Evidence	Disadvantages Side-effects	Advantages
Endometrial ablation	p. 114 May offer a solution where other methods have failed.	Unsuitable for women who wish to have children in the future as fertility is lost. May experience cramping, vaginal discharge, and nausea after the procedure. Vaginal discharge may be present for a few days. Need for further intervention may occur at a later date.	Minimally invasive. Suitable for women who do not wish to remain fertile.
Myomectomy	Myomectomy involves removing uterine fibroids via one of several surgical techniques. Effective in reducing the amount of blood loss, but there is no guarantee that fibroids will not recur, with the need for further treatment at a later date.	Excessive blood loss. Fibroids may recur. Risk of scar tissue formation.	Restores the uterus to normal function. Preserves fertility.
Hysterectomy	Later option for many as newer treatments are now available. Offers complete resolution of symptoms for those who choose to have the procedure.	Wound infection. Prolapse of the bladder or bowel. Depression. Urinary problems.	No risk of recurrence or need for further treatment.

Complications

Despite rarely being life threatening, menorrhagia has significant effects on personal, social, family and work life of women and thereby reduces their quality of life.[71]

More than two thirds of women with menstrual blood loss greater than 80 mL per cycle have evidence of anaemia.[72]

Key reminders

- Common
- May be undiagnosed and therefore untreated
- Debilitating
- Impacts on quality of life
- Numerous treatment options available.

REFERENCES

1. Zondervan KT, Yudkin PL, Vessey MP, *et al.* The community prevalence of chronic pelvic pain in women and associated illness behaviour. *Br J Gen Pract.* 2001; **51**(468): 541–7.
2. Health Protection Agency. *Sexually Transmitted Infections.* Available at: www.hpa.org.uk/web/HPAweb&Page&HPAwebAutoListName/Page/1201094610372#._STI_data_for_the_UK (accessed 1 February 2013).
3. Simon S, Everitt H, van Dorp F. *Oxford Handbook of General Practice.* Oxford: Oxford University Press; 2010.
4. Newsome L. *The Basics – vaginal discharge.* Available at: www.gponline.com/Clinical/article/1033896/the-basics-vaginal-discharge/ (accessed 2 February 2013).
5. Yusef A, Chowdhury M, Shaidul Islam KM, *et al.* Common microbial aetiology of abnormal vaginal discharge among sexually active women in Dhaka, Bangladesh. *South East Asia J Public Health.* 2011; **1**: 35–9.
6. Curren D. *Bacterial Vaginosis.* Available at: http://emedicine.medscape.com/article/254342-overview#a0104 (accessed 5 February 2013).
7. Scott Smith D. *Trichomoniasis.* Available at: http://emedicine.medscape.com/article/230617-overview#a0104 (accessed 5 February 2013).
8. Schwebke JR, Burgess D. Trichomoniasis. *Clin Microbiol Rev.* 2004; **17**(4): 794–803.
9. Spellberg B, Edwards JE. The pathophysiology and treatment of candida sepsis. *Curr Infect Dis Rep.* 2002; **4**(5): 387–99.
10. NM Department of Health Family Planning Programme. *Medical Overview.* Available at: www.health.state.nm.us/phd/fp/medical_overview.htm (accessed 30 March 2013).
11. Todar K. *Neisseria gonorrhoeae, the Gonococcus, and Gonorrhoea.* Available at: http://textbookofbacteriology.net/themicrobialworld/gonorrhea.html (accessed 5 February 2013).
12. FFPRHC and BASHH Guidance. The management of women of reproductive age attending non-genitourinary medicine settings complaining of vaginal discharge. *J Fam Plan Reprod Health Care.* 2006; **32**(1): 33–41.
13. Newsome L. *The Basics – recurrent vaginal candidiasis.* Available at: www.gponline.com/clinical/article/1004744/Basics---Recurrent-vaginal-candidiasis (accessed 20 February 2013).
14. British National Formulary. 2013. Available at: www.bnf.org/bnf/index.htm
15. Duncan S, Sherrard J. *Chlamydia.* Available at: www.gponline.com/Clinical/article/1170834/Clinical-Review---Chlamydia/ (accessed 10 August 2013).

16. Korting HC, Kollman M. Effective single dose treatment of uncomplicated gonorrhoea. *Int J of STD AIDS*. 1994; **5**: 239–43.

17. Spear GT, St John E, Zariffard MR. Bacterial vaginosis and human immunodeficiency virus infection. *AIDS Res Ther*. 2007; **4**: 25.

18. Bailey JV, Farquhar C, Owen C. Bacterial vaginosis in lesbians and bisexual women. *Sex Transm Dis*. 2004; **31**: 691–4.

19. Wiesenfeld HC, Hillier SL, Krohn MA, *et al*. Bacterial vaginosis is a strong predictor of Neisseria gonorrhoea and chlamydia trachomatis infection. *Clin Infect Dis*. 2003; **36**(5): 663–8.

20. Miller M, Liao Y, Gomez AM, *et al*. Factors associated with the prevalence and incidence of Trichomonas vaginalis infection among African American women in New York city who use drugs. *J Infect Dis*. 2008; **97**(4): 503–9.

21. Health Protection Agency. *Gonorrhoea*. Available at: www.hpa.org.uk/web/HPAweb&Page&HPAwebAutoListName/Page/1191942171513 (accessed 5 April 2013).

22. Centres for Disease Control and Prevention. *Bacterial Vaginosis*. Available at: www.cdc.gov/std/bv/stdfact-bacterial-vaginosis.htm (accessed 10 April 2013).

23. Purwar M, Ughade S, Bhagat B, *et al*. Bacterial vaginosis in early pregnancy and adverse pregnancy outcome. *J Obstet Gynaecol Res*. 2001; **27**: 175–81.

24. National Institute of Allergy and Infectious Diseases. *Trichomoniasis*. Available at: www.niaid.nih.gov/topics/trichomoniasis/understanding/pages/complications.aspx (accessed 25 April 2013).

25. New Zealand Dermatological Society Incorporated. *Trichomoniasis*. Available at: www.dermnetnz.org/arthropods/trichomoniasis.html (accessed 5 April 2013).

26. Centres for Disease Control and Prevention. *Trichomoniasis: fact sheet*. Available at: www.cdc.gov/std/trichomonas/stdfact-trichomoniasis.htm (accessed 10 April 2013).

27. Longmore M, Wilkinson I, Turmezei T, *et al*. *Oxford Handbook of Clinical Medicine*. 7th ed. Oxford: Oxford University Press; 2007.

28. Centres for Disease Control and Prevention. *Chlamydia: fact sheet*. Available at: www.cdc.gov/std/chlamydia/stdfact-chlamydia.htm (accessed 5 June 2013).

29. Fleming DT, Wasserheit JN. From epidemiological synergy to public health policy and practice: the contribution of other sexually transmitted diseases to sexual transmission of HIV infection. *Sex Transm Inf*. 1999; **75**: 3–17.

30. Mayo Foundation for Medical Education and Research (MFMER). *Gonorrhoea Complications*. Available at: www.mayoclinic.com/health/gonorrhea/DS00180/DSECTION=complications (accessed 15 March 2013).

31. Royal College of Gynaecologists. *Acute Pelvic Inflammatory Disease (PID): tests and treatment – information for you*. Available at: www.rcog.org.uk/acute-pelvic-inflammatory-disease-tests-treatment (accessed 7 February 2013).

32. Royal College of Obstetricians and Gynaecologists (RCOG). *Management of Acute Pelvic Inflammatory Disease*. Available at: www.rcog.org.uk (accessed 3 February 2013).

33. Moore Shepherd S. *Pelvic Inflammatory Disease Treatment and Management*. Available at: http://emedicine.medscape.com/article/256448-treatment (accessed 2 February 2013).

34. Bongard F, Landers DV, Lewis F. Differential diagnosis of appendicitis and pelvic inflammatory disease. A prospective analysis. *Am J Surg*. 1985; **150**: 90–6.

35. British Association for Sexual Health and HIV. UK national guideline for the management of pelvic inflammatory disease. Available at: www.bashh.org/documents/3572.pdf (accessed 12 August 2013).

36. General Practice Notebook. *Antibiotics and Oral Contraceptive Pill*. Available at: www.gpnotebook.co.uk/simplepage.cfm?ID=-932511690 (accessed 12 September 2013).

37. Centres for Disease Control and Prevention. *Pelvic Inflammatory Disease.* Available at: www.cdc.gov/std/pid/stdfact-pid.htm (accessed 15 March 2013).

38. Calis KA. *Dysmenorrhoea.* Available at: http://emedicine.medscape.com/article/253812-overview (accessed 10 February 2013).

39. Kohle S, Deb S. Dysmenorrhoea. *Obs Gynaecol Rep Med.* 2011; **21**(11): 311–16.

40. Cleveland Clinic. *Dysmenorrhoea.* Available at: http://my.clevelandclinic.org/disorders/dysmenorrhea/hic_dysmenorrhea.aspx (accessed 20 March 2013).

41. Mayo Foundation for Medical Education and Research (MFMER). *Adenomyosis.* Available at: www.mayoclinic.com/health/Adenomyosis/DS00636 (accessed 12 March 2013).

42. Holder A. *Dysmenorrhoea in Emergency Medicine.* Available at: http://emedicine.medscape.com/article/795677-overview (accessed 22 March 2013).

43. Kochhar S, Sinha P. *The Basics: ovarian cysts.* Available at: www.gponline.com/Clinical/article/1101447/Basics---Ovarian-cysts/ (accessed 13 February 2014).

44. Marjoribanks J, Proctor ML, Farquhar C. Nonsteroidal anti-inflammatory drugs for primary dysmenorrhoea. *Cochrane Database Syst Rev.* 2003; **4**: CD001751.

45. Wong CL, Farquhar C, Roberts H, *et al.* Oral contraceptive pill as treatment for primary dysmenorrhoea. *Cochrane Database Syst Rev.* 2009; **2**: CD002120.

46. Proctor M, Farquhar C. Diagnosis and management of dysmenorrhoea: clinical review. *BMJ.* 2006; **332**: 1134–8.

47. Polancczky M, Guarnaccia M. Early experience with the contraceptive use of depomedroxyprogesterone acetate in an inner city clinic population. *Fam Plan Pers J.* 1996; **28**: 174–8.

48. MIMS online. *Tranexamic acid.* Available at: www.mims.co.uk/Drugs/cardiovascular-system/haemophilia-bleeding-disorders/tranexamic-acid/ (accessed 15 February 2013).

49. Wellington K, Wagstaff AJ. Tranexamic acid: a review of its use in the management of menorrhagia. *Drugs.* 2003; **63**(13): 1417–33.

50. Aberdeen Endometrial Ablation Trials Group. A randomised trial of endometrial ablation versus hysterectomy for the treatment of dysfunctional uterine bleeding: outcome at four years. *Brit J Obs Gyn.* 1999; **106**: 360–6.

51. Picket SD. *Endometrial ablation.* Available at: http://emedicine.medscape.com/article/1618893-overview#aw2aab6b2b4 (accessed 28 February 2013).

52. Proctor ML, Smith CA, Farquhar CM. Transcutaneous electrical nerve stimulation and acupuncture for primary dysmenorrhoea. *Cochrane Database Syst Rev.* 2002; **1**: CD002123.

53. Proctor M, Farquhar C. Diagnosis and management of dysmenorrhoea: clinical review. *BMJ.* 2006; **332**: 1134–8.

54. On AY, Colakoglu Z, Hepguler S, *et al.* Local heat effect on sympathetic skin responses after pain of electrical stimulus. *Arch Phy Med Rehab.* 1997; **78**(11): 1196–9.

55. Akin M, Weingand K, Hengehold D, *et al.* Continuous low-level topical heat in the treatment of dysmenorrhoea. *Obs and Gyn.* 2001; **97**(3): 343–9.

56. Coulter A, Kelland J, Peto V, *et al.* Treating menorrhagia in primary care. An overview of drug trials and a survey of prescribing practice. *Int J Technol Assess Health Care.* 1995; **11**: 456–71.

57. NHS CRD. Management of menorrhagia. *Effective Health Care.* 1995; **1**(9): 1–15.

58. Warrilow G, Kirkham C, Ismail K, *et al.* Quantification of menstrual blood loss. *Obs Gynaecol.* 2004; **6**(2): 88–92.

59. Ely JW, Kennedy CM, Clark EC, *et al.* Abnormal uterine bleeding: a management algorithm. *JABFM.* 2006; **19**(6): 590–602.

60. Vilos GA, Lefebvre G, Graves GR. Guidelines for the management of abnormal uterine bleeding: SOGC clinical practice guidelines. *J Obs Gynae Can.* 2001; **106**: 1–6.

61. Mayo JL. A healthy menstrual cycle. *Clin Nut Ins.* 1997; **5**(9): 1–8.

62. Shaw JA. *Menorrhagia*. Available at: http://emedicine.medscape.com/article/255540-overview (accessed 17 February 2013).

63. Hickey M, Higham J, Fraser IS. Progestogens versus oestrogens and progestogens for irregular uterine bleeding associated with anovulation. *Cochrane Database Syst Rev.* 2000; **4**: CD001895.

64. Mounsey AL, Wilgus A, Slawson DC. Diagnosis and management of endometriosis. *Am Fam Physician.* 2006; **74**(4): 594–600.

65. Willacy H. *Endometrial Carcinoma*. Available at: www.patient.co.uk/doctor/Endometrial-Carcinoma.htm#ref-2 (accessed 16 February 2012).

66. Sahdev A. Imaging the endometrium in postmenopausal bleeding. *BMJ.* 2007; **334**(7594): 635–6.

67. National Collaborating Centre for Women and Children's Health. *Heavy Menstrual Bleeding: NICE Clinical Guideline 44*. London: NICE; 2007. Available at: www.nice.org.uk/nicemedia/pdf/CG44NICEGuideline

68. Thaby A, Augood C, Duckitt K, *et al.* Nonsteroidal anti-inflammatory drugs for heavy menstrual bleeding. *Cochrane Database Syst Rev.* 2007; **4**: CD000400.

69. Davis A, Godwin A, Lippman J, *et al.* Triphasic norgestimate-ethinyl estradiol for treating dysfunctional uterine bleeding. *Obs and Gynaecol.* 2000; **96**: 913–20.

70. Lethaby A, Irvine G, Cameron I. Cyclical progestogens for heavy menstrual bleeding. *Cochrane Database Syst Rev.* 2008; **1**: CD001016.

71. Matteson KA, Clark MA. Questioning our questions: do frequently asked questions adequately cover the aspects of women's lives most affected by abnormal uterine bleeding? Opinions of women with abnormal uterine bleeding participating in focus group discussions. *Women & Health.* 2010; **50**(2): 195–211.

72. Ministry of Health Malaysia. *Clinical Practice Guidelines: management of menorrhagia*. Available at: www.moh.gov.my/attachments/3939 (accessed 5 October 2013).

CHAPTER 8

Ear, nose and throat (ENT)

INTRODUCTION

ENT problems cover a wide range of conditions. Many are self-limiting and can be managed at home without the need for medical intervention, while others prompt the affected person to visit their GP surgery, hence accounting for a substantial number of GP consultations that place significant burden on resources.

CONDITIONS COVERED IN THE CHAPTER

- Sore throat
- Tonsillitis
- Otitis media
- Otitis externa
- Sinusitis
- Rhinitis.

COMMON PRESENTING SYMPTOMS

May present with one or several of the following:
- fever
- pain in the affected area
- loss of appetite
- ear discharge
- nasal discharge
- associated symptoms of URTI.

TAKING THE EAR, NOSE AND THROAT HISTORY

Initial history is as described in Chapter 3, followed by a focused enquiry relating to the ears, nose and throat.

TABLE 8.1 Symptoms enquiry and further questioning for specific symptoms

Symptom	Further questioning
Fever	Duration of onset and level of fever? Appetite loss? Associated symptoms?
Pain	OPQRST questions as per Chapter 3 Plus: duration of onset? Unilateral or bilateral? Painful to eat and drink? Any additional symptoms?
Loss of appetite	Duration of onset? What is your normal intake? Is patient hungry but then unable to eat the meal? What is the fluid intake? Any associated symptoms?
Ear discharge	Duration of onset? Is discharge from one ear or both? Any recent swimming, air travel or diving? Any problems previously? Any recent ear syringing? Any deafness? Any associated symptoms?
Nasal discharge	What colour is the discharge? Is there any facial pain or pain around the eyes? Any associated symptoms?

Table 8.2 shows a summary of presenting signs and symptoms and the diseases they may suggest. Each symptom will then be discussed in more detail in the context of each disease.

TABLE 8.2 Signs, symptoms and possible diseases

	Fever	Pain	Loss of appetite	Ear discharge	Nasal discharge	Associated symptoms of URTI
Sore throat	Possible	Yes	Possible	No	Yes, probable if there are symptoms of upper respiratory tract infection	Possible
Tonsillitis	Yes	Yes	Yes	No	Possible	Possible

(continued)

	Fever	Pain	Loss of appetite	Ear discharge	Nasal discharge	Associated symptoms of URTI
Otitis media	Yes	Yes	Yes	Possible if the tympanic membrane perforates	Yes, if there are associated symptoms of URTI	Possible
Otitis externa	Possible	Yes	Possible	Possible	No	No
Sinusitis	Yes	Facial pain	Possible	No	Yes	Possible
Rhinitis	No	No	No	No	Yes	No

FURTHER INVESTIGATIONS

Investigations should be chosen on the basis of the history, signs and symptoms, including the duration of symptom and the overall clinical picture.

Other investigations

Other investigations if referral to a consultant is needed are selected on the basis of history, symptoms and clinical findings:

- nasopharyngoscopy
- endoscopic biopsy
- CT scan
- magnetic resonance imaging (MRI scan)
- positron emission tomography (PET) scan.

Urgent referral to ear, nose and throat physician required

- Sudden onset of hearing loss
- Facial numbness or pain
- Double vision or blurred vision
- Recurrent ear infections.

SORE THROAT AND TONSILLITIS

Sore throats are common and the condition is thought to be one of the most frequent reasons for attendance at GP surgeries, estimated to result in approximately 35 million lost days from school or work each year in the UK.[1] Children and young adults form the largest group of patients seeking advice. Many of these conditions are viral, but for those which are bacterial the commonest causative organism is group A beta haemolytic streptococcus.[2]

Clues to aid the diagnosis

TABLE 8.3 Clues to aid diagnosis

Sore throat (pharyngitis)	Tonsillitis
Often accompanies coryzal symptoms	Pharyngeal oedema
Low-grade fever	Headaches
Loss of appetite	Fever
Hoarse voice	Cervical lymphadenopathy
Malaise	Loss of appetite
Lethargy	Feeling very unwell
Pain on swallowing	Pain on swallowing

Other signs suggesting bacterial infection

These include:

- absence of cough
- tender anterior cervical lymph nodes
- history of fever
- exudate on the tonsils.

CLINICAL ALERT!

The presence of three or four of the symptoms above indicates a 40%–60% risk that the patient has a group A beta streptococcal infection, and absence of three or four of these signs suggests an 80% chance that the infection is viral.[3]

Pathophysiology

Viral sore throat

Viral infections account for approximately 70% of all episodes of pharyngitis, and rhinovirus is the most common cause.[4] The causative organism enters the body through the ciliated epithelium that lines the nose, and this is followed by an increase in secretory activity of the mucous glands, swelling of the mucous membranes of the nasal cavity, Eustachian tubes and pharynx, and narrowing of nasal passages, causing obstructive symptoms.[5]

Bacterial sore throat

Group A beta haemolytic streptococcus has a protein located on the cell wall, and this protein is needed for invasive infection to take place. Once the organism gains entry, exotoxins are released and these act as super antigens promoting the release of pro-inflammatory cytokines, which are then able to block the pharyngeal immune response, allowing proliferation of the infecting organism.[6]

CLINICAL ALERT!

- Group A beta haemolytic streptococcus (GABHS) is responsible for about one third of sore throats in children aged 5–15 years, but is the cause of only 10% in adults and younger children.[7]
- Seventy per cent of sore throats in children aged 5–16 years, and 95% of those in children under the age of 5 years, are viral.[7]

Differential diagnosis

TABLE 8.4 Differential diagnoses: beware of!

Condition	Additional pointers	When to consider
Glandular fever	Most common in those aged 15–30 and presents with fever, malaise and sore throat which has persisted for more than 1 week.[2]	Blood test shows antibodies to Epstein–Barr virus and the symptoms include fatigue and tiredness, which can be marked, particularly in the early stages of the disease.
Malignancy of tonsils, larynx or the pharynx.	Sore throat and difficulty swallowing with unexplained weight loss.	Patient reports changes to the voice, such as hoarseness.
HIV	Non-specific symptoms, headache, fever, sore throat.	Consider where patient also complains of a rash, as the 'triad' of fever, rash and sore throat all occurring together should always suggest possible primary HIV infection requiring an HIV test.[8]
Coxsackie virus infection	Similar symptoms with mild fever, sore throat, discomfort when swallowing and loss of appetite.	There are lesions in the mouth (on the tonsils, soft palate and the uvula).

CLINICAL ALERT!

TABLE 8.5 Non-viral and non-bacterial causes of sore throat

Smoking

Chronic cough

Post-nasal drip

Gastro-oesophageal reflux disease

Allergies

Treatment

The decision to prescribe antibiotics depends on the severity of the patient's illness and the presence of symptoms listed above, which may indicate a bacterial infection. If the decision is made that the likely cause is viral, and that no antibiotics are

needed, symptomatic measures such as analgesia, fluids and gargling may be helpful in relieving symptoms.

A delayed prescription for antibiotics may be offered for use if symptoms worsen
or are not improving. However, a recent review indicated that giving no antibiotics
with advice to return if symptoms do not resolve was shown to be more likely to
result in the least antibiotic use, and achieved similar patient satisfaction and clinical outcomes to delayed antibiotics.[9]

An immediate prescription may be needed for patients who are clinically unwell
or at high risk of complications (e.g. immunosuppressed patients).

If antibiotics are required
- penicillin V, twice or three times daily for 10 days, is recommended[10]
- if allergic to penicillin, erythromycin or clarithromycin may be prescribed.

See **Chapter 16 for further information relating to antibiotics.**

CLINICAL ALERT!

⚠ **BEWARE!**

Beware of prescribing amoxicillin, which in the presence of glandular fever will
cause a rash irrespective of sensitivity to the drug.

Complications
There are a number of complications that are more likely to arise if the cause of the
sore throat is bacterial:
- sinusitis
- peritonsillar abscess which is more frequent in older children, adolescents and
  young adults
- otitis media (more common in children)
- scarlet fever (may occur after throat infection caused by group A streptococcal
  infection)
- glomerulonephritis (can occur after a streptococcal infection).

Key reminders
- Sore throats are very common
- Most resolve without treatment
- Frequently associated with upper respiratory tract infection
- Rarely serious.

OTITIS MEDIA

Otitis media is common in children and as with a number of other conditions the cause may be viral or bacterial. There is no universally accepted definition, but it is generally understood to refer to inflammation of the middle ear and is usually of rapid onset.[11] The condition is rare in adults.

Clues to aid the diagnosis

TABLE 8.6 Clues to aid the diagnosis

Age group	Features
Children	Rapid onset
	Earache
	Fever
	Young children may pull or rub the affected ear
	Irritability
	Very red tympanic membrane on examination
Adults	Earache
	Deafness
	Sore throat

CLINICAL ALERT!

- Acute otitis media is predominantly a disease of young children under 3 years of age with a peak incidence between 6 and 11 months.[12]
- In children symptoms often develop after a flu-like illness or URTI with rapid onset of symptoms of which earache (otalgia) is frequently the cardinal sign.[13]
- Compared with children, adults more often present with otalgia, diminished hearing and sore throat.[14]

Pathophysiology

The URTI that has preceded the onset of otitis media has caused congestion and swelling of several sites including the mucosa of the nasal passages, the nasopharynx and the Eustachian tubes. There is an accumulation of secretions in the middle ear and obstruction of the Eustachian tube, which leads to secondary bacterial or viral infection and the subsequent development of pus and the features of otitis media.[15]

Differential diagnosis

Otitis media with effusion is one which may be frequently encountered and is defined as inflammation of the middle ear, accompanied by the accumulation of fluid in the middle ear cleft without the symptoms and signs of acute inflammation.[11] Table 8.7 shows clinical differences between otitis media with and without effusion.

TABLE 8.7 Findings on examination

Otitis media	Otitis media with effusion
Redness of the tympanic membrane and inflammation.	Often no signs of inflammation or discharge on examination.
Bulging tympanic membrane.	Drum may be retracted.
Tympanic membrane may have an opaque appearance.	There is an abnormal colour to the drum.

TABLE 8.8 Differential diagnoses

Condition	Additional pointers	When to consider
Otitis externa	pp. 134–6.	pp. 134–6.
Compacted ear wax	Earache symptoms accompanied by feeling of deafness.	Wax visible in the ear canal, obscuring the tympanic membrane on examination.
Mastoiditis	Clinically unwell with ear pain which is often worse at night.	Consider if the pain and fever are persistent, with possible marked hearing loss.
Perforated ear drum	Hearing loss.	May be additional symptoms of ringing in the ear and a clear or bloody discharge.[16]

Treatment

In many cases analgesia will be sufficient (paracetamol and/or ibuprofen in appropriate doses) and no antibiotics are required. Delayed prescription may be appropriate for use if there is no improvement or symptoms are worsening after 48 hours. With symptomatic treatment alone, 60% of children will have improved within 24 hours and in 80% the condition will have resolved within 3 days.[12]

CLINICAL ALERT!

⚠ **BEWARE!**

- Otitis media caused by pneumococcal bacteria is least likely to resolve without antibiotics.[17]
- Immediate antibiotics may be needed in the immunocompromised, and in the presence of severe illness.
- Amoxicillin is the drug of choice or clarithromycin if allergic to amoxicillin.[18]

Complications

⚠ **BEWARE OF!**

- Febrile convulsions
- Perforated tympanic membrane
- Mastoiditis

- Chronic suppurative otitis media
- Labyrinthitis
- Meningitis
- Chronic suppurative otitis media.

- There are generally fewer complications with otitis media with effusion because inflammation is absent.[19]
- Chronic suppurative otitis media can occur when there is a perforated tympanic membrane with drainage of fluid from the middle ear.
- Recurrent episodes or persistent effusion requires referral as there is a risk of hearing loss.[19]

Key reminders
- Ear infections are common, especially in children.
- Referral may be needed if the problem is recurring.
- Urgent referral for adults where there may be a suspected underlying malignancy.

OTITIS EXTERNA
Otitis externa is common and can affect people of any age, but the highest occurrence is seen in children around the age of 7–12.[20] In the UK more than 1% of people will be diagnosed with the condition each year,[21] while in the US the condition affects approximately four of every 1000 people each year.[22]

Clues to aid the diagnosis
TABLE 8.9 Clues to aid the diagnosis

Signs	Symptoms
Red, swollen, inflamed ear canal	Ear pain
Purulent or serous discharge	Itching
May be difficult to examine the canal if inflamed and filled with debris	Discharge from the ear
Tenderness along the jaw or on touching the ear	Feeling of deafness

Pathophysiology
The ear canal produces a protective layer of cerumen whose purpose is to protect against infection. When the amount produced is excessive, this can cause retention of water and debris, which provides an ideal environment for bacteria to invade and multiply. Otitis externa is commonly seen in swimmers and divers where the ear is

regularly in contact with water. Once infection develops, symptoms arise in response to inflammation and infection in the ear canal.

Differential diagnosis

TABLE 8.10 Differential diagnoses: beware of!

Condition	Additional pointers	When to consider
Otitis media	pp. 132–4.	pp. 132–4.
Impacted ear wax	p. 133.	p. 133.
Neoplasm	May have a bloodstained discharge if tumour is in the middle ear, or if malignancy is in the outer ear there will be a crusty lesion that may progress to an ulcer.[23]	Consider if there is associated earache, loss of hearing, dizziness and usually painless symptoms. Consider as a possibility for lesions that are not healing.
Mastoiditis	p. 133.	p. 133.
Referred pain: often from the teeth or throat	May have toothache, and/or throat pain.	Consider if ear examination is normal but patient is complaining of sore throat or toothache.
Skin problems such as psoriasis, dermatitis	May be visible elsewhere on the body.	Patient may have a history of either psoriasis or dermatitis and on examination there may be dry scales or plaques in the ear canal, suggesting psoriasis, or dead flaky skin may be visible on examination, causing significant itching, indicating possible dermatitis.

CLINICAL ALERT!

- Beware of foreign bodies inserted in the ears of children.
- Consider cholesteatoma (a cyst-like lump of cells in the middle ear) when there is painless discharge associated with significant deafness.

Treatment

Treatment will depend on severity of symptoms:

- analgesia (paracetamol and/or ibuprofen) for relief of pain
- mild discomfort and itching may be relieved by aluminium acetate solution (inserted using ribbon gauze or sponge wick)[24]
- if there is infection a topical antibiotic (e.g. neomycin) may be needed
- if inflammation and infection are suspected, topical antibiotics with added steroid (e.g. Locorten-vioform) may be helpful in alleviating any swelling and relieving pain in the ear canal.[25]

Prescribing tips
- Drops should be continued for 3 days after symptoms have resolved (usually for 5–7 days).
- A longer course may be needed for severe infections.
- Some preparations require installation into the ear 3–4 times daily.
- Otomize is three times daily and Locorten-vioform is twice daily so the latter may be more suitable for some patients.
- Warming the bottle of drops in the hands before instillation minimises dizziness, and inserting a small piece of cotton wool moistened with the drops may help retain the drops in the ear if the patient cannot lie still long enough to allow absorption.[26]

Complications
Complications are rare but the following can occur:
- cellulitis
- abscess formation
- perforated eardrum, which can occur when pus has developed in the inner ear and caused the tympanic membrane to rupture.

CLINICAL ALERT!

⚠ **BEWARE!**

Malignant otitis externa is a potentially life-threatening complication where infection invades the posterior cranial bone. Often caused by a *Pseudomonas* infection, this complication can be potentially fatal in immunocompromised patients and the elderly, especially elderly diabetics, and requires hospitalisation and intravenous antibiotic therapy.[27]

Key reminders
- More common in children
- Symptoms should resolve within about 7 days with treatment
- Condition can become chronic.

SINUSITIS
Sinusitis is a common unpleasant condition increasing in prevalence around the world and has a prevalence rate as high as 15% in some studies.[28] In many cases the condition is acute, but there are instances where the problem becomes chronic with symptoms lasting for up to 12 weeks.

The underlying cause of the problem may be viral or bacterial.

Clues to aid the diagnosis

There are several guidelines which specify combinations of symptoms likely to suggest a diagnosis of sinusitis.

Several signs or symptoms are consistently cited across all the guidelines as being primary diagnostic:

- nasal congestion
- obstruction, or blockage
- purulent rhinorrhoea
- facial pain or pressure.[29]

Additional symptoms include:

- headaches
- fever
- ear pain
- halitosis
- post-nasal drip
- lethargy
- cough
- discomfort in the ears.

CLINICAL ALERT!

⚠ BEWARE!

Differentiating between viral and bacterial sinusitis may be difficult. The presentations shown below are suggestive.

- Prolonged or persistent symptoms lasting for several days with no signs of improvement.
- Severe symptoms or with high fever purulent nasal discharge or facial pain lasting for at least 3–4 days.[30]
- Worsening symptoms following a URTI, with development of a fever, headaches, or an increase in nasal discharge.
- Bacterial sinusitis becomes more likely when symptoms have not improved or have worsened after a 7–10-day period and are characterised by early improvement followed by worsening with the onset of purulent nasal discharge.[31]

Persistent symptoms

CLINICAL ALERT!

⚠ BEWARE!

Sinusitis can become chronic with more persistent symptoms. This may occur in association with the following:
- blockage of the passages caused by a deviated nasal septum
- nasal polyps
- hay fever where the associated inflammation causes blockage to the passages
- predisposing factors for chronic sinusitis are many and include pollution, allergens, viruses, bacteria and moulds, genetic influences, immune deficiency, cystic fibrosis, and ciliary defects, chronic localised inflammation, anatomic obstruction, polyps and tumours[32]
- the risk of non-infectious chronic sinusitis is increased in patients with cystic fibrosis, gastro-oesophageal reflux, or exposure to environmental pollutants[33]
- children with sinusitis may have less specific symptoms. The most common manifestations of bacterial sinusitis are cough (80%), followed by nasal discharge (76%) and fever (63%), while headache and facial pain are rare.[30]

Pathophysiology

Sinusitis frequently follows a viral URTI and in many cases resolves without any medical treatment. The nasal mucosa responds to the virus by producing mucus and recruiting inflammatory mediators such as white blood cells, which cause congestion and swelling of the nasal passages.[34] The increased production of mucus interferes with the function of the cilia, resulting in failure to clear debris from the nasal passages and therefore increasing the chances of bacterial growth and infection.

Differential diagnosis
- Rhinitis (*see* pp. 140–3)
- Migraine (*see* pp. 201–6).

Treatment
- Analgesia to relieve pain (paracetamol or ibuprofen or a combination of both).
- Antibiotics may be needed if the patient becomes clinically unwell or bacterial infection is suspected or if there is a high risk of complications (consider for patients with comorbid conditions).
- If antibiotics are necessary, choices are amoxicillin (doxycycline or clarithromycin if allergic to penicillin).[24]

See **Chapter 16 for further information relating to antibiotics.**

Other treatment options

- Nasal decongestants have been found to improve symptoms, with less headache and facial pain, as well as significantly lower nasal obstruction.[35]
- Saline irrigations are well tolerated and although minor side-effects are common, the beneficial effect of saline appears to outweigh any side-effects.[36]
- Oral decongestants such as pseudoephedrine can be prescribed, but they have a weaker effect in relieving the nasal obstruction when compared to topical intranasal decongestants.[37]
- Intranasal corticosteroids: various products available but mometasone furoate nasal spray, used as an adjunctive treatment with an oral antibiotic, has been shown to be significantly more effective in reducing the symptoms of acute rhino sinusitis than antibiotic treatment alone.[38]
- If an antibiotic is prescribed, erythromycin, clarithromycin, and doxycycline have limited coverage for streptococcal pneumoniae and haemophilus influenza organisms,[39] which are two of the organisms commonly implicated in acute bacterial sinusitis.[40]

Complications

CLINICAL ALERT!

Complications are rare but are always possible. Table 8.11 gives information relating to possible complications and clues to aid their diagnosis.

TABLE 8.11 Complications and clues to aid their diagnosis

Condition	Signs and symptoms
Orbital cellulitis	A potentially sight-threatening condition that presents with swelling, lid erythema and oedema and frequently follows a URTI, although acute bacterial sinusitis is the commonest cause.[41] The affected person is usually clinically unwell.
Osteomyelitis	Infection of the facial bones, which leads to headaches and fever.
Blood clots	Initially unilateral with swelling of the eye socket, pupil is fixed and dilated, symptoms spreading to both eyes.
Meningitis	Dangerous complication where bacteria have spread to the brain, causing either brain abscesses or meningitis with potentially life-threatening complications.

Key reminders

- Usually self-limiting
- Self-help measures effective in most cases
- Antibiotics only required if bacterial infection is suspected
- When complications do occur they can be potentially serious and in some cases life threatening.

RHINITIS

Rhinitis is caused by inflammation of the nasal membranes and is typically classified as allergic or non-allergic. Allergic rhinitis may be seasonal (hay fever) or perennial (persistent) while non-allergic may be inflammatory as well as non-inflammatory.[42] Both types may have equally unpleasant symptoms, and can potentially result in time away from work or school with an impact on quality of life. Both allergic rhinitis and non-allergic rhinitis are risk factors for the development of asthma,[43] and there is also evidence to suggest that rhinitis coexists in up to 75% of patients with known asthma.[44]

CLINICAL ALERT!

- Allergic rhinitis is the most predominant form in children but accounts for a third of cases in adults.[45]
- Prevalence of perennial rhinitis appears to be increased among patients with obstructive sleep apnoea.[46]

Clues to aid the diagnosis

Allergic rhinitis is characterised by sneezing and itching.

Non-allergic rhinitis is more commonly associated with nasal blockage or nasal discharge (rhinorrhoea).

CLINICAL ALERT!

⚠ **BEWARE!**

- Where rhinorrhoea is a problem the colour of the nasal discharge may be useful in assessing the presence of infection. (If clear infection unlikely, yellow suggests allergy or possible infection; green is usually indicative of infection.)[45]
- Rhinitis and sinusitis can coexist with symptoms of rhinitis as above and additional symptoms of facial pain and loss of smell.[47]

Trigger factors

Table 8.12 shows some of the common trigger factors for each type:

TABLE 8.12 Common trigger factors

Allergic rhinitis	Non-allergic rhinitis
Pollens (tree and grass pollens)	House dust mite
Animals (domestic animals and also horses)	Moulds
House dust mite	Occupational causes such as dust, flour
Occupational causes such as dust, flour	Other irritants such as cigarette smoke, cold air
Moulds	

Pathophysiology

Allergic rhinitis involves inflammation of the mucous membranes of several sites which can include the nose, eyes, sinuses and also the ears (both the Eustachian tubes and the middle ear). The process by which inflammation occurs is highly complex and involves two phases: an early and late phase. During the early phase IgE is released in response to the specific protein that has been inhaled (e.g. a specific pollen grain) and once this specific protein enters the respiratory tract it can bind to the IgE on the mast cells.[48] This then starts the inflammatory process and the onset of symptoms characteristic of rhinitis. This is followed by a late-phase reaction, and whereas histamine appears to be the major mediator of the early phase, the late phase is more closely associated with other mediators, chemokines, and cytokines that have inflammatory and proinflammatory effects, leading to recruitment of inflammatory cells such as eosinophils and basophils, a process which generally subsides in 12–24 hours.[49] Non-allergic rhinitis is less well understood, with unclear pathophysiology, but there is some suspicion that despite non-allergic triggers most of the non-allergic rhinitis patients also have some degree of inflammation.[50]

Differential diagnosis

 BEWARE!

There are a number of conditions where symptoms may mimic those of rhinitis but symptoms would be persistent.

TABLE 8.13 Differential diagnoses

Condition	Additional pointers	When to consider
Deviated septum	Nasal congestion.	Sometimes visible but not always.
Nasal polyps	Similar symptoms of nasal blockage, rhinorrhoea and there may also be post-nasal drip.[51]	Consider if there is chronic or recurrent acute sinusitis symptoms in association with snoring rhinorrhoea and dull headaches.[51]
Nasal tumours	Few if any signs while the tumour is in its early stages. Once tumour progresses there may be symptoms of unilateral epistaxis and nasal obstruction.[52]	There are symptoms such as severe headache and visual disturbance, although these symptoms suggest that the neoplasm is advanced.[52]
Medication induced (rhinitis medicamentosa)	Symptoms of nasal congestion.	Consider as a possibility in patients taking antihypertensives, beta-blockers, phosphodiesterase type 5 inhibitors, such as sildenafil, contraceptives, antidepressants and antipsychotics, gabapentin and NSAIDs.[53]

(continued)

Condition	Additional pointers	When to consider
Sarcoidosis	Can cause symptoms of rhinitis, before the onset of systemic symptoms.	Granulomatous infections in the nose can lead to crusting, bleeding and nasal obstruction.[54]
Hormonal cause	About 30% of women suffer from nasal symptoms during pregnancy.[55]	Consider in women who develop symptoms during the menopause and those using oral contraception where nasal symptoms have been reported.[56]

Treatment

A number of treatment options are available. *See* Table 8.14 for options and evidence for use.

TABLE 8.14 Treatment options

Drug	Evidence
Oral antihistamines	Effective in relieving symptoms and can be given as regular therapy in persistent rhinitis for greater effect.[57]
Topical nasal antihistamines (e.g. azelastine)	Found to be as effective as loratadine in the relief of symptoms.[58]
Topical intranasal steroids (e.g. fluticasone, mometasone)	Intranasal corticosteroids are also considered first line for patients with mild persistent or moderate/severe symptoms and can be used alone or in combination with oral antihistamines.
Antileukotrienes (e.g.) montelukast	Antileukotrienes do not appear to be as effective as intranasal corticosteroids, but they may be an option when oral antihistamines and/or intranasal corticosteroids are not well tolerated or have been ineffective.[59]
Decongestants (e.g. pseudoephedrine)	Can be used for allergic and non-allergic rhinitis and work by reducing swelling of mucosal tissue but also decrease vascular leakage, helping to ease both rhinorrhoea and nasal congestion.[60]

Prescribing tips

- Oral antihistamines: second generation antihistamines (e.g. cetirizine or loratadine) preferred as these have fewer side-effects.
- Topical nasal antihistamines act rapidly and are effective in relieving symptoms, but correct application is needed to avoid poor response, and incorrect use may lead to development of a bitter taste in the mouth.
- Nasal sprays have a similar side-effect profile, the most common being epistaxis with a reported incidence of 17%–23%.[61]
- Antileukotrienes may be a useful addition where patient also has asthma symptoms.
- Decongestants if prescribed have a number of side-effects that may impact on compliance with treatment.

Referral for further investigations suggested

- Lack of response to treatment
- Suspected food allergy
- Where the diagnosis is uncertain
- Where symptoms may be caused by the patient's occupation.

CLINICAL ALERT!

⚠ BEWARE!

Unilateral symptoms of bloody discharge that may be purulent, with nasal blockage and pain, suggest malignancy and require urgent referral.

Complications

- Poorly controlled allergic rhinitis may also contribute to the development of other diseases including acute and chronic sinusitis, recurrence of nasal polyps, otitis media with or without effusion, hearing impairment, and sleep apnoea.[62]
- Non-allergic rhinitis can also lead to complications of sinusitis and middle ear infections but can also cause the growth of nasal polyps, which can develop as a result of chronic inflammation.[63]

Key reminders

- Unpleasant condition
- Very common
- Can occur at specific times of the year or throughout the year
- Can affect adults and children alike.

REFERENCES

1. Stubbs BM. Acute tonsillitis. *InnovAiT.* 2009; **2**(1): 50–5.
2. Simon C, Everitt H, Van Dorp F. *Oxford Handbook of General Practice.* Oxford: Oxford University Press; 2010.
3. National Prescribing Centre. The management of common infections in primary care. *MeReC Bulletin.* 2006; **17**(3). Available at: www.npc.nhs.uk/merec/infect/commonintro/resources/merec_bulletin_vol17_no3_sore_throat.pdf
4. Somro A, Akram M, Ibrahim khan M, *et al.* Pharyngitis and sore throat: a review. *Afr J of Biotechnol.* 2011; **10**(33): 6190–7.
5. Aung K. *Viral Pharyngitis.* Available at: http://emedicine.medscape.com/article/225362-overview#a0104 (accessed 5 May 2012).
6. Halsey E. *Bacterial Pharyngitis.* Available at: http://emedicine.medscape.com/article/225243-overview (accessed 5 May 2012).
7. Worrall GJ. Acute sore throat. *Can Fam Physician.* 2007; **53**(11): 1961–2.
8. National AIDS Trust. *Primary HIV Infection.* Available at: www.nat.org.uk/media/Files/Publications/July-2008-Primary-HIV-Infection.pdf (accessed 25 May 2013).

9. Spurling GK, Del Mar CB, Dooley L, *et al.* Delayed antibiotics for respiratory infections. *Cochrane Database Syst Rev.* 2013; **4**: CD004417.

10. Pelucchi C, Grigoryan L, Galeone C, *et al.* Guideline for management of acute sore throat. *CMI.* 2012; **18**(Suppl. 1): 1–27.

11. Scottish Intercollegiate Guidelines. *Diagnosis and Management of Childhood Otitis Media in Primary Care: SIGN Guideline 66.* Edinburgh: SIGN; 2003.

12. Ah-See K. *Acute Otitis Media in Children.* Available at: www.gponline.com/clinical/article/674679/Acute-otitis-media-children/ (accessed 1 June 2013).

13. Pettigre MM, Gent JF, Pyles RB. Viral-bacterial interactions and risk of acute otitis media complicating upper respiratory tract infection. *J Clin Microbiol.* 2011; **49**(11): 3750–5.

14. Ramakrishnan K, Sparks RA, Berryhill W. Diagnosis and treatment of otitis media. *Am Fam Physician.* 2007; **76**(11): 1650–8.

15. Rovers MM, Schilder AG, Zielhuis GA, *et al.* Otitis media. *Lancet.* 2004; **363**: 465–73.

16. Mayo Foundation for Medical Education and Research (MFMER). *Ruptured Eardrum (Perforated Eardrum).* Available at: www.mayoclinic.com/health/ruptured-eardrum/DS00499/DSECTION=symptoms (accessed 21 May 2013).

17. Dowell SF. Acute otitis media caused by resistant pneumococci. *Am Fam Physician.* 2000; **61**(2): 318–23.

18. Health Protection Agency. *Management of Infection Guidance for Primary Care.* Available at: www.hpa.org.uk/webc/HPAwebFile/HPAweb_C/1194947333801 (accessed 6 May 2013).

19. Thrasher RD. *Otitis Media with Effusion.* Available at: http://emedicine.medscape.com/article/858990-overview (accessed 15 May 2013).

20. Roland PS, Stroman DW. Microbiology of acute otitis externa. *Laryngoscope.* 2002; **112**(7 Pt 1): 1166–77.

21. Rowlands S, Devalia H, Smith C, *et al.* Otitis externa in U.K. general practice: a survey using the U.K. General Practice Research Database. *Br J Gen Pr.* 2001; **51**(468): 533–8.

22. Osguthorpe JD, Nielsen DR. Otitis externa: review and clinical update. *Am Fam Physician.* 2006; **74**(9): 1510–6.

23. Cancer Research UK. *Cancer of the Ear.* Available at: www.cancerresearchuk.org/cancer-help/about-cancer/cancer-questions/about-cancer-of-the-ear#symptoms (accessed 19 May 2012).

24. British National Formulary. 2013. Available at: www.bnf.org/bnf/index.htm

25. Seedat RY. *The Discharging Ear: a practical approach.* Available at: www.ajol.info/index.php/cme/article/download/43968/27486 (accessed 19 June 2013).

26. Sander R. Otitis externa: a practical guide to treatment and prevention. *Am Fam Physician.* 2001; **63**(5): 927–37.

27. Lang R, Palmer S, Kitzes-Cohen R, *et al.* Successful treatment of malignant external otitis with oral ciprofloxacin: report of experience with 23 patients. *J Infect Dis.* 1990; **161**: 537–40.

28. Suh JD, Kennedy DW. Treatment options for chronic rhinosinusitis: proceedings of the American Thoracic Society. *ATS J.* 2011; **8**(1): 132–40.

29. Meltzer EO, Hamilos DL. Rhinosinusitis diagnosis and management for the clinician: a synopsis of recent consensus guidelines. *Mayo Clin Proc.* 2011; **86**(5): 427–43.

30. Chow AW, Benninger MS, Itzhak B, *et al.* IDSA clinical practice guideline for acute bacterial rhinosinusitis in children and adults. *Clin Infect Dis.* 2012; **54**(8): e72–112.

31. Sande MA, Gwaltney JM. Acute community acquired bacterial sinusitis: continuing challenges and current management. *Clin Inf Dis.* 2004; **39**: S151–8.

32. Rosenfeld RM, Andes D, Bhattacharyya N, *et al.* Clinical practice guidelines on adult sinusitis. *Otolaryngol Head Neck Surg.* 2007; **137**: 375–7.

33. Slavin RG, Spector SL, Bernstein IL, *et al*. The diagnosis and management of sinusitis: a practice parameter update. *J Allergy Clin Immunol.* 2005; **116**(6 Suppl.): S13–47.

34. Radojicic C. *Sinusitis.* Cleveland Clinic Centre for Continuing Education. Available at: www.clevelandclinicmeded.com/medicalpubs/diseasemanagement/allergy/rhino-sinusitis/ (accessed 17 May 2013).

35. Bachert C, Hormann K, Mosges R, *et al*. An update on the diagnosis and treatment of sinusitis and nasal polyposis. *Allergy.* 2003; **58**(3): 176–91.

36. Harvey R, Hannan SA, Badia L, *et al*. Nasal saline irrigations for the symptoms of chronic rhinosinusitis. *Cochrane Database Syst Rev.* 2007; **3**: CD006394.

37. Masood A, Moumoulidis I, Panesar J. Acute rhinosinusitis in adults: an update on current management. *Postgrad Med J.* 2007; **83**(980): 402–8.

38. Meltzer EO, Bachert C, Staudinger H. Treating acute rhinosinusitis: comparing efficacy and safety of mometasone furoate nasal spray, amoxicillin, and placebo. *J Allergy Clin Immunol.* 2005; **116**(6): 1289–95.

39. Hughes D. Choosing the best antibiotic for acute bacterial rhinosinusitis. *Respiratory reviews.com.* Available at: www.respiratoryreviews.com/nov00/rr_nov00_antimicrobial.html (accessed 25 September 2012).

40. Poole MD. A focus on acute sinusitis in adults: changes in disease management. *Am J of Med.* 1999; **106**(5 Suppl. 1): 138–47.

41. Jackson K, Baker SR. Clinical implications of orbital cellulitis. *Laryngoscope.* 2009; **96**: 568–74.

42. Kochhar S. *Managing Allergic Rhinitis.* Available at: www.gponline.com/Clinical/article/1140756/Managing-allergic-rhinitis/ (accessed 19 August 2013).

43. Passalacqua G, Ciprandi G, Pasquali M, *et al*. An update on the asthma–rhinitis link. *Curr Opin Allergy Clin Immunol.* 2004; **4**: 177–83.

44. Bachert C, Vignola A, Gevaert P, *et al*. Allergic rhinitis, rhinosinusitis and asthma: one airway disease. *Immunology Allergy Clin North Am.* 2004; **24**: 19–43.

45. Scadding GK, Durham SR, Mirakian R, *et al*. BSACI guidelines for the management of allergic and non-allergic rhinitis. *Clin Exp Allergy.* 2008; **38**: 19–42.

46. Canova CR, Downs SH, Knoblauch A, *et al*. Increased prevalence of perennial allergic rhinitis in patients with obstructive sleep apnoea. *Respiration.* 2004; **71**(2): 138–43.

47. American Academy of Otolaryngology–Head and Neck Surgery. *Fact Sheet: allergic rhinitis, sinusitis and rhinosinusitis.* Available at: www.entnet.org/HealthInformation/rhinitis.cfm (accessed 22 September 2013).

48. Lang DM. *Allergic Rhinitis.* Cleveland Clinic Centre for Continuing Education. Available at: www.clevelandclinicmeded.com/medicalpubs/diseasemanagement/allergy/allergic-rhinitis/ (accessed 12 October 2013).

49. Hansen I, Klimek L, Mosges R, *et al*. Mediators of inflammation in the early and the late phase of allergic rhinitis. *Curr Opin Allergy Clin Immunol.* 2004; **4**: 159–63.

50. Newton JR, Wong AH, See K. A review of nasal polyposis. *Ther Clin Risk Manag.* 2008; **4**(2): 507–12.

51. McClay JE. *Nasal Polyps.* Available at: http://emedicine.medscape.com/article/994274-clinical (accessed 24 September 2013).

52. Klem C. *Malignant Tumours of the Sinuses.* Available at: http://emedicine.medscape.com/article/847189-overview#a0103 (accessed 24 September 2013).

53. Kushnir NM. *Rhinitis Medicamentosa.* Available at: http://emedicine.medscape.com/article/995056-overview (accessed 27 September 2013).

54. Schroer B, Pien LC. *Non-allergic Rhinitis: common problem, chronic symptoms.* Available at: www.ccjm.org/content/79/4/285.full (accessed 22 September 2013).

55. Gani F, Braida A, Lombardi C, *et al.* Rhinitis in pregnancy. *Eur Ann Allergy Clin Immunol.* 2003; **35**(8): 306–13.

56. Philpott CM, Robinson AM, Murty GE. Nasal pathophysiology and its relationship to the female ovarian hormones. *J Otolaryngol Head Neck Surg.* 2008; **37**: 540–6.

57. Leurs R, Church MK, Taglialatela M. H1-antihistamines: inverse agonism, anti-inflammatory actions and cardiac effects. *Clin Exp Allergy.* 2002; **32**: 489–98.

58. McNeely W, Wiseman LR. Intranasal azelastine. A review of its efficacy in the management of allergic rhinitis. *Drugs.* 1998; **56**: 91–114.

59. Small P, Kim H. Allergic rhinitis. *Allergy, Asthma & Clin Imm.* 2011; 7(Suppl. 1): S3.

60. Scarupa MD, Kaliner MA. *Disease Summaries: in depth review of allergic rhinitis.* Available at: www.worldallergy.org/professional/allergic_diseases_center/rhinitis/rhinitis_indepth.php (accessed 15 September 2013).

61. Waddell AN, Patel SK, Toma AG. Intranasal steroid sprays in the treatment of rhinitis: is one better than another? *J Laryngol and Otol.* 2003; **117**(11): 843–5.

62. Settipane RA. Complications of allergic rhinitis. *Allergy Asthma Proc.* 1999; **20**(4): 209–13.

63. Mayo Foundation for Medical Education and Research (MMFER). *Non-allergic Rhinitis.* Available at: www.mayoclinic.com/health/nonallergic-rhinitis/DS00809/DSECTION=complications (accessed 19 September 2013).

CHAPTER 9

Eyes

INTRODUCTION

Eye problems occur in all countries and range from relatively minor and easily treated conditions to more serious problems that can be potentially sight threatening. A number of eye diseases can occur in children as well as adults, while conditions such as diabetic retinopathy, cataracts, macular degeneration, and glaucoma are more commonly found in those aged 50 or over.[1]

CONDITIONS COVERED IN THE CHAPTER

- Conjunctivitis
- Blepharitis
- Styes
- Dry eyes.

PRESENTING SYMPTOMS

May present with one or several of the following:

- pain
- itching
- watery or discharge from the eye
- visual disturbance
- soreness
- redness.

TAKING THE OPHTHALMIC HISTORY

Initial history as described in Chapter 3, followed by a focused enquiry relating to the eyes.

TABLE 9.1 Symptoms enquiry and further questioning for specific symptoms

Symptom	Additional questions
Pain	*See* Chapter 3.
Itching	Unilateral or bilateral?
Watery or discharge from the eye	Are there any aggravating or relieving factors?
	Duration of symptoms?
Soreness	Exposure to irritants at home or at work?
Redness	Any additional symptoms such as headache or foreign-body sensation?
	Have they had anything similar in the past and if so what treatment?
Visual disturbance	Recent changes: gradual or sudden onset?
	Is the vision blurred?
	Are there any floaters in either eye?
	Double vision?

Table 9.2 shows a summary of presenting signs and symptoms and the disease they may suggest.

TABLE 9.2 Presenting signs and symptoms and disease they may suggest

	Pain	Itching	Watery or discharge from the eye	Visual disturbance	Soreness	Redness of the conjunctiva
Conjunctivitis	Gritty sensation	Yes	Yes	Possible (blurred vision)	Yes	Yes
Blepharitis	Possible discomfort/ burning sensation	Yes	Yes	Possible (blurred vision)	Yes of the eyelids	No
Styes	Yes	No	Possible	No	No	No
Dry eyes	Discomfort	Yes	Possible	Possible (blurred vision)	Yes	No

FURTHER INVESTIGATIONS

Investigations should be chosen on the basis of the history and symptoms, including the duration of symptoms and the overall clinical picture.

OTHER INVESTIGATIONS SELECTED ON THE BASIS OF HISTORY, SYMPTOMS AND CLINICAL FINDINGS

There are a number of specialist ocular investigations which include:

- slit lamp examination
- ophthalmoscopy
- MRI
- CT
- ultrasonography
- angiography.

URGENT REFERRAL TO AN OPHTHALMOLOGIST REQUIRED

- Treatment failure
- Worsening symptoms
- Unilateral pain in either eye
- Severe photophobia where the cause is unknown
- Loss of vision
- Abnormal pupil reaction.

CONJUNCTIVITIS

Conjunctivitis is a common condition affecting both males and females and can occur in either sex at any age. It is reported to be the commonest cause of red eye[2] and while the symptoms are unpleasant they are not usually serious.

Clues to aid the diagnosis

Conjunctivitis occurs when there is inflammation of the conjunctiva. The condition can arise as a result of a bacterial or viral infection or as an allergic response to irritants.

Symptoms

Symptoms vary according to the underlying cause but may include:

- itching and soreness of the eyes
- blurred vision
- redness of the whites of the eyes
- watery eyes
- crusting of the lashes especially on waking.

Differentiating between the types can be difficult, but there are some features which may help in making the diagnosis. *See* Table 9.3.

TABLE 9.3 Features helpful in making a diagnosis

Type	Differentiating symptoms	Additional information
Bacterial conjunctivitis	Eye discharge often with crusting of the lashes.	Highly contagious. Redness of the conjunctiva. Eyes stuck together on waking. Usually bilateral.
Viral conjunctivitis	Itchy, watery eyes a predominant feature.	Highly contagious and spread by contact with another infected person, symptoms usually bilateral. Usually self-limiting but tends to follow a longer course, frequently lasting approximately 2–4 weeks.
Allergic conjunctivitis	Itching is the predominant symptom.	May be associated with a history of atopy, asthma, eczema or rhinitis. May be seasonal, occurring in specific months, or perennial (caused by dust mites, cigarette smoke or pets).

CLINICAL ALERT!

⚠ BEWARE!

- Conjunctivitis in newborns can occur as a result of infection caught from the mother as the baby passes through the birth canal during the delivery. Chlamydia is the most common cause of the condition in this age group with symptoms developing during the first months of life.[3]
- *Neisseria gonorrhoeae* is potentially the most dangerous and virulent infectious cause of neonatal conjunctivitis and if untreated, can cause corneal ulceration and rapid progression to corneal perforation.[4]

Pathophysiology

In healthy eyes the epithelial layer covering the conjunctiva acts as the defence mechanism and any disruption to this layer can increase the risk of developing infection. In bacterial conjunctivitis, infection can occur when the normal flora that colonise the conjunctival layer become contaminated. This can occur via cross infection from a contaminated source, and is often acquired when the eyes have been rubbed. Allergic conjunctivitis arises when there is inflammation of the surface of the eyes caused by a hypersensitivity reaction. The inflammation which arises (usually mast cell driven) results in the symptoms described above during the acute phase and can lead to a late-phase response (with associated eosinophilia and neutrophilia) in some patients, which can subsequently become a chronic disease, resulting in remodelling of the ocular surface tissues.[5] When this occurs, symptoms will be more severe.

Differential diagnosis

 BEWARE!

TABLE 9.4 Differential diagnoses

Condition	Additional pointers	When to consider
Uveitis	Eye pain, floating spots and blurred vision.	Consider if there is a history of autoimmune disease such as systemic lupus erythematosus. There may also be photophobia, and sunlight may worsen the discomfort.[6]
Scleritis	Pain that is often severe enough to disturb the sleep.	The eye is tender to palpation but vision is not typically affected, although half of patients who have scleritis have an associated systemic disease, e.g. rheumatoid arthritis (most common), or other autoimmune diseases or infections such as tuberculosis or syphilis.[7]
Glaucoma	Eye pain with blurred vision and possible nausea and vomiting.	Consider in older patients with associated symptoms of reduced peripheral vision and complaining of being able to see halos around objects.
Keratitis	Watery red eye with pain in the eye.	Consider if the pain is severe enough to make opening the eye difficult and there is visual disturbance and dislike of the light.

CLINICAL ALERT!

⚠ **BEWARE!**

- If misdiagnosed or left untreated uveitis is a potentially sight-threatening condition and can affect the adjacent structures such as the retina, vitreous, optic nerve head and retinal blood vessels.[8]
- Scleritis can result in loss of vision, uveitis and glaucoma, most common in necrotising scleritis, which is often associated with underlying systemic collagen vascular disorders such as rheumatoid arthritis.[9] The pain caused by scleritis is not eased by analgesia and can be constant.
- Blindness and loss of vision arise as a result of untreated glaucoma.
- Complications of keratitis include corneal ulceration or corneal inflammation, visual disturbance or blindness.[10]

Treatment

Even if the cause is thought to be bacterial, evidence suggests that self-help measures, such as eye cleansing with sterile water and cotton balls, warm water compresses, and attention to both hand and eyelid hygiene, may be sufficient for symptoms to settle without the need for medication. Delayed prescribing of antibiotics has been shown to give similar duration and severity of symptoms as would be seen with immediate prescribing, and is believed to achieve reduced rates of re-attendance for eye infections.[11]

Treatment of conjunctivitis depends on the type: *see* Table 9.5.

TABLE 9.5 Treatment of conjunctivitis

Type	Treatment	Dose
Bacterial conjunctivitis	Chloramphenicol eye drops or ointment Or	The recommended dosage for all adults, children and infants of all age groups is 2 drops to the affected eye every 3 hours or more frequently if required, and should be continued for at least 48 hours after eye appears normal.[12]
	Fucithalmic	One drop into affected eyes twice daily.[13]
Viral conjunctivitis	Self-limiting	No specific treatment recommended, but patient may find bathing the eyes, use of cold compresses and artificial tears helps relieve symptoms.
Allergic conjunctivitis	Sodium cromoglycate	Adults and children (1 month and over): 1 or 2 drops to be administered into each eye four times daily.[14]

Prescribing tips
- Both bacterial and viral conjunctivitis may clear without treatment.
- Viral conjunctivitis will usually clear up in 7–14 days without treatment, and antibiotic drops if prescribed for bacterial conjunctivitis will shorten the duration of infection and reduce risk of spread to others.[15]
- Avoid contact lens wearing during treatment.
- Maximum duration of treatment with chloramphenicol is 5 days.
- Chloramphenicol available OTC.

Complications
Conjunctivitis is rarely serious and complications are rare. However, the following have been reported:
- the risk of secondary infections, such as pneumonia, meningitis and septicaemia, is higher in babies with chlamydial conjunctivitis which can lead to sepsis and death[3]
- in children with conjunctivitis caused by haemophilus influenza approximately 25% may subsequently develop otitis media.[16]

Key reminders
- Common condition which can occur at any age.
- Treatment depends on type of conjunctivitis.
- Viral type self-limiting.
- Rarely causes complications.

BLEPHARITIS

Blepharitis occurs when there is inflammation of the margin of the eyelids, and the condition can give rise to inflammation around the follicles and eyelashes (anterior blepharitis) or the inflammation may involve the meibomian glands (posterior blepharitis). The disease is common and accounts for about 5% of all ophthalmological problems presenting in primary care[17] and can affect both adults and children alike.

Clues to aid the diagnosis

- Bilateral
- Burning sensation
- Visual disturbance
- Itching
- Crusting of the lashes
- May have asymptomatic periods followed by exacerbations with recurrence of symptoms.

CLINICAL ALERT!

- Soft, oily, yellow scaling or, rarely, brittle scaling around the lashes distinguishes blepharitis from other causes of eyelid inflammation.[18]
- Blepharitis often is associated with other systemic diseases, particularly rosacea and seborrhoeic dermatitis, and is related to other ocular conditions like dry eye, chalazion, conjunctivitis and keratitis.[19]

Pathophysiology

The pathophysiology of blepharitis is poorly understood but is thought to differ between the two types. Anterior lid margin problems are believed to be predominantly associated with either bacterial or dermatological problems and may involve infestation with parasites,[20] which collect in the eyelashes. The normal function of the meibomian glands is then disrupted, with disturbance to the production of oily secretions, resulting in increased tear evaporation and dry eyes.[21] Posterior blepharitis can be caused by irregular oil production by the meibomian glands which creates a favourable environment for bacterial growth, or the condition can arise as a result of other skin conditions such as acne rosacea and scalp dandruff.[22]

Differential diagnosis

⚠ **BEWARE!**

Some of the conditions that may be considered in the differential diagnosis are as follows:

- conjunctivitis: pp. 149–52
- dry eyes: pp. 156–9

- eczema/dermatitis: pp. 173–6
- keratitis: pp. 156–9.

Other possible considerations include:
- chalazion: a slowly developing lump that forms due to blockage and swelling of an oil gland in the eyelid[23]
- basal cell carcinoma.

Treatment

Treatment of blepharitis is an ongoing process and eyelid hygiene forms a vital part of this treatment.
- Heat to the eyelid promotes cleansing of the secretory passages[24] and can be applied using warm facecloths or gauze soaked in warm water.
- Cleansing of the eyelid margins to remove any crusting or debris.
- Once thoroughly cleansed, an antibiotic ointment can be applied. Ointments containing an antibiotic and steroid combination can also be used, but their use is not recommended for longer term management.[25]
- Artificial tears may be useful if the eyes are dry.
- Warm compresses over the closed eyelid may relieve symptoms and speed resolution.[26]

For resistant cases oral antibiotics may be needed. If other treatments have failed, a course of either oxytetracycline or doxycycline is recommended for approximately 4 months and may be effective because it changes the composition of meibomian gland secretions.[25]

Complications

Complications of blepharitis may affect either the eyelids or the eye itself and are shown in Table 9.6.

TABLE 9.6 Complications of blepharitis

Complication	Additional information
Stye	pp. 155–6.
Meibomian cyst (chalazion)	Painless swelling unless it becomes infected when pain will develop.
Eyelash problems	Abnormal growth of eyelashes, which grow towards the eye, or loss of eyelashes.
Scarring or ulceration of the eyelid	May lead to entropion (where the eyelid turns inwards towards the eyeball or ectropion (where the eyelid turns outwards or away from the eyeball).
Dry eyes	pp. 156–9.
Conjunctivitis	pp. 149–52.
Watering eyes	May be worsened in windy conditions.
Corneal inflammation	Leading to ulceration and scarring of the cornea.

- Referral required if patient develops pain and visual disturbance.
- Urgent referral if vision deteriorates rapidly and there is pain and redness of the cornea.
- Blepharitis can become recurrent and chronic and resistant to treatment.

Key reminders

- Symptoms are bilateral.
- Often associated with underlying pathology.
- Eyelid hygiene important as part of treatment and future prevention.
- Complications can involve the eyelid or the eye itself.

STYES

Styes (or hordeolum) are an acute infection of the eyelid and may be described as external or internal. External styes occur as a result of infection in the hair follicle of sebaceous glands and are generally seen along the eyelid. Internal styes arise as a result of an infection of the meibomian glands.

Clues to aid the diagnosis

Frequently presents with the following symptoms:

- unilateral symptoms
- swollen eyelid
- painful eyelid
- crusting on the eyelid
- may cause excess tear production.

An external hordeolum arises from a blockage and infection of sebaceous glands; an internal hordeolum is a secondary infection of meibomian glands. Both types can arise as a secondary complication of blepharitis.[27] Infections are often caused by organisms from the staphylococcus group and risk is increased with make-up use, in those with poor lid hygiene and in contact lens wearers.[28]

TABLE 9.7 Differential diagnoses

Condition	Additional pointers	When to consider
Blepharitis	pp. 153–5.	pp. 153–5.
Chalazion	Tend to develop further from the edge of the eyelid than styes.	If the lump is painless.
Neoplasm of the eyelid	Several types of malignant neoplasms, but basal cell carcinoma is the commonest.	Eyelashes may be missing at the site of the neoplasm. Sebaceous carcinoma can mimic chalazion or blepharitis and is commonest among middle aged to elderly men.[24]

Treatment

- Warm compresses to the affected eye may help.
- The condition is often self-limiting, requiring no treatment. In some patients the stye will burst, releasing pus, and if this occurs pain and discomfort resolve quickly.
- Antibiotics may be required if infection is spreading and cellulitis of the eyelid develops.

Complications

- Progression to chronic granulation can occur with untreated styes with formation of a chalazion, which exists as a painless lump that can become large and cause visual disturbance.[27]
- Complications may include the simultaneous development of more than one stye on the same lid, disruption of eyelash growth, possible lid deformity and risk of recurrence particularly in individuals with blocked glands in the eyelids, chronic eyelid infections (such as blepharitis), and immune disorders.[29]
- Cellulitis of the lid can also develop.

Key reminders

- Common condition.
- Painful.
- Often self-limiting.
- Complications are rare.

DRY EYES

Dry eye syndrome (DES), also known as keratoconjunctivitis sicca (KCS) or keratitis sicca, and is a multifactorial disease of the ocular surface and tear film that results in ocular discomfort, visual disturbances and tear instability with potential damage to the cornea and conjunctiva.[30] The problem is reported to be common, with increasing prevalence with older age. Among those 65 years or older reported prevalence rates are 10%–30% with the condition being 50% more common in women than men.[31]

Clues to aid the diagnosis

Symptoms vary according to the severity of the problem but frequently include:
- feeling of dryness and a gritty sensation
- patient may complain they feel there is something in the eye
- blurred vision
- patients may complain symptoms seem worse in certain environments (after reading, or after computer use).

⚠ BEWARE!

As well as older adults (females particularly) the following factors are also more likely to be associated with development of the problem:

- smokers
- contact lens wearers
- postmenopausal women who use hormone replacement therapy (HRT), especially those using oestrogen alone[32]
- Sjögren's syndrome is an autoimmune disease affecting saliva and tear production, causing symptoms of both dry mouth and dry eyes.

Pathophysiology

The pathophysiology of dry eye syndrome is highly complex. In health the moisture of the eye, which is essential for optical and physiological reasons, is maintained by the secretions of lipids, aqueous humour and mucus, with lipids playing a role in preventing evaporation and stabilising the tear film.[33] Any dysfunction to any component of the lacrimal unit leads to disruption of the delicate balance between secretion and degradation of tear components,[34] and there are now believed to be two distinct components of the disease that have been identified as tear evaporation and insufficient tear production, which may occur individually or together. In older persons, ageing of the tear film is characterised by its destabilisation and is associated with significant changes in the tear lipid layer producing reduced protection from evaporation in the older population.[35] Other mechanisms include inflammation of the ocular surface, and in patients with Sjögren's syndrome there is inflammation of tear-secreting glands and a reduction in tear production, and changes in the composition of tears resulting in chronic dry eye.[36] Other mechanisms include disruption of oil secretion, which results in increased evaporation and destabilisation of the tear film, and reduced aqueous secretion due to decreased production or increased evaporation, which normally protects the ocular surface by carrying bacteriolytic enzymes and proteins, and providing the ocular surface with moisture,[32] both of which are important factors in the development of dry eye syndrome.

Table 9.8 shows some important causes of dry eyes.

TABLE 9.8 Causes of dry eyes

Causes of decreased tear production	Causes of increased evaporation of tears	Causes of abnormality to the ocular system or problems with the afferent nerve pathway (which supplies the cornea, conjunctiva and the meibomian glands)
Blepharitis	Central heating or air conditioning	Bell's palsy
Allergic conjunctivitis	Allergic conjunctivitis	Problems with contact lens use
Sjögren's syndrome	Drugs such as antihistamines	Ocular manifestations of HIV[37]
Drugs such as anticholinergics, antihistamines, antidepressants (both selective serotonin reuptake inhibitors (SSRIs) and tricyclic types), and beta-blockers[38]	Reduced rate of blinking	Complications of contact lens use

Differential diagnosis

⚠ **BEWARE OF!**

- Blepharitis: pp. 153–5.
- Allergic conjunctivitis: pp. 149–52.
- Problems with contact lenses.
- Ocular manifestations of HIV. Some of those detected include cytomegalovirus (CMV) retinitis, ocular toxoplasmosis, and varicella zoster virus retinitis; however, one study found that of these possible problems CMV retinitis represented a major sight-threatening problem.[39]

Treatment

- Treatment usually involves the use of artificial tears; for mild or moderate symptoms the use of these products may be sufficient to relieve symptoms.
- Hypromellose is one of the most frequently prescribed.
- If symptoms are severe, eye gels or ointments may be useful.

Prescribing tips

- Hypromellose requires frequent use.
- If gels or ointments are prescribed because of their greater viscosity they may cause blurring of vision; therefore, it may be safer and more acceptable to the patient to use them at bedtime.

Complications

The following have been reported.[40]

- Increased susceptibility to irritation, allergy, and infection.
- Secondary conjunctivitis/keratitis.
- Squamous metaplasia of the conjunctiva, which may be initiated by instability of the tear film.
- Corneal ulceration.

CLINICAL ALERT!

Referral is needed if patient develops or complains of:
- deteriorating vision or visual disturbance
- eye pain
- photophobia
- marked redness of the eye
- non-response to treatment.

Key reminders

- Varies in severity from person to person.
- Highly complex underlying pathophysiology.
- Increased prevalence in older age.
- More common in females.

REFERENCES

1. Department of Health and Human Services. Prevalence of visual impairment and selected eye diseases among persons aged ≥50 years with and without diabetes in United States, 2002. *MMWR Weekly.* 2004; **53**(45): 1069–71.
2. GP Notebook. *Conjunctivitis.* Available at: www.gpnotebook.co.uk/simplepage.cfm?ID=-1905590270&linkID=557&cook=no&mentor=1 (accessed 1 October 2012).
3. Mallika PS, Asok T, Aziz S, *et al.* Neonatal conjunctivitis – a review. *Malay Fam Physician.* 2008; **3**(2): 77–81.
4. McCourt E. *Neonatal Conjunctivitis.* Medscape. Available at: http://emedicine.medscape.com/article/1192190-overview#aw2aab6b2b4 (accessed 20 January 2014).
5. Ono SJ, Abelson MB. Allergic conjunctivitis: update on pathophysiology and prospects for future treatment. *J Allergy and Clin Immunol.* 2005; **115**(1): 118–22.
6. Levinson RD. *Uveitis, Anterior, Granulomatous.* Available at: http://emedicine.medscape.com/article/1209505-clinical (accessed 21 October 2012).
7. Galor A, Jeng BH. Red eye for the internist. When to treat, when to refer. *Cleveland Clin J Med.* 2008; **75**(2): 137–44.
8. Sudharshan S, Ganesh SK, Biswas J. Current approach in the diagnosis and management of posterior uveitis. *Indian J Ophthalmol.* 2010; **58**(1): 29–43.
9. Galor A, Thorne JE. Scleritis and peripheral ulcerative keratitis. *Rheum Dis Clin North Am.* 2007; **33**(4): 835–54.
10. Mayo Foundation for Medical Education and Research (MFMER). *Keratitis.* Available at:

www.mayoclinic.com/health/keratitis/DS01190/DSECTION=complications (accessed 27 July 2013).

11. Everitt HA, Little PS, Smith PWF. A randomised controlled trial of management strategies for acute infective conjunctivitis in general practice. *BMJ*. 2006: **333**(7563): 321.

12. Electronic Medicines Compendium. *Chloramphenicol Eye Drops*. Available at www.medicines.org.uk/emc/medicine/22536/spc (accessed 13 July 2013).

13. Electronic Medicines Compendium. *Fucithalmic*. Available at: http://xpil.medicines.org.uk/ViewPil.aspx?DocID=2994 (accessed 19 July 2011).

14. The College of Optometrists. *Sodium Cromoglycate*. Available at: www.college-optometrists.org/en/CPD/Therapeutics/prescribing-network/optometrists-formulary/ophthalmic-drugs/antiinflammatory/sodium-cromoglicate.cfm (accessed 19 August 2013).

15. Centres for Disease Control and Prevention. *Conjunctivitis (Pink Eye)*. Available at: www.cdc.gov/conjunctivitis/about/treatment.html (accessed 13 February 2014).

16. Wald ER. Conjunctivitis in infants and children. *Pediatr Infect Dis*. 1997; **J16**(2 Suppl.): S17–20.

17. Manners T. Managing eye conditions in general practice. *BMJ*. 1997; **315**(7111): 816–17.

18. Papier A, Tutle DJ, Mahar TJ. Differential diagnosis of the swollen red eyelid. *Am Fam Physician*. 2007; **76**(12): 1815–24.

19. Bernardes TF, Bonfioli AA. Blepharitis. *Semin Opthalmol*. 2010; **25**(3): 79–83.

20. Jackson WB. Blepharitis: current strategies for diagnosis and management. *Can J Opthalmol*. 2008: **43**(2): 170–9.

21. Miller KV, Odufuwa TOB, Liew G, *et al*. Interventions for blepharitis (protocol). *Cochrane Database of Syst Rev*. 2005; **4**: CD005556.

22. American Optometric Association. *Blepharitis*. Available at: www.aoa.org/Blepharitis.xml (accessed 19 August 2013).

23. American Optometric Association. *Chalazion*. Available at: www.aoa.org/x9762.xml (accessed 21 October 2012).

24. Carter SR. Eyelid disorders: diagnosis and management. *Am Fam Physician*. 1998; **57**(11): 2695–702.

25. Scott Lowery R. *Adult Blepharitis*. Available at: http://emedicine.medscape.com/article/1211763-overview#showall (accessed 24 August 2013).

26. The Merck Manual. *Eyelid and Lachrymal Disorders*. Available at: www.merckmanuals.com/professional/eye_disorders/eyelid_and_lacrimal_disorders/blepharitis.html (accessed 29 April 2013).

27. Bessette MJ. *Hordeolum and Stye in Emergency Medicine*. Available at: http://emedicine.medscape.com/article/798940-overview#a0104 (accessed 6 March 2012).

28. Family Practice Notebook. *Hordeolum*. Available at: www.fpnotebook.com/eye/Lid/Hrdlm.htm (accessed 10 March 2012).

29. Medical Disability Guidelines. *Stye*. Available at: www.mdguidelines.com/stye (accessed 15 May 2013).

30. Kastelan S, Tomic M, Salopek-Rabatic J, *et al*. Diagnostic procedures and management of dry eye. *Biomed Res Int*. Available at: www.hindawi.com/journals/bmri/2013/309723/

31. Report of the International Dry Eye Workshop (DEWS). *Ocular Surface*. 2007; **5**(2): 65–204.

32. Schaumberg DA, Buring JE, Sullivan DA, *et al*. Hormone replacement therapy and dry eye syndrome. *JAMA*. 2001; **286**(17): 2114–19.

33. Gayton JL. Aetiology, prevalence, and treatment of dry eye disease. *Clin Ophthalmol*. 2009; **3**: 405–12.

34. Bhavsar AS, Bhavsar SG, Jain SM. A review on recent advances in dry eye: pathogenesis and management. *Oman J Ophthalmol*. 2011; **4**: 50–6.

35. Maissa C, Guillon M. Tear film dynamics and lipid layer characteristics: effect of age and gender. *Cont Lens Anterior Eye*. 2010; **33**(4): 176–82.

36. Sjögren's Syndrome Foundation. *Dry Eyes: a hallmark symptom of Sjögren's syndrome.* Available at: www.sjogrens.org/home/about-sjogrens-syndrome/symptoms/dry-eyes (accessed 19 May 2013).

37. American Academy of Ophthalmology. *Dry Eye Syndrome: preferred practice pattern.* Available at: one.aao.org/asset.axd?id=54c358de-eb12-4024-b34c-2b0d09f9b659 (accessed 25 April 2013).

38. Wong J, Lan W, Ong LM, *et al.* Non-hormonal systemic medications and dry eye. *Ocul Surf.* 2011; **9**(4): 212–26.

39. Jabs DA. Ocular manifestations of HIV infection. *Trans Am Ophthalmol Soc.* 1995; **93**: 623–83.

40. American Optometric Association. *Care of the Patient with Dry Eye*. Available at: www.aoa.org/documents/QRG-10B.pdf (accessed 10 March 2013).

CHAPTER 10

Skin

INTRODUCTION

Consultations for skin problems form a huge component of the workload in primary care. There are an estimated 13 million consultations for skin diseases each year, and over half of the UK population (both adults and children alike) are affected by a skin disease of some type each year.[1]

CONDITIONS COVERED IN THIS CHAPTER

- Scabies
- Impetigo
- Fungal skin infections (tinea)
- Eczema
- Psoriasis
- Cellulitis
- Acne
- Chickenpox
- Shingles.

COMMON PRESENTING SYMPTOMS

- Rash
- Itching
- Inflammation
- Infection
- Oozing.

TAKING THE DERMATOLOGICAL HISTORY

Initial history as described in Chapter 3, followed by a focused enquiry relating to the skin.

For symptoms enquiry and further questioning for specific symptoms *see* Table 10.1.

TABLE 10.1 Symptoms enquiry and further questioning for specific symptoms

Symptom	Further questioning
Rash	When did the rash appear?
	Has the patient had anything similar before?
	Is it localised and if so where?
	Is it all over the body?
	Does anything make the rash worse?
Itching	If itching is present is it constant?
	Is the itching at particular sites or more generalised?
	More severe at night when in bed?
Inflammation	Does patient think there is any swelling?
	Is there tenderness on examination?
Infection	Is there redness and inflammation?
	Has patient felt feverish?
	Has patient had any tenderness or pain?
	Any visible sign of pus?
Oozing/discharge	What colour is the discharge?

Table 10.2 shows a summary of presenting signs and symptoms and the diseases they may suggest.

TABLE 10.2 Summary of presenting signs and symptoms and diseases they may suggest

	Rash	Itching	Inflammation	Infection	Oozing/discharge
Scabies	Yes	Yes	Only if infected	Possible if skin becomes damaged through scratching	No
Impetigo	Yes	Possible	Possible	Yes	Yes
Fungal infections (tinea)	Yes	Yes	Yes	No pus	Occurs with tinea pedis
Eczema	Yes	Yes	Yes	Possible	Yes if infected

(continued)

	Rash	Itching	Inflammation	Infection	Oozing/discharge
Psoriasis	Yes	Possible with plaque and pustular psoriasis Intense itching with erythrodermic psoriasis	Occurs in pustular psoriasis	No	No
Cellulitis	No	No	Yes	Yes	Possible
Acne	Yes	No	Possible	Yes	No
Chicken-pox	Yes	Yes	Possible	Can occur if skin is broken with intense scratching	No
Shingles	Yes	Possible prior to appearance of the rash	Possible	Possible	Possible

FURTHER INVESTIGATIONS

Investigations should be chosen on the basis of the history and symptoms, including the duration of symptoms and the overall clinical picture.

- Biopsy.

Further tests if malignancy suspected to exclude spread:

- CT scan
- MRI scan
- lymph node biopsy.

URGENT REFERRAL TO DERMATOLOGIST REQUIRED

- Any skin condition not responding to treatment.
- Suspected skin cancer.

SCABIES

Scabies is an extremely common condition resulting in approximately 300 million cases worldwide each year.[2] It is caused by the parasitic mite *Sarcoptes scabiei* and is highly contagious, spreading easily from person to person by physical contact. The condition is particularly common in crowded areas such as nursing homes, schools and shelters.

Clues to aid the diagnosis

- Intense itching

- Burrows visible between the fingers
- Rash never spreads to the face in adults
- Rash appears as tiny red intensely itchy bumps commonly seen on the limbs and trunk in adults
- Infants and small children may develop lesions more diffusely, with lesions appearing on the face, scalp, neck, palms and soles.

Pathophysiology

The scabies mite is predominantly spread from person to person by skin to skin contact, and spread is still possible even if the person is asymptomatic. From the time of primary infection, there is an interval of up to 10 weeks until clinical manifestations appear.[3] Once fertilised, the females burrow into the upper layers of the epidermis where they lay eggs that will hatch in approximately 3–5 days. New burrows are created by the larvae who will reach maturity in a further 4 days. The cycle is then repeated.

Differential diagnosis

⚠ **BEWARE!**

There are a number of differential diagnoses including:
- eczema/dermatitis (*see* pp. 173–6)
- chickenpox (*see* pp. 185–8)
- folliculitis (infection affecting the hair follicles of the skin)
- insect bites
- urticaria (itchy rash that may occur in response to a trigger or can have no known cause)
- lichen planus (itchy rash with inflammation of the skin).

CLINICAL ALERT!

⚠ **BEWARE!**

- Norwegian scabies is a variant type that occurs more frequently in those with an impaired immune system, which allows mites to proliferate and multiply so that their number can reach millions. Those at risk include the elderly and patients with leukaemia, lymphoma or HIV.[4]
- Infected patients may present with atypical lesions and often are misdiagnosed, which can potentially lead to serious consequences, such as spreading of the infestation and super-infection of the lesions.[5] This type is very contagious, with crusted lesions appearing at multiple sites on the body.
- The risk of secondary infection is high and the condition is more difficult to treat than traditional scabies.

Treatment

Table 10.3 shows pharmacological and non-pharmacological treatments.

TABLE 10.3 Pharmacological and non-pharmacological treatments

Treatment type	Recommendation	Additional information
Pharmacological	Permethrin 5% cream can be safely used in young children and has virtually no allergic side-effects and cosmetically it is highly acceptable.[6] Malathion is an alternative to permethrin 5% cream, especially when treatment of the scalp or hairy areas is needed.[7]	Applied to the whole body and left for 12 hours before rinsing. Reapply to the hands if hand washing is necessary.[8]
Non-pharmacological	All bed linen, clothing and towels should be washed.	High-temperature washes to avoid reinfestation.
Norwegian scabies	Treatment as above.	Should be applied on 2–3 consecutive days.

Prescribing tips

- Treatment is repeated in 1 week.
- All family members should be treated.
- Avoid application after a hot bath as advice now states that this increases absorption of treatment, leaving less at the site.[9]
- Benzyl benzoate is also available as a treatment option but is regarded as too irritant.[6]

CLINICAL ALERT!

- Itching does not resolve immediately after treatment and may persist for at least 2 weeks.
- Additional topical treatment to alleviate itching may help: Eurax can be applied 2–3 times daily (once daily in children under 3 years of age).[10]
- Emollients may soothe symptoms.
- If lesions become infected a course of antibiotics may be needed.

Complications

- Intense itching leading to scratching may result in secondary bacterial skin infection.
- Scabies may cause a flare-up of eczema or dermatitis.
- Scabies is associated with the risk of post-streptococcal glomerulonephritis.
- Other complications of scabies include impetigo, furunculosis and cellulitis.[11]
- Staphylococci or streptococci in the lesions can lead to pyelonephritis, abscesses, pyogenic pneumonia, sepsis and death.[11]

CLINICAL ALERT!

⚠ **BEWARE!**

In the immunosuppressed, crusted scabies has a high mortality rate because of secondary sepsis.

Key reminders

- Very common.
- Highly contagious.
- Often occurs where people reside in group situations, such as nursing homes, or where close contact is common (e.g. schools).
- Symptoms do not resolve immediately with treatment.

IMPETIGO

Impetigo is a highly contagious infection of the skin which can occur in people of any age, but occurs most frequently in young children. The infection may be primary (affecting healthy skin) or secondary, where the infection arises in the presence of another skin problem such as eczema or dermatitis. In the UK one study reported the annual incidence of impetigo to be nearly 2.8% in children up to 4 years of age and 1.6% among children 5–15 years of age.[12]

There are predominantly two forms of impetigo (*see* Table 10.4).

TABLE 10.4 Types of impetigo

Type	Description	Additional information
Bullous	Painless fluid-filled blisters, which may be large.	Less common type. Most commonly affects neonates but also can occur in older children and adults.[13]
Non-bullous	More contagious than bullous type and is characterised by sores which develop a yellow, crusty, scabbed appearance.	Commonest type accounting for the majority of cases, frequently found on skin affected by another skin condition.

The two commonest causative organisms are Group A Streptococcus, and *Staphylococcus aureus.*

Clues to aid the diagnosis

Non-bullous impetigo is characterised by:
- vesicles or pustules that rupture to ooze fluid followed by crusting at the site
- sores are painless
- frequently seen around the nose and mouth but can occur anywhere on the body.[14]

Bullous impetigo is characterised by:
- fluid-filled blisters, usually on the trunk, the arms or legs which quickly spread and then burst so that a crust is formed
- sores are painless, but there may be itching
- other symptoms, such as fever and swollen glands, are more common in bullous impetigo.[14]

Pathophysiology

Healthy skin is usually able to resist infection or colonisation by bacteria, but any unbroken skin allows bacteria to gain entry via receptors that are only accessible on damaged skin and hence set up the process of infection. Lesions are most common in warm, moist areas of the body and predisposing factors which may facilitate colonisation by bacteria include warm ambient temperatures, humidity, poor hygiene and crowded living conditions.[15]

Differential diagnosis

⚠ BEWARE OF!

- Eczema/dermatitis (*see* pp. 173–6).
- Scabies (*see* pp. 164–6).
- Chickenpox (*see* pp. 185–8).

Treatment

Level of treatment will depend on the severity of the infection. Topical antibiotic cream may be sufficient in some cases, or a combination of oral antibiotics and a topical agent may be needed.
- Topical agent: fusidic acid applied 2–3 times daily is an effective treatment for impetigo, with very few side-effects.[16]
- Oral antibiotics: flucloxacillin is often a first-line choice or clarithromycin for those with penicillin allergy, for a duration of 7 days.[9]

Hygiene measures

- Any weeping or oozing of the area may need to be covered to avoid spread of infection.
- Avoid touching the lesions unless needed (i.e. for application of antibiotic cream) and wash hands as needed.
- Avoid close contact with others.
- Keep separate towels and face cloths.
- Children should stay away from school until crusts have dried out.

Complications

- In rare cases, impetigo caused by *Streptococcus* infection can result in glomerulonephritis, scarlet fever or erythema multiforme.[17]

- Cellulitis (*see* pp. 179–82).
- Scarlet fever (rare infection that is associated with a rash).

⚠ BEWARE!

- Although rare, septicaemia is a potentially life-threatening complication.
- Acute post-streptococcal glomerulonephritis is a serious complication that affects 1%–5% of patients with non-bullous impetigo.[12]

Key reminders

- Impetigo is very common, particularly in children.
- Highly contagious and easily spread.
- Easy to treat.
- Good hygiene to avoid spread to others.

FUNGAL SKIN INFECTIONS (TINEA)

Fungal infections can affect both adults and children alike, with some types more common in children and others more prevalent among adults. Ringworm (tinea) is a common infection of the skin that can affect people of any age but is particularly prevalent among children. The causative fungi are commonly called dermatophytes, and once infection is present it is easily spread from person to person by skin to skin contact or from infected objects such as bedding, towels or from pets.

Tinea is classified according to the site of infection as shown in Table 10.5.

TABLE 10.5 Tinea classified according to site of infection

Name	Site	Additional information
Tinea capitas	Ringworm occurring on the scalp.	May cause hair loss.
Tinea corporis	Ringworm of the trunk.	Often seen on exposed areas such as the arms.
Tinea barbae	Fungal infection of the beard.	Neck may also be involved.
Tinea cruris	Fungal infection of the groin and pubic area.	Often occurs in conjunction with *Tinea pedis* and/or *Tinea unguium*.
Tinea pedis	Fungal infection that occurs between the toes and plantar surface.	Often unilateral, causing fissuring of the skin and maceration.

(continued)

Name	Site	Additional information
Tinea unguium	Fungal nail infection.	Characterised by thick, discoloured nails. This type is more common in adults and is more likely to develop in older people, diabetics and in those with poor venous and lymphatic drainage, ill-fitting shoes and also in those who actively engage in sport; however, in many cases there is no underlying cause.[18]
Tinea manuum	Fungal infection affecting the palm and between the fingers.	Often unilateral and may occur with *Tinea pedis*.

CLINICAL ALERT!

- *Tinea pedis*, generally known as 'athlete's foot', is the most common dermatophyte infection in adults, with men 20–40 years of age most frequently affected.[18]
- *Tinea capitas* is the most common dermatophyte infection seen in children.[19]

Clues to aid the diagnosis

Appearance of a rash with itching is common in fungal skin infections, with nail discolouration the dominant feature of nail involvement. Pruritus is the main symptom in most forms of tinea affecting the skin and it takes about 2 weeks from inoculation to the development of skin changes that are clinically visible.[20] When the fungus affects the nails, toenails are commonly affected and a brownish tinge becomes apparent.

Pathophysiology

Fungi can cause infection on any area of the skin, and the nails, hair and warm moist skin provide the perfect environment for fungi to set up infection. Pathophysiology varies slightly for each tinea type.

Tinea capitas

From the time the infection is acquired the fungus invades the outer layer of the epidermis and continues downward growth into the hair, invading the keratin as it does so. One or two patches of hair loss appear on the scalp and the hair is usually broken off just above the surface, producing an appearance similar to seborrhoeic dermatitis.[21]

Tinea corporis

Dermatophytes invade the epidermis and lesions appear as single or multiple lesions. Each lesion has a scaly appearance with a central clearing, and an elevated reddened edge commonly appearing on the extremities, trunk or face.[22]

Tinea barbae

Similar mechanism to *Tinea capitas*.

Tinea cruris

The causative dermatophytes produce keratinases, which allow invasion of the corni-fied cell layer of the epidermis.[23] Invasion to deeper layers is usually prevented by activation of an immune response.

Tinea pedis

Similar mechanism to *Tinea corporis*. *Tinea pedis* infections, most often the inter-digital type, may be complicated by cellulitis, with maceration and fissuring of the skin developing in the infected interspaces, weakening the natural barrier of the skin.[24] This process then provides a route of entry for pathogenic bacteria, allowing infection to develop.

Tinea unguium

Usually starts as discoloured yellowish streaks in the nail, spreading to involve the whole nail. Occurs more frequently in adults and often the toenails are the first to be involved with the fingernails less frequently affected.[21]

Differential diagnosis

⚠ BEWARE!

- Dermatitis/eczema (*see* pp. 173–6).
- Psoriasis (*see* pp. 177–9).
- Erythema multiforme (an acute, self-limiting and sometimes recurring skin condition that is associated with certain infections, medications and other various triggers.[25]
- Candida (skin infection caused by candida).

Treatment

Treatment type depends on the site and severity of the infection, but successful treatment of superficial tinea infections of the skin may be achieved with antifun-gal cream applied twice daily. Suitable choices are Daktacort HC or Canesten HC.

Prescribing tip

It is advisable for topical treatment to be continued for 7 to 10 days after the rash has disappeared.[26] This reduces the risk of recurrence, which can occur if treatment is discontinued too early.

CLINICAL ALERT!

More extensive infections and difficult to treat infections such as scalp or nail infections may require oral treatment with terbinafine.

Duration of oral treatment varies according to the site of infection

Terbinafine is commonly prescribed, but duration of treatment varies according to the site of the infection.

- *Tinea pedis* requires treatment for 2–6 weeks, *Tinea corporis* for 4 weeks and *Tinea cruris* for 2–4 weeks.[27] *Tinea capitas* requires treatment for 4 weeks.[28]
- In adults, dose is 250 mg daily for duration that treatment is required.
- In children, dose prescribed is calculated according to body weight. Daily dose of 62.5 mg for children 10–20 kg, 125 mg for children 20–40 kg, and 250 mg for children greater than 40 kg.[9]
- For fungal nail infections, treatment is generally needed for 12 weeks to treat toenail infections and for 6 weeks to treat fingernail infections.[29]
- *Tinea barbea* is treated for up to 4 weeks with terbinafine 250 mg daily.[30]

Complications

- Spread of infection to other sites.
- Risk of infection when the skin has been broken by scratching.

CLINICAL ALERT!

⚠ BEWARE!

- Scalp ringworm can cause hair loss and scarring of the skin.
- Fungal infections rarely spread below the surface of the skin to cause serious illness, but immunocompromised patients, such as those with HIV or AIDS, may find it difficult to get rid of the infection.[31]

Key reminders

- Can affect people of any age.
- Common all over the world.
- There are several types, some more common than others.
- Infection at some sites can be difficult to treat.
- Oral treatment may be required for some cases.

ECZEMA

Eczema is an extremely common condition affecting both adults and children. In the UK one in 30 GP consultations is for eczema in children,[32] and statistics indicate that 15%–20% of school-aged children and 2%–10% of adults will be affected by the condition at some time in their life.[33]

Clues to aid the diagnosis

Often presents first in young children with symptoms that flare up at intervals and settle again in between these episodes.

Commonly presents with

Eczema commonly presents with the following:
- areas of skin redness
- intense itching
- often evidence of scratching
- skin lesions with thickening of the epidermis.

CLINICAL ALERT!

⚠ **BEWARE!**

The condition is not normally associated with other features, so the presence of fever and/or other symptoms point to an alternative diagnosis.

Pathophysiology

Atopic eczema is associated with a reduction in the lipid barrier of the skin, which leads to an increased amount of water loss and subsequently dry skin.[34] The exact pathophysiology of the condition is extremely complex, but is believed to involve a number of elements including genetic factors, environmental triggers, defects in the skin barrier and in the immunoglobulin responses, although the influence of the latter is poorly understood.[35]

Differential diagnosis

⚠ **BEWARE OF!**

- Fungal infections (*see* pp. 169–72).
- Psoriasis (*see* pp. 177–9).
- Scabies (*see* pp. 164–6).

Treatment

Treatment often uses a stepwise approach to management based on the severity of symptoms at presentation.

CLINICAL ALERT!

Emollients play a vital part in the management of eczema and should be used even when the patient is asymptomatic. Regular use of an emollient helps to restore the skin's barrier function, preventing penetration of irritants, allergens and bacteria, thereby reducing or preventing the development of eczema.[36]

There are many types of emollients and they can be classified according to how they are applied (*see* Table 10.6).

TABLE 10.6 Emollient choices

Type of emollient	Examples	Additional information
Lotions	Dermol Aveeno Eurax	Lotions have a higher water content and less fat than creams.[36]
Creams	Aqueous cream Epaderm Diprobase cream E45 cream Oilatum Dermol Aveeno Eurax	Contain a mixture of fat and water and may be useful when the skin is sore but must be used frequently to avoid skin becoming dry. Creams contain preservatives, which some people can become sensitive to, although this is rare.
Ointments	Diprobase ointment Liquid and white soft paraffin Emulsifying ointment Epaderm	Ointments can become contaminated; the use of pump dispensers minimises the risk,[37] but if the emollient is in a pot, to avoid contamination from inserting the fingers into the pot, the cream should be removed from the pot using a clean spoon or spatula before applying to the skin.
Bath and shower oils	Diprobase shower gel Double base shower gel Oilatum shower emollient Aveeno bath oil E45 bath oil Cetraben bath additive Oilatum bath additive	Both oils serve to leave a film of oil on the skin, which helps to trap water in the skin, therefore keeping skin hydrated.
Soap substitutes	E45 emollient wash cream	Some soaps are highly scented and may serve as an irritant; soap substitutes provide a non-irritant alternative.

Prescribing tips

- Lotions have the advantage of spreading easily across large areas of skin and may therefore be useful where the eczema affects a large area, but are not as effective for very dry skin.

- Creams are less greasy than some of the other emollient choices and may therefore be more acceptable to some patients.
- Ointments can be very greasy, which some patients may find off-putting, but they are useful for very dry and thickened skin as they help with water retention and therefore have a good moisturising effect.

Additional topical steroid treatments may be needed when emollients are not enough to control symptoms and are often required intermittently for recurrence of symptoms. Table 10.7 presents some steroid preparations.

TABLE 10.7 Steroid preparations

Product	Available as	Potency
Hydrocortisone	Cream or ointment	Mild
Eumovate (Clobetasone butyrate)	Cream or ointment	Moderate
Betnovate (Betamethasone valerate RD)	Cream or ointment	Moderate
Betnovate (Betamethasone valerate)	Cream or ointment Scalp application	Potent
Locoid (Hydrocortisone butyrate)	Cream	Potent
Elocon Mometasone	Cream or ointment Scalp application	Potent
Dermovate Clobetasol propionate	Cream or ointment Scalp application	Very potent

Prescribing tips for steroids
- Recommended for short-term use only.
- Should be used with caution in children.
- Not recommended for use for more than 5–7 days in children.
- Cream often best for moist or weeping areas.
- Ointment best for dry, scaly, thickened areas.

Other treatments for eczema are shown in Table 10.8.

TABLE 10.8 Other treatments for eczema

Treatment	Additional information
Medicated dressings	Improve hydration and increase the penetration of topical corticosteroids, also have an anti-inflammatory effect and suppress itching.[38] The intact dressing prevents the patient from scratching and also reduces the risk of infection.
Topical immunosuppressants	Creams such as tacrolimus ointment and pimecrolimus cream are initiated by a dermatologist (or GP with specialist knowledge). They may be useful when eczema is not responding to other treatments or to areas where side-effects are more likely (e.g. the eyes or face).[39] They are associated with an increased risk of skin infections and should not be applied to infected or weeping skin.[40]
Phototherapy	May be helpful where other treatments have failed but has been found to achieve only about 50% complete clearance rates in atopic dermatitis patients.[41]
Antihistamines	May be helpful if itching is severe (sedating antihistamine may be needed for children if symptoms are causing sleep disturbance).

Complications

Common complications include skin infections, boils and folliculitis. If the skin infection is severe, septicaemia may develop.

CLINICAL ALERT!

⚠ BEWARE!

- Erythroderma is a potentially fatal skin condition causing a severe redness of the skin and can arise in patients with worsening eczema. Requires hospitalisation.
- Eczema herpeticum is a potentially fatal condition caused by viral infection, usually *Herpes simplex* virus, and occurs in association with pre-existing skin disease, usually atopic dermatitis.[42] The patient becomes unwell with fever and requires urgent treatment with antiviral drugs.
- In patients with severe eczema there is a risk of eye symptoms that can lead to permanent damage and loss of vision.[43] Requires urgent referral to a dermatologist and ophthalmologist if necessary.

Key messages

- Eczema is very common
- Can occur at any age
- Emollients used with or without symptoms form the cornerstone of treatment
- Complications are rare.

PSORIASIS

Psoriasis can occur at any age and primarily affects the skin, the nails and occasionally the joints.[44] Prevalence rates are difficult to determine because of the relapsing and remitting nature of the condition, but in the general population estimates range between 0.6% and 4.8%.[45] There is some indication that the condition has a genetic link and twin studies have shown a concordance rate for monozygotic twins to be 62%–70% compared to 21%–23% for dizygotic twins.[46] Similarly, a familial link has also been noted, with one study reporting a 14% risk if one parent was affected, 41% risk if both parents are affected, and a 6% risk if one sibling is affected, compared to only a 2% risk when no parent or sibling was affected.[47]

Clues to aid the diagnosis

There are several types of psoriasis (*see* Table 10.9). Plaque psoriasis is the commonest.[48]

TABLE 10.9 Types of psoriasis

Type	Recognition	Additional information
Plaque psoriasis	Lesions can vary both in size and number. There are ring-like lesions with varying degrees of thickness. Plaques are usually redder around the edges with a paler centre and are usually symmetrical, affecting elbows or knees, although they can occur anywhere on the body.	Often improves during periods of warmer weather with exposure to sun.
Guttate psoriasis	This type appears as small scattered lesions. It is commonest in children and young adults and often disappears without treatment, although this may take several weeks.[49]	Often preceded by a streptococcal infection of the throat or upper respiratory tract.[49]
Erythrodermic psoriasis	Rare form of psoriasis that can affect any age. Trauma, infections and drugs, such as lithium, antimalarials, trimethoprim and sulfamethoxazole, as well as environmental, psychological and metabolic factors can trigger psoriasis and the erythrodermic form of the disease.[50]	This is a medical condition requiring urgent admission. The condition can be fatal.
Pustular psoriasis	Pustular psoriasis is an uncommon form of psoriasis. Onset is often rapid with a widespread rash affecting any area of the body, consisting of small pustules on a red base, and accompanied by fever.[51]	Patients are usually systemically unwell and require admission to hospital for treatment and observation.
Psoriatic arthritis	This type is characterised by inflammation and painful swollen joints.	Inflammatory type of psoriasis that tends to run a relapsing and remitting course.

Pathophysiology

The pathophysiology of psoriasis is poorly understood, but it is thought that the psoriatic skin lesions are the result of inflammation in the dermis and hyperproliferation with abnormal differentiation of the epidermis, and overproduction of proinflammatory cytokines such as interferon and tumour necrosis factor (TNF).[52] Trigger factors are thought to play a part in the condition and these are thought to include infectious episodes, and stressful life events with as many as 60% of patients describing stress as being a key 'exacerbator' or trigger of their disease.[53]

Differential diagnosis

Because of the variable types of psoriasis there are many possible differential diagnoses, so only the most common will be discussed here.
- Eczema/dermatitis: *see* pp. 173–6.
- Pityriasis rosea starts with a single area (herald patch), which progresses to form a Christmas-tree-shaped distribution. Disappears without treatment, although this may take several weeks.
- Lichen planus is characterised by an itchy rash of unknown cause, more common in adults over 30 years of age.
- Discoid lupus erythematosus appears with a rash that usually affects the face and scalp but is occasionally more widespread and consists of red scaly patches, which tend to clear eventually, but can leave some thinning and scarring or colour change in the skin.[54]

Treatment

As with eczema, emollients play an important role in the treatment and management of psoriasis and should be applied regularly on a daily basis. When used correctly they can be very effective in reducing dryness, keeping the skin moist, and reducing itching. (*See* p. 174 for information relating to suitable emollients.) Table 10.10 sets out some treatment options.

TABLE 10.10 Treatment options

Type	Treatment	Additional information
Plaque psoriasis	Regular use of emollients.	Apply emollients at least 3–4 times daily.
	Short-term use of a topical steroid.	Short-term use of a potent topical steroid (e.g. Dermovate) or a combined potent corticosteroid plus calcipotriol (e.g. Dovobet) is recommended.[55] Additional treatment, such as coal tar, may be added to augment the effect of the topical steroid, or may be used in isolation, or alternatives such as vitamin D analogues (e.g. calcipotriol) may be added to steroids or used alone.[56]
Guttate psoriasis	Often resolves without any treatment.	May take several weeks and can recur.

Type	Treatment	Additional information
Erythrodermic psoriasis	Emergency admission.	Hospital care involves bed-rest, emollients and treatment of any complications.
Pustular psoriasis	Emergency admission.	Difficult to treat and often needs treatment with a combination of drugs, which potentially have unpleasant side-effects.
Psoriatic arthritis	Treatment should be aimed at treating both skin and joint problems.	Methotrexate, retinoids and psoralen combined with ultraviolet A (PUVA) treatment appears to be most effective at treating skin and joints together.[57]

Complications
- Secondary infections
- Possible increased risk of lymphoma
- Possible increased risk of cardiovascular and ischaemic heart disease
- Psoriatic arthritis.

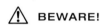

⚠ BEWARE!

There is increasing evidence that psoriasis is a risk factor for AF and stroke, with risk highest among young patients with severe psoriasis.[58]

Key reminders
- Occurs at various sites on the body including the scalp and nails
- Various types
- Some variants require treatment in hospital
- Plaque psoriasis is the most common type.

CELLULITIS
Cellulitis in adults is a common medical condition that can occur with varying degrees of severity. Milder cases can be successfully managed in primary care; however, more severe cases lead to hospital admission and are believed to account for approximately 2%–3% of hospital admissions.[59]

Clues to aid the diagnosis
Usually unilateral, the condition presents with:
- redness and swelling of the leg
- spreading erythema
- fever
- pain.

⚠ BEWARE!

- The majority of patients with cellulitis have a raised WCC count and elevated ESR or CRP.[60] Normal results, therefore, make the diagnosis less likely.
- The infection can potentially spread rapidly with resulting fever and malaise, and the patient will be clinically unwell.

Pathophysiology

Cellulitis occurs as a result of an infection of the dermis and subcutaneous tissues.

Where the skin is healthy and intact, it provides an excellent barrier to any organisms that are present either on the skin or externally in the environment, successfully preventing them from entering the tissues and causing disease. Even when micro-organisms gain access to soft tissues, the body's defence mechanism would normally be able to kill any invading intruder. However, when this fails the organisms are able to multiply to progress to the signs and symptoms of cellulitis. Bacteria can gain entry via a break in the skin, such as a laceration, insect bite or cut. Once entry to the dermis has been gained, bacteria multiply to cause the typical signs and symptoms of cellulitis. The condition can also occur where no obvious route of entry exists and this is common in dry and irritated skin where bacteria gain entry through microscopic breaks in the skin. Group A streptococci are the most common bacterial contaminants responsible for soft-tissue infections, and *Staphylococcus aureus* is the second most common; both are present in natural skin flora.[61] Less common organisms include *Streptococcus pneumoniae*, *Haemophilus influenzae*, gram-negative bacilli and anaerobes.[62] The condition is commonest in patients with lymphoedema, leg oedema, venous insufficiency, leg ulcers and the obese.[63] When these additional problems exist there is a risk of infections becoming recurrent. The leg is the commonest site of infection and accounts for 70% of cases.[64]

Differential diagnosis

⚠ BEWARE!

There are a number of differential diagnoses and just the more commonly found are listed here. These include:

- infected insect bites
- erythema multiforme, which is characterised by the presence of small spots that have a dusky red centre, a paler area around this, and a red ring around the edge that is generally darker in colour
- erysipelas, an infection of the skin, which because the infection is nearer to the skin surface, is more superficial than cellulitis
- infected burns
- Stevens–Johnson syndrome, which is characterised by a painful red or

purplish rash that spreads and blisters, eventually causing the top layer of skin to die and shed

- varicose eczema, which causes a rash of the lower limbs arising as a result of venous disease and stasis of blood.

Treatment

The decision to treat at home or in hospital is based on the severity of illness and the presence of comorbid illnesses, which may interfere with the healing process and make response to treatment more difficult. CREST guidance[59] offers advice on grading symptom severity (*see* Table 10.11) and suggests that only patients assessed as class 1, where there are no unstable comorbidities and no signs of severe sepsis, are suitable for treatment in the primary care setting; the remainder will require admission to hospital.

Prescribing information.

- Antibiotics are effective in 90% of cases of cellulitis[65] but more severe infections will require intravenous rather than oral treatment.
- Local antibiotics guidelines may guide choice of antibiotics prescribed but penicillin V with or without flucloxacillin, or amoxicillin with clavulanic acid, are often used, with treatment continued for 10 to 14 days or until signs of infection have resolved.[66]
- In addition to antibiotics, analgesia (e.g. paracetamol or ibuprofen) may be required for pain relief.

TABLE 10.11 CREST (Now GAIN) Guidance[59] Reproduced with kind permission

Class 1	No signs of systemic toxicity. No uncontrolled comorbidities. Suitable for management on an outpatient basis.
Class 2	Either systemically unwell or systemically well, but with comorbid illness which may interfere with ability to resolve the infection.
Class 3	Systemically unwell with acute confusion, tachycardia, tachypnoea, hypotension or may have unstable and poorly controlled comorbidities that may interfere with response to treatment or may have a severe limb-threatening infection as a result of vascular compromise.
Class 4	Severe life-threatening infection such as necrotising fascitis and sepsis.

Complications

⚠ **BEWARE OF!**

- Extension of the redness and increase in severity of the symptoms may signal a deeper infection.
- Spread of the bacteria can lead to development of septicaemia.
- Recurring cellulitis may cause damage to the lymphatic system that over time can progress to lymphoedema.[67]

- Necrotising fasciitis can occur; this is a more serious infection affecting the soft tissue and fascia.

CLINICAL ALERT!

⚠ BEWARE!

Necrotising fasciitis is an insidiously advancing soft-tissue infection characterised by widespread fascial necrosis leading to severe systemic toxicity, septicaemia and rapid death unless appropriately treated.[68]

Urgent admission required
Urgent admission is required in the event of the following.
- Onset of nausea and vomiting
- Failure to respond to treatment
- Worsening symptoms and/or deterioration in any comorbid condition.

Key reminders
- Early recognition is important to prevent potentially life-threatening outcomes.
- Potentially serious if left undiagnosed and untreated.
- Diagnosis can be made on assessment of the patient and clinical findings alone.
- Patient education is important in preventing recurrence, and information regarding foot care and skin care should form part of the treatment plan.

ACNE
Acne can be very distressing for the affected person and has the potential to cause considerable anxiety and psychological distress. Symptoms can range from mild to severe, and it is estimated that approximately 15% of those aged 15–17 years old suffer with moderate to severe acne in the UK.[69] Although often thought of as primarily a condition affecting teenagers, this is not always the case and an estimated 12% of adults may suffer with the condition, which may persist into middle age.[70] As a result there are an estimated 3.5 million visits to GP surgeries each year in the UK for advice and treatment.[71]

Clues to aid the diagnosis
Diagnosis is usually made on appearance of the skin and the presence of comedones that generally form two types, either closed (whiteheads) or open (blackheads). Pustules and papules also develop, appearing in varying number and at various sites: commonly the face, back, chest and sometimes the upper arms.

Pathophysiology

The process is thought to originate from obstruction of the pilosebaceous gland, which is comprised of the hair follicle, hair shaft and the sebaceous gland.[72] During adolescence there is increased production of sebum and this increased sebum production is an important factor in the development of acne. The initial event in the development of an acne lesion is abnormal desquamation of the keratinocytes that line the sebaceous follicle.[73] Excessive sebum production together with a disturbance of the maturation of the keratinocytes increases adhesion between cells lining the pilosebaceous gland.[74] This accumulation of adherent keratinised cells causes obstruction to the flow of sebum within the canal that subsequently leads to obstruction of the pilosebaceous gland itself, which manifests itself as the development of comedones. Colonisation of the pilosebaceous duct with *Propionibacterium acnes* occurs, which leads to inflammation of lesions, a complex process that occurs through activation of various processes that may subsequently lead to rupture of the comodone.[75]

CLINICAL ALERT!

- Acne tends to appear earlier in females than in males, possibly reflecting the earlier onset of puberty, but it is often more severe in adolescent males than females, which may be caused by androgen production that stimulates sebum production.[76]
- When onset of acne is at an older age, more females than males are affected.[77]

Differential diagnosis

There are several differential diagnoses but only the commonest are shown in Table 10.12.

TABLE 10.12 Differential diagnoses

Condition	Additional information	When to consider
Folliculitis	There are papules and pustules that occur as a result of inflammation and infection of the hair follicles.	Multiple or single lesions appear and may be seen on the head, neck, trunk, buttocks and extremities.[78] Superficial folliculitis is the commonest type and presents with painless or tender pustules that heal without leaving scarring.[79]
Rosacea	Often seen in those over the age of 20 years, affecting three females to every male.[80]	Patient relates symptoms to certain triggers such as extremes in weather conditions, stress, anxiety, hot baths, beverages (e.g. alcohol, hot drinks) and certain foods (e.g. liver, dairy products, hot or spicy foods).[81]

CLINICAL ALERT!

- Folliculitis may be complicated by staphylococcal infection, which will lead to the development of painful lesions that have the potential to cause scarring.
- *Acne fulminans* is a rare variant of acne characterised by a sudden, violent onset of tender, nodulo-cystic and ulcer-crusted lesions over the back and chest, with fever, arthralgia and weight loss.[82] The condition predominantly affects young adolescent males and is difficult to treat.

Treatment

There are various treatment options, often commenced on a trial and error basis. *See* Table 10.13.

TABLE 10.13 Treatment options

Acne severity	Treatment	Additional information
Mild	Medicated face washes	Little evidence to support their use and some products can be expensive.
	Topical benzoyl peroxide	Benzoyl peroxide can be purchased over the counter and is available in various strengths. It is a powerful antimicrobial agent that rapidly destroys *P. acnes* and is able to reduce the number of comedones.[83]
Moderate	Topical antibiotics, e.g. clindamycin	Topical antibiotics are another option for mild-to-moderate acne and are effective in treating *P. acnes* and reducing any inflammation. Topical clindamycin and erythromycin have been shown to be effective against inflammatory acne vulgaris with or without the addition of zinc but none of those tested was more effective than benzoyl peroxide.[84] Products containing a combination of clindamycin 1% and benzoyl peroxide 5% have been proven to be superior to each individual component used alone and have been found to be effective in reducing inflammatory lesions.[85]
	Topical retinoids (e.g. tretinoin or adapalene)	Effective in reducing inflammation and reducing the formation of new comedones.
Moderate to severe	Oral antibiotics	Tetracycline or oxytetracycline is often prescribed, but local guidelines may suggest alternative choices.
Oral contraceptives	Yasmin, Celeste	Combined COCs suppress androgens secreted from the ovary that in turn will decrease the amount of free, biologically active androgens, which will subsequently reduce the negative action of androgens on sebaceous glands and hair follicles.[86]

Prescribing tips

- Benzoyl peroxide may cause skin irritation, although this is thought more likely when higher strengths are used.[87]

- Benzoyl peroxide should be used for a minimum of 2 months before switching to topical antibacterial agent.[9]
- Similarly, topical antibiotics should also be continued for 6 months until full effect is achieved.
- Topical retinoids may cause side-effects such as peeling, erythema, dryness, burning and itching, particularly at the onset of treatment.[88]
- Oral antibiotics can potentially cause several problems. Tetracycline may cause vaginal candida infections and dyspepsia, while erythromycin can cause dyspepsia or abdominal discomfort even when taken with food, and the resistance of *P. acnes* to the drug develops more frequently (in up to 60% of isolates) than with other systemic antibiotics.[89]

Complications

One of the most unpleasant after effects of acne is the scarring that may occur. It is permanent and can therefore be extremely distressing for those affected. Little information is known on accurate prevalence rates, but estimates generally suggest the problem affects 1%–11% of those affected.[90] Treatment is available but requires specialist dermatological referral. Unfortunately, results can be unpredictable and the person should therefore be advised that success is not guaranteed prior to starting any treatment.

CLINICAL ALERT!

Facial scarring affects both sexes equally and occurs in 95% of cases,[90] although the degree of scarring varies from patient to patient and may be mild in some cases and more severe in others.

Key reminders

- Common in adolescents but can affect adults
- Commonest on the face but can affect the back, chest and upper arms
- Associated with psychological distress
- Can occur in relatively mild forms or be severe
- Numerous treatments available.

CHICKENPOX

Chickenpox is a highly contagious infectious disease caused by the varicella-zoster virus. It is easily spread from person to person via droplet infection or from infected items such as bedding or clothing. The time from contracting the infection to onset of symptoms is 10–21 days, with the patient infectious 48 hours before onset of the rash.[91] It is very common in young children, especially those under 10 years of age, with more than 90% of cases occurring in this age group.[92] It is usually a mild disease in children but there is increased morbidity if it occurs in adults or in those who are immunocompromised. It is not possible to develop shingles from exposure to a person with chickenpox. It is, however, possible to develop chickenpox as a result of exposure to a person with shingles.

Clues to aid the diagnosis

In most cases the disease is easily recognised and there may have been contact with others who have also developed symptoms (usually classmates or siblings). Before the rash appears the child may appear unwell, with headache, nausea and loss of appetite. Other typical symptoms include:

- rash that appears as small red macules on the trunk, arms, legs and face, which progress to vesicles with a blister-like appearance, over the next day or so; these are then intensely itchy
- there may be a mild fever
- spots can also appear on the hands, feet and in the mouth in more severe cases
- chickenpox is most infectious from 1–2 days before the rash starts, and remains contagious until all the blisters have crusted over, which is generally 5–7 days after the onset of the rash.

CLINICAL ALERT!

⚠ BEWARE!

- Adults who develop chickenpox tend to have more severe symptoms and are more unwell than children who contract the disease.
- Women who develop chickenpox in pregnancy up to week 28 are at risk of foetal damage occurring to the eyes, legs, arms, brain, bladder or bowel (estimated to affect around 1–2 of every 100 babies).[93]
- If a woman develops varicella 5 days before to up to 2 days after delivery, the newborn will be at risk for neonatal varicella, and there is a risk that these newborns may develop severe neonatal varicella infection.[94]

Pathophysiology

Once the virus gains entry to the body, it is able to infect the mucosa of the respiratory tract. Multiplication of the virus takes place in the lymph nodes in the early days after contracting the infection. This process is then followed by a second round of viral replication that occurs in the internal organs of the body, most notably the liver and the spleen, with further viraemia (virus in the bloodstream) 14–16 days after contracting the virus.[92] This process is then followed by the invasion of the virus into the capillary endothelial cells and the epidermis, which then leads to the development of the characteristic vesicles that are seen in chickenpox.

Differential diagnosis

⚠ **BEWARE OF!**

- Drug reactions.
- Erythema multiforme (*see* p. 180). Infections are thought to be associated with the development of at least 90% of cases of this condition, with the single most common trigger for developing it being infection with *Herpes simplex* virus.[95]
- Insect bites.
- Bullous pemphigoid, which is characterised by blisters on the skin.

Treatment

Chickenpox will often resolve without any treatment, but the measures described in Table 10.14 may help to alleviate any unpleasant symptoms.

TABLE 10.14 Treatment to alleviate symptoms of chickenpox

Age and health status	Treatment	Additional information
Healthy child	Analgesia.	Ibuprofen or paracetamol.
	Calamine lotion.	Applied to rash.
	Antihistamine.	Stop the itching.
Adults	Usually same treatment as for children.	Antiviral treatment needs to be commenced within 24 hours of the onset of the rash.
	In adults with severe symptoms or who have risk factors that may raise the risk of complications, antiviral treatment may be helpful.	Acyclovir 800 mg five times daily for 7 days.[9]
Pregnant	Symptomatic treatment.	Seek specialist advice regarding further treatment.
Immunocompromised adults	Acyclovir.	If presenting within 24 hours of onset of the rash.
		For immunocompetent individuals presenting more than 48 hours after the development of the rash symptomatic treatment only is advised, but patient should be monitored for signs of severe infection.[96]

Complications

In healthy individuals the risk of complications is rare. Risk is increased in certain patients.

- In adults the condition is more likely to cause severe systemic manifestations leading to a high frequency of complications with increased mortality rate, particularly in the older age group and in smokers.[97]

- Neonates (infants within the first 4 weeks of life) and those who are immunocompromised due to illness or treatments such as chemotherapy or high-dose steroids, may experience more serious complications that include viral pneumonia, secondary bacterial infections and encephalitis.[98]

CLINICAL ALERT!

⚠ BEWARE!

- In adults the most frequent serious complication is pneumonia.[99]
- The mortality rate in children who are immunocompromised is much higher than that seen in otherwise healthy children and is estimated at 7% among children with leukaemia.[100]
- Chickenpox results in the death of approximately 25 people each year in England and Wales and 75% of these deaths occur in adults.[101]
- Pneumonia can occur in up to 10% of pregnant women with chickenpox; the severity of this complication seems increased in later gestation.[102]

Key reminders
- Very common, particularly in children
- Usually mild
- Complications are rare
- More serious disease with problems more likely in adults and the immunocompromised.

SHINGLES

Following chickenpox infection, the virus can lay dormant in the nervous tissue for several years but may reappear at any time following reactivation of the virus, presenting as shingles (*Herpes zoster*). It is not known what causes the virus to reactivate, but it is thought to be associated with conditions that depress the immune system such as old age, immunosuppressive therapy or HIV infection.[103] About 250 000 people in the UK get shingles every year, with prevalence increasing among the elderly, statistics indicating that approximately 10%–20% of the British population will experience shingles at some point in their lifetime.[103]

Clues to aid the diagnosis
Before the appearance of the rash there may be a sensation of pain or discomfort along the affected nerve, with possible numbness or itching. This may be present for 1–2 days before the appearance of skin lesions but in some cases may be evident for up to 3 weeks.[104] There may be mild fever and headaches, but this initial phase is then followed by development of the characteristic skin lesions, which are painful and typically follow a dermatomal distribution.

⚠ BEWARE!

- Shingles affecting the trigeminal (fifth cranial) nerve has potentially devastating consequences, putting the person at risk of ophthalmic complications including lid ulceration, conjunctivitis, keratitis, uveitis, optic neuritis, secondary glaucoma, and, in severe cases, blindness.[105]
- When the facial and auditory nerves are affected the patient may develop Ramsay Hunt syndrome, which may cause deafness, vertigo and facial palsy with symptoms mimicking those of Bell's palsy.[106]

Pathophysiology

The reactivated virus causes inflammation in the dorsal root ganglion, but the virus can potentially spread to any area of the nervous system. If this occurs other symptoms can develop and will be influenced by the portion of the nerve that is affected.

Differential diagnosis

- Impetigo (*see* pp. 167–9).
- Coxsackie virus, which is a viral infection, more common in children but can occur at any age.
- *Herpes simplex* (viral infection).
- *Eczema herpeticum*, which is a viral infection characterised by clusters of itchy blisters, and can occur as a complication of eczema.
- Pleurisy.
- Pathology in the underlying bone, muscles or the vertebra, which may be caused by a malignancy, infection, inflammation or possible trauma.

Treatment

For those who are normally healthy and at low risk of complications pain relief may be all that is required. Table 10.15 shows suggested treatment for pain relief and additional treatment for those at risk of complications.

TABLE 10.15 Treatment options

Treatment	Drug and dose	Additional information
Pain relief	Co-codamol: 8/500 mg 30/500 mg Dihydrocodeine 30 mg	Simple analgesia (paracetamol, codeine) should be tried before progressing to stronger alternatives such as tramadol, oxycodone or morphine.[107]
Antiviral treatment	Acyclovir 800 mg	*See* p. 190. Effectively suppresses viral replication and has been shown to have a beneficial effect on both acute and chronic pain.[108] *See* prescribing tips below.

Prescribing tips

- It is recommended that acyclovir is prescribed for those aged 60 or older presenting within 72 hours of appearance of rash.
- Acyclovir should also be considered for patients below this age experiencing severe pain within 72 hours of onset of the rash.
- Patients of any age with ophthalmic involvement presenting within the first 72 hours of onset of the rash and those with active zoster affecting the cervical, lumbar and sacral dermatomes should also be offered acyclovir.[109]

Complications

The development of complications and the symptoms experienced depends on the severity of the disease and the site of the dermatome affected.

- Postherpetic neuralgia (PHN) is a frequent complication of *Herpes zoster*, with the risk of developing this increasing in older age.[110]
- Bacterial skin infections can develop at the affected site.

CLINICAL ALERT!

Antiviral agents have been shown to decrease the duration of *Herpes zoster* rash and the severity of pain associated with the rash.[111]

TABLE 10.16 Treatment of postherpetic neuralgia

Drug	Additional information
Simple analgesia, e.g. paracetamol or co-codamol.	May not provide sufficient pain relief.
Gabapentin started at 300 mg at night and increased if needed. Lower starting dose of 100 mg recommended for the elderly because of the greater risk of adverse effects.	Studies have shown gabapentin improves sleep and reduces pain.[112]
Pregabalin usually started at 75 mg 12 hourly, increased up to 300 mg twice daily if needed.	Similar benefits to gabapentin.
Capsaicin cream.	Can be applied to area up to four times daily but must not be used on broken or irritated skin and effect may not be evident for up to 4 weeks.
Amitriptyline or nortriptyline may be started as 25 mg at night (10 mg for frail elderly patients, with weekly increments to a maximum of 75 mg, although side-effects (drowsiness, unsteadiness) may reduce compliance.[107]	Both are unlicensed for use in postherpetic neuralgia but both have been found to be effective in relieving pain. My take up to 3 weeks to start to relieve symptoms.
Tramadol.	Compared with placebo tramadol may be more effective at reducing pain after 6 weeks in people with postherpetic neuralgia but evidence is limited.[113]

Drug	Additional information
Oxycodone or morphine.	Oxycodone and morphine are effective at reducing pain associated with postherpetic neuralgia, although oxycodone has been linked to increased adverse effects such as constipation, nausea and sedation,[114] which may affect compliance.

In severe pain a combination of drugs may be needed to achieve adequate pain relief.
A combination of morphine and gabapentin, or oxycontin and gabapentin, has demonstrated better pain relief than single agents.[115]

CLINICAL ALERT!

⚠ BEWARE!

- In the elderly and immunocompromised, encephalitis can develop, which is potentially life threatening.
- Ophthalmic *Herpes zoster* is a severe complication that is difficult to manage, and even after aggressive management, patients may have long-term sequelae, including vision loss and pain related to the location of the rash.[116]

Key reminders
- Caused by reactivation of the *Herpes zoster* virus
- Increased prevalence among the elderly
- Early symptom is pain before the appearance of the rash
- Postherpetic neuralgia is the most common after-effect.

REFERENCES

1. Schofield JK, Grindlay D, Williams HC. *Skin Conditions in the UK: a health needs assessment.* University of Nottingham; 2009. Available at: www.nottingham.ac.uk/research/groups/cebd/documents/hcnaskinconditionsuk2009.pdf (accessed 24 July 2013).
2. McCarthy JS, Kemp DJ, Walton SF, *et al.* Scabies: more than just an irritation. *Post Grad Med J.* 2004; **80**(945): 382–7.
3. Currie BJ, McCarthy JS. Permethrin and ivermectin for scabies. *N Engl J Med.* 2010; **362**(8): 717–25.
4. Centres for Disease Control and Prevention. *Parasites: scabies.* Available at: www.cdc.gov/parasites/scabies/ (accessed 24 June 2012).
5. Sugimoto T, Kashiwagi A. A case of scabies masquerading as drug eruption. *Eur J Intern Med.* 2007; **18**: 445–6.
6. Karthikeyan K. Treatment of scabies: newer perspectives. *Postgrad Med J.* 2005; **81**: 7–11.
7. Idriss S, Levitt J. Malathion for head lice and scabies: treatment and safety considerations. *J Drugs Dermatol.* 2009; **8**(8): 715–20.
8. American College of Dermatologists. *A–Z of Skin: scabies.* Available at: www.dermcoll.asn.au/public/a-z_of_skin-scabies.asp (accessed 12 July 2013).

9. British National Formulary. 2013. Available at: www.bnf.org/bnf/index.htm

10. Electronic Medicines Compendium. *Eurax Cream.* Available at: www.medicines.org.uk/emc/medicine/13272/spc (accessed 19 July 2013).

11. McCroskey AL. *Scabies in Emergency Medicine.* Available at: http://emedicine.medscape.com/article/785873-overview#a0199 (accessed 26 June 2012).

12. George A, Rubin G. A systematic review and meta-analysis of treatments for impetigo. *Br J Gen Pract.* 2003; **53**: 480–7.

13. Cole C, Gazewood J. Diagnosis and treatment of impetigo. *Am Fam Physician.* 2007; **75**(6): 859–64.

14. Health Protection Agency. *Impetigo.* Available at: www.hpa.org.uk/web/HPAweb&HPAwebStandard/Page/1230626089375 (accessed 20 May 2013).

15. Nichols RL, Florman S. Clinical presentations of soft-tissue infections and surgical site infections. *Clin Infect Dis.* 2001; **33**(Suppl. 2): S84–93.

16. Koning S, van Suijlekom-Smit LWA, *et al.* Fusidic acid cream in the treatment of impetigo in general practice: double blind randomised placebo controlled trial. *BMJ.* 2002; **324**: 203.

17. Medical Disability Guidelines. *Impetigo Complications.* Available at: www.mdguidelines.com/impetigo/complications (accessed 12 June 2013).

18. Noble SL, Forbes RC, Stamm PL. Diagnosis and management of common tinea infections. *Am Fam Physician.* 1998; **58**(1): 163–74.

19. Andrews MD, Burns M. Common tinea infections in children. *Am Fam Physician.* 2008; **77**(10): 1415–20.

20. Miller AC. *Tinea in Emergency Medicine.* Available at: http://emedicine.medscape.com/article/787217-overview (accessed 25 May 2013).

21. Graham Brown R, Burns T. *Dermatology.* 7th ed. London: Blackwell Science; 2002.

22. Hainer BL. Dermatophyte infections. *Am Fam Physician.* 2003; **67**(1): 101–9.

23. Wiederkehr M. *Tinea Cruris.* Available at: http://emedicine.medscape.com/article/1091806-overview#a0104 (accessed 29 July 2013).

24. Al Hasan M, Fitzgerald SM, Saoudian M, *et al.* Dermatology for the practicing allergist: tinea pedis and its complications. *Clin Mol Allergy.* 2004; **2**: 5.

25. Sokumbi O, Wetter DA. Clinical features, diagnosis, and treatment of erythema multiforme: a review for the practicing dermatologist. *Int J Dermatol.* 2012; **51**(8): 889–902.

26. The Merck Manual Home Health Handbook. *Ringworm: tinea.* Available at: www.merckmanuals.com/home/skin_disorders/fungal_skin_infections/ringworm_tinea.html (accessed 29 July 2013).

27. Electronic Medicines Companion. *Lamisil Tablets.* Available at: www.medicines.org.uk/emc/medicine/1290 (accessed 20 August 2013).

28. Higgins EM, Fuller LC, Smith CH. Guidelines for the management of tinea capitas. *Brit J Dermatol.* 200; **143**: 53–8.

29. Rodgers P, Bassler M. Treating onychomycosis. *Am Fam Physician.* 2001; **63**(4): 663–73.

30. Szepietowski JC. Tinea barbae. Available at: http://emedicine.medscape.com/article/1091252-treatment (accessed 5 August 2013).

31. Mayo Foundation for Medical Education and Research (MFMER). *Ringworm (Body): complications.* Available at: www.mayoclinic.com/health/ringworm/DS00489/DSECTION=complications (accessed 13 February 2014).

32. Purdy, S. *Atopic Eczema in Children: guidelines in practice.* Available at: www.eguidelines.co.uk/eguidelinesmain/gip/vol_11/feb_08/purdy_eczema_feb08.php#refs (accessed 26 June 2012).

33. Green C, Colquitt JL, Kirby J, *et al. Clinical and Cost-effectiveness of Once-daily Versus More*

Frequent Use of Same Potency Topical Corticosteroids for Atopic Eczema: a systematic review and economic evaluation. Available at: www.hta.ac.uk/execsumm/summ847.shtml

34. National Institute for Health and Clinical Excellence. *Atopic Eczema in Children: management of atopic eczema in children from birth up to the age of 12 years. NICE guideline 57.* London: NICE; 2007. Available at: www.nice.org.uk/cg057

35. Akdis CA, Akdis M, Bieber T, *et al.* Diagnosis and treatment of atopic dermatitis in children and adults: European Academy of Allergy and Clinical Immunology/American Academy of Allergy, Asthma and Immunology: Consensus Report. *Allergy.* 2006; **61**(8): 969–87.

36. National Eczema Society. *Emollients Factsheet.* Available at: www.eczema.org/emollients (accessed 23 July 2012).

37. Scottish Intercollegiate Guidelines Network. *Management of Atopic Eczema in Primary Care. SIGN guideline 125.* Edinburgh: SIGN; 2011. www.sign.ac.uk/pdf/sign125.pdf

38. Schwartz RA. *Paediatric Atopic Dermatitis: treatment and management.* Available at: http://emedicine.medscape.com/article/911574-treatment (accessed 30 September 2012).

39. National Institute for Health and Clinical Excellence. Tacrolimus and pimecrolimus for atopic eczema. *NICE guideline 82.* London: NICE; 2004. www.nice.org.uk/nicemedia/live/11538/32902/32902.pdf

40. British Association of Dermatologists. *Eczema: patient information leaflet.* Available at: www.bad.org.uk/site/796/default.aspx (accessed 26 April 2013).

41. Pavlovsky M, Baum S, Shpiro D, *et al.* Narrow band UVB: is it effective and safe for paediatric psoriasis and atopic dermatitis? *J Eur Acad Dermatol Venereol.* 2011; **25**: 727–9.

42. Liaw FY, Huang CF, Hsueh JT. Eczema herpeticum. *Can Fam Physician.* 2012; **58**(12): 1358–61.

43. Mayo Foundation for Medical Education and Research (MFMER). *Atopic Dermatitis (Eczema): complications.* Available at: www.mayoclinic.org/diseases-conditions/eczema/basics/complications/con-20032073 (accessed 7 May 2013).

44. Icen M, Crowson CS, McEvoy MT, *et al.* Trends in incidence of adult-onset psoriasis over three decades: a population based study. *J Am Acad Dermatol.* 2009; **60**(3): 394–401.

45. Naldi L. Epidemiology of psoriasis. *Curr Drug Targets Inflamm Allergy.* 2004; **3**(2): 121–8.

46. Elder JT, Nair RP, Guo SW, *et al.* The genetics of psoriasis. *Arch Dermatol.* 1994; **130**: 216–24.

47. Brandrup F, Holm N, Grunnet N, *et al.* Psoriasis in monozygotic twins: variations in expression in individuals with identical genetic constitution. *Acta Derm Venereol.* 1982; **62**: 229–36.

48. Luba KM, Stulberg DL. Chronic plaque psoriasis. *Am Fam Physician.* 2006; **73**(4): 636–44.

49. The Psoriasis Association. *Guttate Psoriasis.* Available at: www.psoriasis-association.org.uk/pages/view/about-psoriasis/types-of-psoriasis/guttate (accessed 25 April 2013).

50. Fry L, Baker BS. Triggering psoriasis: the role of infections and medications. *Clin Dermatol.* 2007; **25**(6): 606–15.

51. Kangesan B. Psoriasis. *InnovAiT.* 2013; **6**(7): 437–41.

52. Camisa C. *Psoriasis.* Available at: www.clevelandclinicmeded.com/medicalpubs/disease management/dermatology/psoriasis-papulosquamous-skin-disease/#cesec3 (accessed 25 July 2012).

53. Fortune DG, Richards HL, Main CJ, Griffiths CE. What patients with psoriasis believe about their condition. *J Am Acad Dermatol.* 1998; **39**: 196–20.

54. British Association of Dermatologists. *Discoid Lupus Erythematosus.* Available at: www.bad.org.uk/site/812/default.aspx (accessed 14 July 2013).

55. Scottish Intercollegiate Guidelines Network. *Diagnosis and Management of Psoriasis and Psoriatic Arthritis in Adults. SIGN guideline 121.* Edinburgh: SIGN; 2010. Available at: www.sign.ac.uk/guidelines/fulltext/121/contents.html

55. Tettey S, Sahota A. *Clinical Review of Managing Psoriasis in Primary Care*. Available at: www. gponline.com/Clinical/article/1128473/Clinical-review-managing-psoriasis-primary-care (accessed 17 June 2013).

56. Al Hamadi A. *Psoriatic Arthritis*. Available at: http://emedicine.medscape.com/article/ 331037-overview (accessed 21 June 2012).

57. Ole Ahlehoff O, Gunnar H, Gislason CH, *et al*. Psoriasis and risk of atrial fibrillation and ischaemic stroke: a Danish nationwide cohort study. *Eur Heart J*. 2012; **33**(16): 2054–64.

58. Cox NH, Colver GB, Paterson WD. Management and morbidity of cellulitis of the leg. *J Royal Soc Med*. 1998; **91**(12): 634–7.

59. Clinical Resource Efficiency Support Team. *CREST Management of Cellulitis in Adults*. 2005. Available at: www.acutemed.co.uk/docs/Cellulitis%20guidelines,%20CREST,%2005. pdf (accessed 25 June 2012).

60. Lazzarini L, Conti E, Tossiti G, *et al*. Erysipelas and cellulitis: clinical and microbiological spectrum in an Italian tertiary care hospital. *J Inf*. 2005; **51**(5): 383–9.

61. Dupuy A, Benchikhi H, Roujeau JC, *et al*. Risk factors for erysipelas of the leg (cellulitis): case control study. *BMJ*. 318(7198): 1591–4.

62. Gabillot-Carré M, Roujeau JC. Acute bacterial skin infections and cellulitis. *Curr Opin Infect Dis*. 2007; **20**(2): 118–23.

63. Björnsdóttir S, Gottfredsson M, Thórisdóttir AS, *et al*. Risk factors for acute cellulitis of the lower limb: a prospective case-control study. *Clin Infect Dis*. 2005; **41**(10): 1416–22.

64. Herschline T. *Cellulitis Treatment and Management*. Available at: http://emedicine. medscape.com/article/214222-treatment (accessed 12 July 2012).

65. Powell J. *Clinical Review: cellulitis and erysipelas*. Available at: www.gponline.com/Clinical/ article/1106149/Clinical-Review---Cellulitis-erysipelas (accessed 17 July 2013).

66. Al-Niaimi F, Cox N. Cellulitis and lymphoedema: a vicious cycle. *J of Lymphoedema*. 2009. Available at: www.lymphormation.org/journal/content/0402_cycle.pdf (accessed 20 December 2012).

67. Eagle M. *Understanding Cellulitis of the Lower Limb*. Available at: www.woundsinternational. com/pdf/content_183.pdf (accessed 21 January 2014).

68. Schwarz RA. *Dermatologic Manifestations of Necrotising Fasciitis*. Available at: http:// emedicine.medscape.com/article/1054438-overview (accessed 1 July 2012).

69. Ghodsi SZ, Orawa H, Zouboulis CC. Prevalence, severity and severity risk factors of acne in high school pupils: a community-based study. *J Invest Dermatol*. 2009; **129**: 2136–41.

70. Goulden V, Stables GI, Cunliffe WJ. Prevalence of facial acne in adults. *J Am Acad Dermatol*. 1999; **41**(4): 577–80.

71. Purdy S, De Berker D. Acne. *BMJ*. 2006; **333**(7575): 949–53.

72. Stathakis V, Kilkenny M, Marks R. Descriptive epidemiology of acne vulgaris in the community. *Australas J Dermatol*. 1997; **38**(3): 115–23.

73. Webster GF. The pathophysiology of acne. *Cutis*. 2005; **76**(2 Suppl.): S4–7.

74. Courtenay LI. A practical approach to the treatment of acne vulgaris. *Nursing Standard*. 2011; **25**(19): 55–64.

75. Eichenfield LF, Leyden JJ. Acne: current concepts of pathogenesis and approach to rational treatment. *Paediatrician*. 1991; **18**: 218–23.

76. Stuhlberg DL, Penrod MA, Blatny RA. Common bacterial skin infections. *Am Fam Physician*. 2002; **66**(1): 119–25.

77. Collier CN, Harper JC, Cantrell WC, *et al*. The prevalence of acne in adults 20 years and older. *J Am Acad Dermatol*. 2008; **58**(1): 56–9.

78. Zaenglein AL, Thiboutot DM. Expert committee recommendations for acne management. *Paediatrics*. 2006; **118**: 1188–99.

79. Jaworsky C, Gilliam AC. Immunopathology of the human hair follicle. *Dermatol Clin*. 1999; **17**: 561–8.

80. Cuevas T. Identifying and treating rosacea. *Nurse Pract*. 2001; **26**: 13–15, 19–23.

81. Barankin B, Guenther L. Rosacea and atopic dermatitis. Two common oculocutaneous disorders. *Can Fam Physician*. 2002; **48**: 721–4.

82. Mendiratta V, Harjai B, Koranne RV. Successful management of acne fulminans with combination of minocycline and dapsone. *Indian J Dermatol*. 2006; **51**: 128–30.

83. Ravenscroft J. Evidence based update on the management of acne. *Arch Dis Child Educ Pract Ed*. 2005; **90**: ep98–101.

84. Dreno B. Topical antibacterial therapy for acne vulgaris. *Drugs*. 2004; **64**(21): 2389–97.

85. Shalita AR, Smith EB, Bauer E. Topical erythromycin v clindamycin therapy for acne. A multicenter, double-blind comparison. *Arch Dermatol*. 1984; **120**: 351–5.

86. Schindler AE. Non-contraceptive use of hormonal contraceptives for women with various medical problems. *J Paediat Obstet Gynecol*. 2008; **34**: 183–200.

87. Sagransky M, Yentzer BA, Feldman SR. Benzoyl peroxide: a review of its current use in the treatment of acne vulgaris. *Expert Opin Pharmacother*. 2009; **10**(15): 2555–62.

88. Phillips TJ. An update on the safety and efficacy of topical retinoids. *Cutis*. 2005; **75**(2 Suppl.): 14–22.

89. Johnson BA, Nunley JR. Use of systemic agents in the treatment of acne vulgaris. *Am Fam Physician*. 2000; **62**(8): 1823–30.

90. Layton AM, Henderson CA, Cunliffe WJ. A clinical evaluation of acne scarring and its incidence. *Clin Experimental Dermatol*. 1994; **19**(4): 303–8.

91. Health Protection Agency (HPA). *Chicken pox*. Available at: www.hpa.org.uk/Topics/InfectiousDiseases/InfectionsAZ/ChickenpoxVaricellaZoster/GeneralInformation/ (accessed 24 January 2014).

92. Papadopoulios AJ. *Chicken pox*. Available at: http://emedicine.medscape.com/article/1131785-overview (accessed 14 July 2012).

93. Royal College of Obstetricians and Gynaecologists. *Chicken Pox in Pregnancy: what you need to know*. Available at: www.rcog.org.uk/files/rcog-corp/Chickenpox%20in%20Pregnancy.pdf (accessed 8 July 2012).

94. Centres for Disease Control and Prevention. *Chicken Pox (Varicella): people at high risk for complications*. Available at: www.cdc.gov/chickenpox/hcp/high-risk.html (accessed 8 June 2013).

95. Oakley A. *Erythema Multiforme*. Available at: www.dermnetnz.org/reactions/erythema-multiforme.html (accessed 25 February 2013).

96. Tunbridge AJ, Breuer J, Jeffery KLM. Chickenpox in adults: clinical management. *J of Infection*. 2008; **57**: 95–102.

97. Hassan Abro A, Ustadi AM, Das K, *et al*. Chickenpox: presentation and complications in adults. *J Pak Med Ass*. 2009; **59**(12): 828–31.

98. Miller E, Marshall R, Vurdien J. Epidemiology, outcome and control of varicella-zoster infection. *Rev Med Microbiology*. 1993; **4**: 222–30.

99. Ho BCH, Tai DYH. Severe adult chickenpox requiring intensive care. *An Acad Med*. 2004; **33**: 84–8.

100. Katsimpardi K, Papadakis V, Pangalis A, *et al*. Infections in a paediatric patient cohort with acute lymphoblastic leukemia during the entire course of treatment. *Support Care Cancer*. 2006; **14**(3): 277–84.

101. Rawson H, Crampin A, Noah N. Deaths from chickenpox in England and Wales. 1995–7: analysis of routine mortality data. *BMJ*. 2001; **323**: 1091–3.

102. Tan MP, Koren G. Chickenpox in pregnancy: revisited. *Reprod Toxicol*. 2005; **21**: 410–20.

103. National Shingles Foundation. *The VZV Initiative: combating the Varicella-Zoster virus in the United Kingdom.* Available at: www.vzvfoundation.org/UK.html (accessed 15 July 2012).

104. Stankus SJ, Dlugopolski M, Packer D. Management of Herpes Zoster (shingles) and post-herpetic neuralgia. *Am Fam Physician.* 2000; **61**(8): 2437–44.

105. Weaver BA. The burden of herpes zoster and postherpetic neuralgia in the United States. *J Am Osteopath Assoc.* 2007; **107**(Suppl. 1) S2–7.

106. Kumar P, Clark ML. *Clinical Medicine.* 8th ed. London: Elsevier; 2009.

107. Duckworth J. *The Basics – shingles.* Available at: www.gponline.com/Clinical/article/1013802/the-basics-shingles (accessed 19 August 2013).

108. Thakur R, Philip AG. Treating herpes zoster and postherpetic neuralgia: an evidence-based approach. *J Fam Pract.* 2012; **61**(9 Suppl.): S9–15.

109. British Infection Society. *Guidelines for the Management of Shingles.* Available at: www.eguidelines.co.uk/eguidelinesmain/guidelines/summaries/infection/bis_shingles.php (accessed 14 July 2012).

110. Opstelton W, Mauritz JW, de Wit NJ, *et al.* Herpes zoster and postherpetic neuralgia: incidence and risk indicators using a general practice research database. *Fam Practice.* 2002; **19**(5): 471–5.

111. Schmader K. Management of herpes zoster in elderly patients. *Infect Dis Clin Pract.* 1995; **4**: 293–9.

112. Rowbotham M, Harden N, Stacey B, *et al.* Gabapentin for the treatment of postherpetic neuralgia: a randomized controlled trial. *JAMA.* 1998; **280**(21): 1837–42.

113. Wareham DW. *Post herpetic neuralgia.* Available at: www.ncbi.nlm.nih.gov/pmc/articles/PMC2943822/ (accessed 21 July 2012).

114. Watson CP, Babul N. Efficacy of oxycodone in neuropathic pain: a randomized trial in post-herpetic neuralgia. *Neurology.* 1998; **50**: 1837–41.

115. Gilron I, Bailey JM, Tu D, *et al.* Morphine, gabapentin or their combination for neuropathic pain. *NEJM.* 2005; **352**: 1324–34.

116. Weaver BA. Herpes zoster overview: natural history and incidence. *J Am Osteopath Assoc.* 2009; **109**(6 Suppl. 2): S2–6.

CHAPTER 11

Neurology

INTRODUCTION

Statistics suggest that approximately 10% of visits to accident and emergency departments are for a neurological problem and an estimated 17% of GP consultations each year are for neurological symptoms that result in an estimated 600 000 people being newly diagnosed with a neurological condition.[1]

CONDITIONS COVERED IN THE CHAPTER

Headaches:
- migraine (with or without aura)
- tension type headache
- chronic tension type headache
- cluster headache
- TIAs.

COMMON PRESENTING SYMPTOMS

- Pain
- Numbness
- Weakness of the limbs
- Muscle spasms
- Memory problems
- Cognitive dysfunction
- Poor attention span and difficulty concentrating.

TAKING THE NEUROLOGICAL HISTORY

Initial history as described in Chapter 3, followed by a focused enquiry relating to the neurological system.

Table 11.1 presents the symptoms enquiry and further questioning for specific symptoms.

TABLE 11.1 Symptoms enquiry and further questioning for specific symptoms

Symptom	Further questioning
Pain	Site of the pain if present? How long have they had pain? Further questions as per Chapter 3.
Numbness	What does patient mean by numbness? Do they mean loss of feeling/sensitivity? Again the OPQRST route may be helpful to determine aggravating or relieving factors, frequency of symptoms. Are there any additional symptoms?
Weakness of the limbs	What does the patient mean by 'weakness'? Not to be confused with generalised weakness, lack of energy. Is there a problem with a particular limb? Does the patient have a problem performing certain tasks, such as lifting objects? Are there any associated symptoms, tingling visual disturbance or numbness?
Muscle spasms	What does the patient mean by 'spasms'? Which muscles are affected? When does the problem occur?
Memory problems	May need support in obtaining a good history from a family member. Is the problem of recent onset or has the memory been worsening for some time? Can they remember recent events or more distant events? Are there any additional symptoms, such as poor concentration? Is the memory loss intermittent or there all the time? Any history of falls or head injury? Any additional symptoms such as mental confusion?
Cognitive dysfunction	Again input from a close family may be useful in assessing the symptoms. What has changed? Is their ability to carry out daily living activities affected?
Poor attention span and difficulty concentrating	The MMSE can be used to assess a number of different mental abilities, including: short- and long-term memory, attention span, concentration, language and communication skills, ability to plan, ability to understand instructions.[2]

Table 11.2 shows a summary of presenting signs and symptoms and the diseases they may suggest.

TABLE 11.2 Presenting signs and symptoms and diseases they may suggest

	Pain	Numbness	Weakness of the limbs	Visual disturbance	Memory problems	Cognitive dysfunction	Poor attention span/ difficulty concentration
Migraine (with or without aura)	Yes	No	No	Yes	No	No	No
Tension type headache	Yes	No	No	No	No	No	No
Chronic tension type headache	Yes	No	No	Yes	No	No	Possible
Cluster headache	Yes	No	No	May have redness of the eye, possible drooping of the eyelid	No	No	No
TIA	No	Yes	Yes	Yes	Yes	Yes	Yes

FURTHER INVESTIGATIONS

Investigations should be chosen on the basis of the history and symptoms, including the duration of symptoms and the overall clinical picture.

- Brain imaging
- CT scan
- MRI scan
- Carotid imaging.

URGENT REFERRAL TO A NEUROLOGIST REQUIRED

- Headaches presenting with vomiting or visual disturbance
- Headaches that have changed in frequency
- Headaches causing sleep disturbance
- New onset of headaches with a history of malignancy elsewhere in the body
- Headache with any additional neurological symptoms
- Memory loss, mental confusion or altered level of consciousness
- Recurrent TIAs.

HEADACHES

Headaches are a relatively common problem and can be potentially disabling, resulting in days lost from school or work. They are a frequent cause of GP consultations and neurological referrals and are estimated to account for around 4.4% of all GP appointments,[3] and 30% of neurology appointments.[4] There are now a number of recognised headache types, some more common than others, each with different signs and symptoms and different treatment options. Tension headaches are the most common headache type, affecting an estimated 3% of adults.[5]

Clues to aid the diagnosis

Table 11.3 shows the nature of symptoms for each headache type.

TABLE 11.3 Symptoms for headache types

Type	Signs and symptoms	Additional information
Migraine (with or without aura)	Patients often describe recurrent episodes which vary in duration but can persist for up to 3 days. In younger children the pain usually affects the front or both sides of the head, while in adolescents and adults the pain usually affects one side of the head only.[6]	Often associated with nausea and vomiting and patients may get some relief from lying in a darkened room. Patients who have migraine with aura may complain of visual disturbance before pain becomes a problem.

Type	Signs and symptoms	Additional information
Tension headache	Headache is often generalised and occurs in an episodic fashion with often short-lived symptoms.	May be described by the patient as feeling like a tight feeling or band around the head. Can be related to stress.
Chronic tension-type headache	Similar symptoms to tension-type headache.	Characterised by frequent episodes which can be daily in some cases. Potentially disabling.
Cluster headache	Characterised by a daily headache, which often occurs at night, waking the patient from sleep. There is intense severe pain usually centred in or around one eye, although pain may spread to a wider area.[7]	Cluster headaches are more common in men often in their twenties or older (very rarely children) and are more common in smokers.[8] The name is derived from the fact that cluster headaches typically occur in bouts which can last for several weeks, and may recur on a yearly or 2-yearly basis, often following a pattern where they occur at around the same time of the year.

Pathophysiology

The pathophysiology of migraine, cluster and tension-type headaches is not well understood, although migraine and cluster headaches are believed to initially begin in the brain as a neurologic dysfunction, with subsequent involvement of the trigeminal nerve and cranial vessels.[9]

Cluster headaches

In cluster headaches both extracranial and temporal artery blood flow are increased, but this only occurs after the onset of pain and it is also thought that histamine may play a part as increased numbers of mast cells have been detected at painful sites in some patients,[10] but this has not been found consistently.

Tension-type headache

Tension-type headache can be primarily a central neurologic disturbance similar to migraine or can occur as the result of increased cervical and pericranial muscle activity, which may be caused by flexion-extension injury of the neck, poor posture, or anxiety with increased clenching or grinding of the teeth.[9]

Migraine

There have been a number of theories suggested to explain the pathophysiology of migraine-type headaches. The first is a vascular theory, which suggests that extracranial blood vessels become distended and develop a pulsing action during a migraine attack, and in a person who is awake, stimulation of intracranial blood vessels induces the headache.[11] However, this theory has not been shown to explain the fact that some treatments effective in treating migraine do not have any effect on blood vessels. The second theory suggests that a migraine is initiated in response to a complex series of neural and vascular events and changes in cerebral perfusion.[12]

Diagnosis

Diagnosis of headache type can usually be made from the history and the pattern of symptoms.

 CLINICAL ALERT!

 BEWARE OF!

Warning signs of other pathology include:
- progressively worsening headaches over months
- change in headache type/symptoms
- headache of new onset after the age of 50 years
- presence of neurological symptoms such as visual disturbances or vomiting
- additional symptoms, such as weight loss or fever, which may indicate an alternative cause.

Differential diagnosis

⚠ **BEWARE!**

As well as the possibility that the headache may be a result of one of the other types of headache discussed, there a number of other causes where there is potentially an underlying problem causing the symptoms. *See* Table 11.4.

TABLE 11.4 Secondary causes

Common secondary causes	Additional information	Additional information
Otitis media	*See* pp. 132–4.	*See* pp. 132–4.
Acute sinusitis	*See* p. 141.	*See* p. 141.
Dental problems (dental caries or dental abscess)	Characterised by toothache, pain on eating and drinking and the breath may have an unpleasant smell.	May present with sudden onset of severe headache, or may have a mild headache prior to the onset of a more severe one.
Medication overuse	Poorly understood but is associated with frequent intake of analgesics.	Often at its worst on waking in the morning, and pain increases after physical exertion and can be characterised by a headache that persists all day, fluctuating with medication use, which patient is repeatedly taking every few hours.[8]
Menstrual headache	Occurs monthly in association with the onset of menstruation.	Early signs and symptoms are non-specific but later the patient may complain of variable symptoms such as early morning headaches, dizziness, nausea and vomiting.

Common secondary causes	Additional information	Additional information
Stroke	Accompanied by speech problems, drooping of the face, unilateral paralysis of limbs.	The nature of the headache varies according to the type of stroke. When the cause is ischaemic there is sudden onset of severe headache, which may worsen with physical activity, coughing or straining, while with an ischaemic stroke pain occurs at the site where blood flow is blocked and is often felt in the eyes or on the side of the head.[13]
Pre-eclampsia	Occurs after the twentieth week of pregnancy.	Blood pressure elevated, with protein in the urine.

Table 11.5 shows rarer underlying causes of headache.

TABLE 11.5 Rarer underlying causes of headache

Rare secondary causes	Additional information
Brain tumour	Severe headache associated with vomiting, and may be worse first thing in the morning and made worse by activities such as bending, coughing and sneezing, exercising or even shouting.[14]
Meningitis	Severe headache accompanied by rash, stiff neck, fever and photophobia.
Brain abscess	Commonest symptoms are headache, changes in mental state, may indicate cerebral oedema, fever, seizures and nausea and vomiting.[15]
Carbon monoxide poisoning	Arises as a result of faulty gas appliances. Headache may be accompanied by other symptoms of nausea, poor concentration and poor memory.
Trigeminal neuralgia	Characterised by bouts of sudden, severe, episodic pain typically felt on one side of the jaw or cheek that generally last several seconds and may repeat in quick succession, coming and going throughout the day with episodes lasting for days, weeks or months at a time and then disappearing for months or years.[16]
Acute glaucoma	Acute attacks are characterised by pain, redness in the eye, blurred vision and haloes around lights.

Treatment

Treatment will depend on the type of headache the person is suffering from. In some cases patients may be able to reduce the frequency of attacks where they are able to recognise specific trigger factors. Palliative measures such as sleep and ice packs to the forehead may be useful for some patients.

Medication options are shown in Table 11.6.

TABLE 11.6 Medication options (migraine with or without aura)

Drug treatment

Aspirin 900 mg or ibuprofen is recommended for acute treatment in patients with all severities of migraine (avoid in patients with asthma) or paracetamol 1000 mg for acute treatment of mild to moderate migraine attacks.[17]

Triptans (e.g. sumatriptan) have been found to achieve significant pain relief for patients suffering from acute migraine within 2 hours of administration.[18]

Preventative treatment

Patients suffering regular migraine headaches may require medication aimed at preventing attacks. Beta-blockers such as propranolol and metoprolol are effective for migraine prevention.[19]

Children

As for adults: simple analgesia is first line.

Addition of an anti-emetic such as domperidone or metoclopramide may be helpful in reducing nausea.

Prescribing tips

ADULTS

- Addition of anti-emetic may help to relieve nausea and vomiting if this is a problem.
- If a triptan is prescribed, a return of symptoms occurs in up to 50% of patients within 48 hours,[8] which may make them a reluctant option for some patients.

CHILDREN AND ADOLESCENTS

- Use of anti-emetics, while helpful in treating nausea, has not been shown to have any efficacy in reducing the frequency of attacks.[20]
- In adolescents whose symptoms are not controlled with analgesia, sumatriptan nasal spray (10 mg) may be beneficial for use in those aged 12–17 years.[21]
- Other possible options available for prophylaxis include amitriptyline, and pizotifen and gabapentin, but none of these is currently licensed for use in migraine prevention.[22]

TABLE 11.7 Treatment of other headache types

Headache type	Drug	Additional information
Tension type	Antidepressants (amitriptyline at a dose of 25–150 mg daily) has shown benefits.	Amitriptyline in combination with stress management has been shown to provide more benefit than monotherapy for management of chronic tension type headache.[23]
Cluster headache	Both zolmitriptan and sumatriptan are effective in the acute treatment of cluster headaches. Sumatriptan 6 mg is first-line choice with nasal sumatriptan or nasal zolmitriptan second line.[17]	Sumatriptan is available in oral, subcutaneous or intranasal forms. Zolmitriptan is available as an oral or intranasal product.
	Preventative treatment: verapamil 240–960 mg daily.	During two weeks of treatment, 80% of patients receiving verapamil had a greater than 50% reduction in headache frequency, with a substantial number having a vast improvement in symptoms within the first week of treatment.[24]

CLINICAL ALERT!

 BEWARE OF!

Medication-overuse headache can occur in any patient with frequent use of any symptomatic treatment for headache, with symptoms resembling those of chronic tension-type headache or migraine. Symptoms resolve when the causative medication is stopped; however, the original symptoms for which the medication was originally prescribed may recur.

Non-pharmacological treatment options

Some patients may prefer to explore other treatment options rather than take medication. Table 11.8 shows some of the options and their benefits.

TABLE 11.8 Non-pharmacological treatment options

Treatment	Aims of treatment	Additional information
Acupuncture	Acupuncture is a treatment where needles are inserted into the skin at defined points.	A Cochrane review reported that there is now consistent evidence to suggest that acupuncture provides additional benefit to treatment of acute migraine attacks and available studies suggest that acupuncture is at least as effective as, or possibly more effective than, prophylactic drug treatment, and has fewer adverse effects.[25]

(continued)

Treatment	Aims of treatment	Additional information
Stress management	Although studies have identified a number of potential trigger factors to the onset of migraine such as certain foods, one of the most common triggers reported by individuals with migraine is stress,[26] therefore the purpose of teaching patients to cope with stress more effectively is to ultimately alleviate its influence as a trigger factor.	Stress management techniques have been found to achieve improvement in symptoms better than a placebo and comparable with some pharmacological treatments without the risk of the side-effects often associated with pharmacological therapy.[27]
CBT	CBT teaches patients how to recognise and cope with stressors in their life so that they understand how their symptoms may be affected by their behaviour patterns and thought processes.	Research indicates that CBT is most effective when combined with relaxation training or biofeedback.[28]
Hypnosis	Under hypnosis the person is induced into a trance during which the mind is open to suggestions that enable negative reactions to be removed and allowing positive ones to be prominent and enhanced.	Hypnosis has been shown to be cost-effective, virtually free of side-effects or risk of adverse reactions, and does not have the ongoing expense associated with regular medication.[29]
Biofeedback	This treatment teaches the patient to monitor and modify symptoms such as muscle tension.	Variable results with some studies suggesting beneficial effects, others less conclusive. Biofeedback has been reported as a costly and time-consuming treatment and one study reported that there was no additional benefit when compared to simple relaxation techniques alone.[30]
Relaxation therapy	Aims to teach relaxation techniques and breathing exercises.	Relaxation techniques and breathing exercises may be an option for some patients and can be practised at home.

Complications

 BEWARE!

- Frequent headaches are often accompanied by additional symptoms such as sleep disturbance, overuse of analgesia, anxiety, depression, and impaired physical, social and occupational functioning.[31]

Key messages
- Very common, tension type being the commonest
- Various types
- Can be debilitating, resulting in time off work or school
- Often occur in conjunction with other symptoms
- Important to exclude any possible underlying cause
- Numerous treatment options available.

TRANSIENT ISCHAEMIC ATTACK (TIA)

Approximately 150 000 patients per year in the UK suffer a TIA,[32] while in the US between 200 000 and 500 000 events are diagnosed each year.[33] TIAs are regarded as a serious warning sign of an impending stroke and the 90-day risk of stroke after a TIA has been reported as being as high as 17%, with the greatest risk apparent in the first week.[34]

Clues to aid the diagnosis

TIAs are characterised by several signs that may be variable from patient to patient. These are generally recognised as:
- sudden onset of unilateral numbness which may affect the face, arms or legs
- visual disturbance which may affect one or both eyes
- loss of balance and lack of coordination
- difficulty speaking
- mental confusion
- sudden onset of headache.

CLINICAL ALERT!

The difference between a TIA and an ischaemic stroke (the commonest type) is that following a TIA the symptoms disappear completely within 24 hours and in 75% of cases the symptoms clear within 1 hour, but often within a few minutes.[35] Following a stroke, however, the severity of the initial deficit is inversely proportional to the prognosis for recovery, with most of the spontaneous recovery occurring during the first 3–6 months after the event.[36]

Pathophysiology

A TIA occurs as a result of a temporary reduction or cessation of blood flow through the cerebral blood vessels. Small areas of infarction of the brain tissue follow the development of a thrombosis, or less commonly symptoms can arise as a result of a haemorrhage. Where an embolism or emboli are the cause the principal sources are thrombi and atheromatous plaques from within the great vessels, the carotid and vertebral systems or in the heart.[37] Cardiac causes are most commonly secondary to AF or LV disease, while small-vessel events are due to stenosis of one of the intracranial vessels, anterior from the middle cerebral artery or its branches, and posteriorly from the vertebro-basilar system, usually caused by atherosclerosis driven by risk factors such as hypertension and hypercholesterolaemia.[38]

Differential diagnosis

⚠ BEWARE!

Symptoms may be vague and history may have to be provided by someone who witnessed the episode. Common conditions that may mimic TIA include:
- hypo and hyperglycaemia
- space-occupying lesions
- seizures
- haemorrhagic stroke
- ischaemic stroke
- subarachnoid haemorrhage.

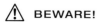

⚠ BEWARE!

- Symptoms of insidious onset are not indicative of TIA.
- Symptoms that are intermittent are less suggestive of TIA and may represent other diagnoses such as migraine, tumours or demyelination.[38]

TABLE 11.9 Risk factors for TIA

Risk factor	Additional information
Increasing age	Stroke risk is known to increase with increasing age and nearly three-quarters of all strokes occur in people over the age of 65.[39]
Smoking	Smoking is also associated with an approximate doubling of ischaemic stroke risk, and is also implicated in a two to fourfold increased risk for haemorrhagic stroke.[40] Furthermore, there is evidence that smokers who cease smoking will over time reduce the risk of both of these forms of stroke to never-smoking levels.[41]
Diabetes	Diabetes is an independent risk factor for stroke, increasing the overall risk by approximately 25%–50%.[42]
Hypertension	Hypertension is the most important modifiable risk factor for stroke and TIA.[43]
Obesity (high waist to hip ratio)	Obesity, particularly abdominal adiposity, is now regarded as having a significant association with risk of TIA and stroke, independent of other vascular risk factors.[44]
Hyperlipidaemia	A German study reported an increased risk for TIA in subjects with hyperlipidaemia.[45]
Excessive alcohol intake	Alcohol in excess of more than two drinks per day may increase stroke risk by as much as 50%.[46]

BEWARE!

Where a combination of risk factors are present, TIA risk is also increased with the presence of two or more risk factors increasing the risk twofold, while the presence of four or five risk factors increases TIA risk fivefold.[45]

Treatment

Prevention of further TIA episodes and stroke is at the forefront of treatment and management. The ABCD 2 calculator[47] is another tool useful for identifying those at high risk of stroke following a TIA. Points are awarded for each risk factor (age, diabetes, duration of symptoms and presence of symptoms of TIA) and those with a score of four or more are regarded as being at high risk of an early stroke.[48] However, concerns have been expressed that patients with a lower score may still be at risk of stroke as a result of cerebral ischaemia, or they may already have radiographic evidence of acute infarction.[49]

Royal College of Physicians guidance recommends that all patients with suspected TIA are referred for specialist assessment and investigation which should be within 24 hours for patients at high risk of subsequent stroke and within 1 week for patients at lower risk of subsequent stroke.[50]

Drug treatment

- Aspirin 300 mg should be commenced immediately.[51]
- NICE guidance suggests modified release dipyridamole in combination with aspirin to prevent ischaemic stroke.[51]

Prescribing tips

- Clopidogrel is an alternative to aspirin for patients not able to tolerate aspirin.
- Consider addition of PPI for gastro protection when commencing aspirin.

Further investigations

Brain imaging may be needed where the pathology underlying the patient's neurological symptoms is uncertain, and for patients suspected of intracerebral haemorrhage, such as those on anticoagulants or those with a long duration of symptoms.[50]

Complications

- Risk of stroke after experiencing a TIA is 4% at two days, 8% at 30 days, and 9% at 90 days; however, prospective day-to-day follow-up has shown the 7-day incidence of stroke to be as high as 11%.[52]
- There is a high incidence of CHD in patients having TIAs that indicate an increased likelihood of disability or death from cardiac disease in the future.[53]

Key messages

- Increased prevalence with increasing age
- Warning sign of impending stroke
- Treatment aimed at stroke prevention
- Potentially life threatening if stroke occurs.

REFERENCES

1. The Neurological Alliance. *Neuro Numbers: a brief review of the numbers of people in the UK with a neurological condition.* Available at: www.neural.org.uk/store/assets/files/20/original/NeuroNumbers.pdf (accessed 2 September 2013).
2. NHS Choices. *Dementia Diagnosis.* Available at: www.nhs.uk/Conditions/Dementia/Pages/Diagnosis.aspx (accessed 9 February 2013).
3. Latinovic R, Gulliford M, Ridsdale L. Headache and migraine in primary care: consultation, prescription, and referral rates in a large population. *J Neurol Neurosurg Psychiatry.* 2006; **77**(3): 385–7.
4. Larner AJ. Guidelines for primary headache disorders in primary care: an 'intervention' study. *Headache Care.* 2006; **3**(1): 1–2.
5. World Health Organization. *Headache Disorders. Fact sheet number 277.* Available at: www.who.int/mediacentre/factsheets/fs277/en/ (accessed 20 February 2013).
6. Cleveland Clinic Foundation. *Migraines in Children and Adolescents.* Available at: http://my.clevelandclinic.org/disorders/headaches/hic_migraines_in_children_and_adolescents.aspx (accessed 20 March 2013).
7. The Migraine Trust. *Cluster Headache.* Available at: www.migrainetrust.org/factsheet-cluster-headache-10908 (accessed 24 September 2013).
8. British Association for the Study of Headache. *Guidelines for All Healthcare Professionals in the Diagnosis and Management of Migraine, Tension-Type, Cluster and Medication-Overuse Headache.* 3rd ed. Available at: www.migraineclinic.org.uk/wp-content/uploads/2009/08/Bash-Guidelines.pdf (accessed 2 September 2013).
9. Kunkel RS. *Headache.* Available at: www.clevelandclinicmeded.com/medicalpubs/disease management/neurology/headache-syndromes/ (accessed 4 September 2013).
10. Blanda M. *Cluster Headaches.* Available at: http://emedicine.medscape.com/article/792150-overview#a0104 (accessed 3 October 2013).
11. Chawla J. *Migraine Headache.* Available at: http://emedicine.medscape.com/article/1142556-overview#a0104 (accessed 5 October 2013).
12. Cutrer FM, Charles A. The neurogenic basis of migraine. *Headache.* 2008; **4**(89): 1411–4.
13. National Institute of Neurological Disorders and Stroke. *Headache: hope through research.* Available at: www.ninds.nih.gov/disorders/headache/detail_headache.htm (accessed 24 September 2013).
14. Cancer Research UK. *Brain Tumours.* Available at: www.cancerresearchuk.org/cancer-help/type/brain-tumour/about/brain-tumour-symptoms#common (accessed 7 October 2013).
15. Levy RM. Brain abscess and subdural empyema. *Curr Opin Neurol.* 1994; **3**: 223–8.
16. National Institute of Neurological Disorders and Stroke. *Trigeminal Neuralgia Fact Sheet.* Available at: www.ninds.nih.gov/disorders/trigeminal_neuralgia/detail_trigeminal_neuralgia.htm#171433236 (accessed 24 October 2013).
17. Scottish Intercollegiate Guidelines Network. *Diagnosis and Management of Headache in Adults: a national clinical guideline. SIGN guideline 107.* Edinburgh: SIGN; 2008. Available at: www.sign.ac.uk/pdf/sign107.pdf

18. Loder E. Fixed drug combinations for the acute treatment of migraine: place in therapy. *Drugs*. 2005; **19**(9): 769–84.
19. Silberstein SD, Holland S, Freitag F, *et al*. Evidence based guideline update: pharmacologic treatment for episodic migraine prevention in adults. *Neurology*. 2012; **78**(17): 1337–45.
20. Victor S, Ryan SW. Drugs for preventing migraine headaches in children. *Cochrane Database Syst Rev*. 2003; **4**: CD002761.
21. Natarajan S, Jabbour JT, Webster CJ, *et al*. Long-term tolerability of sumatriptan nasal spray in adolescent patients with migraine. *Headache*. 2004; **44**(10): 969–77.
22. British National Formulary. 2013. Available at: www.bnf.org/bnf/index.htm
23. Holyroyd KA, O'Donnell FJ, Stensland M, *et al*. Management of chronic tension-type headache with tricyclic antidepressant medication, stress management therapy, and their combination: a randomized controlled trial. *JAMA*. 2001; **285**(17): 2208–15.
24. Ashkenazi A, Schwedt T. Cluster headache: acute and prophylactic therapy. *Headache*. 2011; **51**: 272–86.
25. Allais LK, Brinkhaus GB, Manheimer B, *et al*. Acupuncture for migraine prophylaxis. *Cochrane Database Syst Rev*. 2009, **1**: CD001218.
26. Hung CI, Liu CY, Wang SJ. Precipitating or aggravating factors for headache in patients with major depressive disorder. *J Psychosom Res*. 2008; **64**: 231–5.
27. Sauro KM, Becker WJ. The stress and migraine interaction. *Headache: the Journal of Head and Face Pain*. 2009; **49**(9): 1378–86.
28. University of Maryland Medical Centre. *Migraine Headaches: non-drug treatments and lifestyle changes*. Available at: www.umm.edu/patiented/articles/what_specific_drugs_used_prevent_migraines_000097_9.htm (accessed 30 September 2013).
29. Hammond DC. Review of the efficacy of clinical hypnosis with headaches and migraines. *Int J Clin Exp Hypn*. 2007; **55**(2): 207–19.
30. Mullally WJ, Hall K, Goldstein R. Efficacy of biofeedback in the treatment of migraine and tension type headaches. *Pain Physician*. 2009; **12**(6): 1005–11.
31. Farooq K, Williams P. Headache and chronic facial pain. *Contin Educ Anaesth Crit Care Pain*. 2008; **8**(4): 138–42.
32. Giles MF, Rothwell PM. Risk of stroke early after transient ischaemic attack: a systematic review and meta-analysis. *Lancet Neurol*. 2007; **6**(12): 1063–72.
33. Kleindorfer D, Panagos P, Pancioli A, *et al*. Incidence and short-term prognosis of transient ischaemic attack in a population-based study. *Stroke*. 2005; **36**(4): 720–3.
34. Rothwell PM, Warlow CP. Timing of TIAs preceding stroke: time window for prevention is very short. *Neurology*. 2005; **64**: 817–20.
35. Brain Foundation. *Stroke*. Available at: http://brainfoundation.org.au/a-z-of-disorders/107-stroke (accessed 9 October 2013).
36. Doblin BH. Rehabilitation after stroke. *New Eng J Med*. 2005; **352**(16): 1677–84.
37. Kumar P, Clark M. *Clinical Medicine*. 8th ed. London: Elsevier; 2009.
38. Qureshi S, Clarke A, Rudd A. *Clinical Review: transient ischaemic attack*. Available at: www.gponline.com/Clinical/article/1148540/Clinical-Review---Transient-ischaemic-attack/ (accessed 3 October 2013).
39. Internet Stroke Centre. *Stroke Statistics*. Available at: www.strokecenter.org/patients/about-stroke/stroke-statistics/ (accessed 15 October 2013).
40. Kurth T, Kase CS, Berger K, *et al*. Smoking and risk of haemorrhagic stroke in women. *Stroke*. 2003; **34**: 1375–81.
41. Paul SL, Thrift AG, Donnan GA. Smoking as a crucial independent determinant of stroke. *Tobacco Induced Diseases*. 2004; **2**(2): 67–80.

42. Burchfiel CM, Curb JD, Rodriguez BL, *et al*. Glucose intolerance and 22 year stroke risk. The Honolulu heart programme. *Stroke.* 1994; **25**: 951–97.

43. Zhang WW, Cadhilac DA, Donnan GA, *et al*. Hypertension and TIA. *Int J Stroke.* 2009; **4**(3): 206–14.

44. Winter Y, Rohrmann S, Linselsen J, *et al*. Contribution of obesity and abdominal fat mass to risk of stroke and transient ischaemic attacks. *Stroke.* 2008; **39**(12): 3145–51.

45. Weikert C, Berger K, Heidemann C, *et al*. Joint effects of risk factors for stroke and transient ischaemic attacks in a German population: the EPIC Potsdam study. *J Neurol.* 2007; **254**(3): 315–21.

46. National Stroke Association. *Alcohol Use*. Available at: www.stroke.org/site/PageServer? pagename=alcohol (accessed 9 October 2013).

47. Johnston SC, Rothwell PM, Huynh-Huynh MN, *et al*. Validation and refinement of scores to predict very early stroke risk after transient ischaemic attack. *Lancet.* 2007; **369**: 283–92.

48. Worster A. ACP Journal Club. Review: 3 prediction rules particularly ABCD, identify ED patients who can be discharged with low risk for stroke after TIA. *Ann Int Med.* 2009; **151**(6): JC3–15.

49. Cucchiara BL, Messe SR, Taylor RA, *et al*. Is the ABCD score useful for risk stratification of patients with acute transient ischaemic attack? *Stroke.* 2006; **37**(7): 1710–14.

50. Royal College of Physicians. *Diagnosis and Initial Management of Transient Ischaemic Attack.* Available at: www.rcplondon.ac.uk/sites/default/files/transient-ischemic-attack-concise-guideline.pdf (accessed 12 October 2013).

51. National Institute for Health and Clinical Excellence. *Clopidogrel and Modified Release Dipyridamole for the Prevention of Occlusive Vascular Events: review of NICE technology appraisal guidance 90. NICE technology appraisal guidance 210.* London: NICE; 2010. Available at: www.nice.org.uk/nicemedia/live/13285/52030/52030.pdf

52. Wu CM, McLaughlin K, Lorenzetti DL, *et al*. Early risk of stroke after transient ischaemic attack: a systematic review and meta-analysis. *Arch Intern Med.* 2007; **167**(22): 2417–22.

53. Adams RJ, Chimowitz MI, Alpert AS, *et al*. Coronary risk evaluation in patients with transient ischaemic attack and ischaemic stroke. *Circulation.* 2003; **108**: 1278–90.

CHAPTER 12

Musculoskeletal

INTRODUCTION

Musculoskeletal problems are reported to be common and are the most frequent cause of severe long-term pain and physical disability, affecting hundreds of millions of people around the world, significantly affecting the psychosocial status of affected people as well as their families and carers.[1] Although not usually life threatening, they are a cause of concern for their impact on a wide range of issues such as impaired quality of life for the sufferer, cost of care and cost to the economy. However, it is also likely that the true numbers of people affected may be inaccurate because many sufferers may choose to self-medicate and therefore do not seek medical advice or treatment from their GP.

CONDITIONS COVERED IN THE CHAPTER

- Gout
- Osteoarthritis
- Low back pain
- Polymyalgia rheumatica (PMR) and giant cell arteritis (GCA)
- Fibromyalgia.

COMMON PRESENTING SYMPTOMS

- Joint pains
- Swelling
- Stiffness
- Reduced function
- Nodules
- Inflammation.

TAKING THE MUSCULOSKELETAL HISTORY

Initial history as described in Chapter 3, followed by a focused enquiry relating to the musculoskeletal system.

Table 12.1 presents a symptoms enquiry and further questioning for specific symptoms. Table 12.2 gives findings on examination and the diseases they may suggest.

TABLE 12.1 Symptoms enquiry and further questioning for specific symptoms

Symptom	Further questioning
Joint pains	Use the suggested questions in Chapter 3.
Swelling	When did patient first notice any swelling?
	Is it a single joint or several?
	Is the swelling increasing?
Stiffness	Is stiffness in one joint (if so which) or in several?
	How long does it take for stiffness to wear off during the day?
	Is the stiffness worse on waking?
Reduced function	Is the problem affecting daily living activities?
	Are there problems washing, dressing and cooking, climbing stairs if needed?
Nodules	Where are they?
	When did patient first notice them?
	Are they painful?
Inflammation	Is one joint affected or several?
	Is the onset of swelling sudden?
	Is there pain?
	Is movement of the joint limited?
	Are there other symptoms (i.e. fever or general malaise)?

TABLE 12.2 Findings on examination and diseases they may suggest

	Pain	Swelling	Stiffness	Reduced function	Nodules	Inflammation
Gout	Yes	Yes	No	Possible	No	Yes
Osteoarthritis	Yes	Possible	Yes	Yes	Possible	May be swelling and tenderness
Low back pain	Yes	No	No	Possible	No	No
Polymyalgia	Yes	Possible	Yes	Yes	No	Possible
Giant cell arteritis	Yes if polymyalgia also present	No	Yes if polymyalgia also present	Yes if polymyalgia also present	No	Yes
Fibromyalgia	Yes	No	Yes	Yes	No	No

FURTHER INVESTIGATIONS

Investigations should be chosen on the basis of the history and symptoms, including the duration of symptoms and the overall clinical picture, and include:

- X-rays
- MRI scan
- blood tests.

URGENT REFERRAL TO AN ORTHOPAEDIC SURGEON REQUIRED

- Pain at night
- Associated neurological symptoms
- Presence of sweats and/or fever
- Suspected malignancy.

GOUT

Gout is an extremely painful condition that is estimated to affect at least 1% of the population in Western countries[2] and around 1.5% of the UK population.[3] The condition appears to be more common in males than females and rarely affects anyone under the age of 25 years of age.

Clues to aid the diagnosis

The condition typically presents with:

- sudden onset of acute pain
- inflammation
- redness
- swelling
- oedema.

Pathophysiology

Gout occurs as a result of urate crystals that settle in a joint, causing an inflammatory response. One of the commonest sites is the metatarsal-phalangeal joint of either great toe. High serum uric acid levels are thought to precede the onset of symptoms and the development of elevated blood levels has been linked to a number of factors including alcohol intake, and the inclusion of seafood and meat in the diet. Other factors thought to contribute are reduced renal clearance of uric acid, which may occur as a result of the use of diuretics, or the presence of comorbid conditions such as hypertension and chronic renal impairment.[4]

CLINICAL ALERT!

 BEWARE OF!

Increased risk associated with:
- high BMI
- chronic renal impairment, which potentially doubles the risk of developing gout due to reduced excretion of urate[5]
- diuretic use, particularly those on treatment for 1 year or longer who have a threefold increased risk of gout[5]
- as many as 50% of untreated hypertensive persons have hyperuricaemia, which often precedes hypertension.[6]

Differential diagnosis
- Osteoarthritis (*see* pp. 219–21).
- Rheumatoid arthritis.
- Pseudogout (a condition similar to gout in that crystals are deposited in the joint but they are composed of a salt called calcium pyrophosphate dihydrate (CPPD) not uric acid.
- Psoriatic arthritis (this type of arthritis occurs in conjunction with psoriasis); *see* pp. 177–9.
- Septic arthritis, which occurs when inflammation of a joint is caused by a bacterial infection.

CLINICAL ALERT!

⚠ **BEWARE!**

Septic arthritis has similar symptoms and is potentially fatal if left untreated.

Treatment
Alongside treatment with medication, lifestyle modification may also be helpful and should include:
- weight reduction where obesity is a problem
- avoidance of foods rich in purine such as meats and shellfish, anchovies, herring, kidney, liver, mackerel, meat extracts, mincemeat, mussels, sardines, and yeast
- increase intake of dairy products as high intake may possibly reduce risk
- reduce alcohol intake if this is above the recommended levels
- increase intake of water if needed.

Although lifestyle modification may not drastically reduce serum uric acid levels, it carries benefits in controlling other components of metabolic syndrome (such as hypertriglyceridaemia, hypertension, type 2 diabetes, hyperlipidaemia and obesity) which are frequently associated with gout.[7]

Treatment for acute episodes is shown in Table 12.3.

TABLE 12.3 Treatment for acute episodes

Drug	Dose
Indomethacin	Indomethacin (50 mg 3–4 times daily), has previously been the NSAID of choice for acute attacks of gout; however, other NSAIDs have been shown to be effective and indomethacin might be associated with more adverse effects, including central nervous system disturbances in the elderly (e.g. headaches, confusion).[8]
Naproxen	Naproxen 750 mg (initial dose), then 250 mg every 8 hours.[9] Naproxen is as effective as other choices but as with other NSAIDs there are concerns about GI effects.
Diclofenac	Diclofenac 50 mg three times daily. Diclofenac has similar actions and side-effects to naproxen, but studies have shown a fourfold increased risk of death from CV causes with diclofenac use.[10]
Colchicine	500 mg tablets. Recent evidence has suggested that low-dose colchicine (two tablets followed by one tablet 1 hour later) is effective when prescribed within 12 hours of onset of an acute gout flare, with a low incidence of GI adverse effects.[11] Maximum of 6 mg per course of treatment is recommended.
Prednisolone	30 mg daily for 5 days has been shown to be a safe and effective alternative when NSAIDs are contraindicated.[12]

Prescribing tips

- Aspirin is not recommended because it can alter uric acid levels and prolong and intensify an acute attack.[13]
- May need to add proton pump inhibitor for gastric protection.
- Colchicine is now a second-line choice because of its narrow therapeutic window and risk of toxicity but if prescribed must be initiated within 36 hours of onset of the acute attack to be effective.[14]
- Prednisolone is suggested as an option where NSAIDs and colchicine are unsuitable and when prescribed in combination with paracetamol, pain relief has been shown to be similar to that achieved with naproxen.[15]

CLINICAL ALERT!

⚠ BEWARE!

- Caution needed when prescribing for the elderly who have a higher risk of potentially serious side-effects.
- Several conditions (IHD, PAD and poorly controlled hypertension) limit the use of NSAIDs and they should therefore be used with extreme caution for patients with these additional conditions.
- Length of treatment with NSAIDs is generally for approximately 4 to 8 days which minimises potential adverse side-effects.[16]
- Colchicine can be prescribed if other treatments are contraindicated, poorly tolerated or have failed to resolve symptoms previously. Colchicine dose should be reduced by at least half if the GFR is less than 50 mL/min and should be avoided in patients with hepatic dysfunction, or biliary obstruction.[13]
- NSAID use is associated with the risk of renal impairment.

TABLE 12.4 Prophylactic treatments

Drug	Dose
Allopurinol	Commenced at 100 mg daily and increased by 100 mg every 1–2 weeks titrated against serum acid levels (maximum dose is 900 mg).[17]
Febuxostat	80 mg once daily increased to 120 mg once daily if serum uric acid remains greater than 6 mg/100 mL after 2–4 weeks.[9]

Prescribing tips
- Prophylactic treatment should not be commenced until the acute phase of gout has completely resolved because fluctuations in serum uric acid levels will exacerbate the inflammatory process.[18]
- Concurrent administration of low-dose NSAIDs (e.g. naproxen 250 mg, twice daily) or colchicine (0.5 mg daily or twice daily) should continue for the following 3–6 months to help prevent flare-ups.[19]
- Febuxostat is recommended as an option for the management of chronic hyperuricaemia in gout for people who are intolerant of allopurinol.[20]

Complications
- Although rare, about 25% of patients with chronic hyperuricaemia develop progressive kidney disease, which can result in kidney failure, although some experts believe that the kidney disease occurs first and is the cause of high concentrations of uric acid rather than the other way around.[21]
- If attacks become frequent, high levels of uric acid in the blood can form crystals that deposit in the kidneys, causing kidney stones.[22]

Key reminders
- Common condition
- Rarely serious but can be debilitating
- Complications are rare
- Prophylactic treatment may be needed if flare-ups are frequent.

OSTEOARTHRITIS

Osteoarthritis is very common and can occur in varying degrees of severity, ranging from relatively mild joint pains to more severe symptoms, potentially leading to disability and a reduced quality of life. Frequently described as 'wear and tear', its prevalence increases steadily with age, and according to one report more than seven million adults in the UK have long-term health problems associated with arthritis and related conditions, and nearly nine million visited their GP in the past year for arthritis and related conditions.[23] As the population ages, it is expected that the number of people with osteoarthritis will increase further and it is expected that by 2030 a projected 67 million people will have doctor-diagnosed arthritis.[24]

Clues to aid the diagnosis

The progression of the condition is generally very slow, with symptoms becoming worse over a period of years. Once symptoms become troublesome they may include:
- pain in the affected joint/joints made worse by activity
- stiffness of the joint at rest may be reported
- pain may be relieved by rest and analgesia, although as further deterioration occurs simple analgesia may become ineffective in relieving pain
- the range of movement in affected joints will be reduced.

Pathophysiology

There is some indication that there is ongoing inflammation and synovitis that results in permanent joint damage.[25] In the early stages of osteoarthritis, swelling of the cartilage usually occurs, because of the increased synthesis of proteoglycans that arises as a result of the attempt by chondrocytes to repair any damage to cartilage.[26] This stage may last for years or decades as the body attempts to rectify any problems. Mechanical or inflammatory injury to cartilage and surrounding structures can lead to irreparable damage and to further inflammation and injury to the cartilage as the body tries to heal itself; however, the repair mechanism fails to function correctly, resulting in scarring, thinning and erosion of the articular cartilage in the joints of those affected by the condition.[27] As the cartilage becomes more eroded bone continues to articulate with the opposing surface, which gives rise to thickening of the subchondral bone as a result, which once damaged may undergo further changes with the formation of cysts. Formation of new bone at the joint margins can also occur, and fragmentation of osteophytes or of the articular cartilage itself results in the presence of intra-articular loose bodies.[26]

Differential diagnosis

⚠ **BEWARE!**

There are many differential diagnoses as shown below:
- gout and pseudogout: *see* pp. 215–18
- rheumatoid arthritis (RA), typically associated with more prolonged morning stiffness than osteoarthritis, and patients with acute RA may also feel generally unwell, with fatigue and low mood[28]
- psoriatic arthritis: *see* pp. 177–9
- fibromyalgia: *see* pp. 228–30
- tendonitis, which is a condition caused by inflammation of the tendons and characterised by pain at sites where tendons insert into the bone.

Treatment

Treatment options include non-pharmacological as well as pharmacological, with the level of treatment chosen with consideration for the severity of the condition and patient choice. NICE guidance suggests a holistic approach and that advice should include self-management strategies as well as consideration for its impact on social life, mood, quality of life, sleep pattern, exercise levels, as well as an assessment of pain levels.[29]

Non-pharmacological treatments
- **Exercise**: Patients with established osteoarthritis have been shown to derive benefit from improving physical functioning, using a variety of exercise types, including aerobic, muscle strengthening, aquatic, and physiotherapy-based exercise with a subsequent reduction in pain and disability.[30]
- **Weight loss**: Obesity and excess weight puts additional stress on joints, therefore weight loss may be beneficial in reducing unnecessary stress on affected joints. Evidence is limited but studies have indicated that weight loss reduced the risk of developing symptomatic osteoarthritis in women, reduced pain and improved ability to function.[31]
- **TENS machine**: The use and effectiveness of the TENS machine to relieve arthritis pain has been evaluated in several studies, but there is insufficient evidence to support its use for relieving pain in arthritic joints.
- **Heat or cold packs**: Although evidence is limited, the use of heat or cold may offer short-term pain relief.[32]

Pharmacological treatment

Table 12.5 shows some of the pharmacological treatments available.

TABLE 12.5 Pharmacological treatments

Treatment
Paracetamol taken regularly up to four times daily.
NSAIDs (e.g. ibuprofen, naproxen, diclofenac)
Corticosteroid injections

Prescribing tips
- Use of a topical NSAID has been shown to achieve good levels of pain relief, with topical diclofenac found to be as effective as oral NSAIDs in knee and hand osteoarthritis.[33]
- Corticosteroids injections should be considered as an adjunct to treatment for relief of moderate to severe pain.[34]
- Cox-2 inhibitors (e.g. celecoxib, etoricoxib) are contraindicated in patients with IHD or a history of stroke and should be prescribed with caution for patients with risk factors for CHD, including hypertension, hyperlipidaemia, diabetes, PAD and current smokers,[35] which would therefore exclude them from use for many patients.

CLINICAL ALERT!

Referral for joint replacement surgery may be an option for those patients whose symptoms are not relieved with available treatments and for those in whom the condition is having a significant impact on their quality of life.

Complications

Osteoarthritis is a progressive condition which worsens over time and can potentially lead to severe debility and mobility problems.

Key reminders
- Very common with increasing prevalence in older age
- Can affect daily life when mobility becomes impaired
- Worsens progressively over time.

LOW BACK PAIN

Low back pain is a common problem and it is estimated that around one third of the UK adult population is affected each year.[36] The condition is often acute, with symptoms lasting less than 6 weeks for many people, with 90% of those affected being symptom-free by this time.[37] For some patients symptoms fail to resolve and the condition becomes chronic with a greater impact on quality of life. This is generally the term used if symptoms last for 3 months or longer, and if they persist for 12 months or more, prognosis worsens significantly.[37]

Clues to aid the diagnosis

Patient may be able to recall a particular event that has led to the development of symptoms. Commonly reported events are:

- history of heavy lifting (causing muscle strain or sprain)
- history of a fall
- onset of pain following a road traffic accident
- may follow a period of prolonged sitting or standing.

CLINICAL ALERT!

 BEWARE!

Suspect other pathology if presentation includes red flags. Table 12.6 shows red flags and possible cause or reason for concern.

TABLE 12.6 Red flags and possible cause/reason for concern

Red flag	Possible cause/reason for concern
HIV positive	Risk factor for spinal infection.[38]
Older age	In patients with osteoporosis there is an increased susceptibility to fractures and these are much more common in females, and at age 50 years, the proportion of women with osteoporosis who will fracture their hip, spine, or forearm or proximal humerus in the next 10 years is estimated at approximately 45%.[39]
Young age	In young adults suspect spondylolysis which is a defect in the connection between vertebrae, which can lead to small stress fractures in the vertebrae that can weaken the bones, allowing for one to slip out of place.[40]
Worsening pain at night or when lying flat	A primary tumour or metastases can cause persistent back pain which is often worse at night.
IV drug users	Risk factor for spinal infection.[41]
Immunocompromised	Increased risk of vertebral osteomyelitis, which usually follows infection such as pneumonia, dental abscess or infection of the urinary tract.[42]
Unexplained weight loss, fever, past history of malignancy	Possible bone metastases.
Corticosteroid therapy	Increased risk of fracture in patients receiving long-term corticosteroids.

Pathophysiology

Pathophysiology is difficult to determine because of the non-specific cause and the number of sites from which pain can arise, which can include tendons, ligaments, muscles, fascia and the vertebral column itself. Damage from events such as heavy lifting may lead to stretching or bruising of tissues, resulting in considerable pain. Following a sprain or strain of either muscles or ligaments a disc may rupture, which will then place pressure on surrounding nerves, resulting in back pain.

Differential diagnosis

The number of possible differential diagnoses is large so only the commonest will be mentioned here. Some are mentioned in Table 12.7.

TABLE 12.7 Differential diagnoses

Condition	Additional pointers	When to consider
Osteomyelitis	Pain is not relieved by analgesia, rest or other measures such as application of heat, but where the problem occurs in the hip, pelvis or back there may be no symptoms.[43]	There may be redness and warmth and swelling at the affected site.
Spondylolisthesis	Can occur in both adults and children. A congenital cause should be considered in children; age-related changes more likely to be the cause in adults.[44]	There is low back pain and back stiffness, with patient complaining that pain worsens with any physical activity.
Metastases	Pain may radiate elsewhere and may be worse at night.	If there are associated symptoms of sensory and motor dysfunction, and possible loss of bladder and/or bowel continence.[45]
Multiple myeloma	May be asymptomatic in the early stages. Patient may then complain of pain, often in the back.	Hypercalcaemia occurs as excess calcium is released into the bloodstream, leading to symptoms of thirst, nausea, lethargy, and passing large amounts of urine.[46] Infections may be difficult to clear.
Ankylosing spondylitis	Commoner in young males than females and usually occurs in the late teens or early twenties.	Early signs and symptoms may include pain, stiffness in the lower back and hips, often worse in the morning and after periods of inactivity.[47]
Cauda equina syndrome	Difficult to diagnose but is often sudden in onset, progressing rapidly within hours or days and is caused by herniation of a lumbar disc.[48]	There may be low back pain, with pain in the legs and lower limb weakness. There may also be bladder and bowel dysfunction such as retention or overflow incontinence, constipation or incontinence of faeces.[49]
Fibromyalgia	*See* pp. 228–30.	*See* pp. 228–30.
Polymyalgia rheumatica	*See* pp. 226–8.	*See* pp. 226–8.
Herpes zoster	*See* pp. 188–91.	*See* pp. 188–91.

CLINICAL ALERT!

⚠ BEWARE!

- Most low back pain follows injury or trauma to the back, but pain may also be caused by degenerative conditions such as arthritis or disc disease, osteoporosis or other bone diseases, viral infections, irritation to joints and discs, or congenital abnormalities of the spine.[50]
- Other factors associated with the condition are obesity, poor physical condition, poor posture and poor sleeping position, all of which may contribute.
- Repeated back injuries can lead to the development of scar tissue that will eventually lead to weakening of the spine and more serious injury.[50]

Treatment

For the majority of patients symptomatic treatment will be sufficient to alleviate symptoms and allow recovery to take place. About 60% of patients with low back pain report improvement in 7 days with conservative therapy, and most report improvement within 4 weeks from onset.[51] There are a number of treatment options available, both pharmacological and non-pharmacological.

Non-pharmacological options

NICE guidance suggests consideration for referral to an exercise programme, a course of manual therapy or a course of acupuncture.[36]

- **Exercise**: A Cochrane review reported that for sub-acute low back pain there is some evidence that a graded activity programme improves absenteeism outcomes.[52] Supervised, controlled home exercises have also shown benefit with symptom improvement with positive effects preserved for more than 5 years.[53]
- **Manual therapy**: This is a specialised area of physiotherapy for the management of some neuro-musculoskeletal problems and recent randomised clinical trials found it to be more effective than other methods of conservative management for low back and neck pain.[54]
- **Acupuncture**: There is some evidence to support acupuncture as more effective than no treatment, but no conclusions can be drawn about its effectiveness over other treatments as the evidence is conflicting.[55]

Pharmacological treatment options

Table 12.8 suggests pharmacological treatment options.

TABLE 12.8 Pharmacological treatment options

Drug	Additional information
Paracetamol	Regular use recommended and this is generally regarded as a first-line treatment option.
If pain relief insufficient add in NSAID	May require proton pump inhibitor for gastric protection.
Weak opioids (e.g. co-codamol co-dydramol)	If simple analgesia does not achieve satisfactory pain relief, a weak opioid such as codeine or dihydrocodeine can be offered as an alternative.[36]
Tricyclic antidepressants	A small number of studies have indicated that these drugs appear to produce a moderate reduction in symptoms irrespective of whether the patient is depressed or not.[56]
Strong opioids (e.g. tramadol, oxycodone, fentanyl and diamorphine)	Option for short-term use if pain is very severe.

Prescribing tips
- Risk of dependence with opioids if use continues longer term.
- Antidepressants may be considered if pain not controlled and should be started at a low dose and titrated upwards. Clinical trials have supported the use of antidepressants for the management of chronic pain.[57]

CLINICAL ALERT!

Patients should be instructed to watch for worsening symptoms such as an increasing loss of motor or sensory functions, increasing pain and the loss of bladder or bowel function which may indicate a more serious problem.

Complications
Rarely causes complications but can affect quality of life if problem persists.

Key messages
- Common
- Often self-limiting
- Potential cause of long-term health problems if problem becomes chronic
- Non-pharmacological treatments often effective
- If symptoms persist underlying cause should be sought.

POLYMYALGIA RHEUMATICA (PMR) AND GIANT CELL ARTERITIS (GCA)

PMR and GCA (also called temporal arteritis) are closely related inflammatory disorders with shared symptoms. Compared with GCA, PMR is much more common; GCA, however, is more dangerous and has more serious consequences.[58] Both conditions are more prevalent in men and women over the age of 50, with the mean age of diagnosis estimated to be approximately 75 years of age.[59]

TABLE 12.9 Clues to aid the diagnosis

Symptoms of PMR	Symptoms of GCA
Onset of pain can be abrupt	Headaches and weight loss
Symptoms may begin as unilateral, becoming bilateral within a few weeks of onset of symptoms	Myalgias
Pain and stiffness of the shoulders and the hip girdle	Fever
Patient may report problems getting up from a sitting position, and raising their arms above their head because of the degree of stiffness	Scalp pain and jaw pain
One third of patients have flu-like symptoms described as fever, malaise, anorexia, or weight loss[58]	Vision problems

CLINICAL ALERT!

- Both conditions almost exclusively affect people over the age of 50 and the incidence of both peaks at 70–80 years of age.[60]
- Both PMR and GCA will result in raised ESR and CRP on blood testing.
- Approximately 15% of patients with PMR will go on to develop GCA, and 40%–50% of patients with GCA will have associated symptoms of PMR.[61]

Pathophysiology

The underlying pathophysiology of PMR is poorly understood, but research has revealed many of the same immunologic responses and processes that occur in GCA. The latter results in inflammation of arteries of the scalp, often the temporal arteries, but inflammation can also occur in the arteries of the neck and arms. This inflammation causes the arteries to narrow, impeding adequate blood flow.[60]

Differential diagnosis

 BEWARE!

A number of conditions have shared symptoms. Some of the more frequently seen are shown in Table 12.10.

TABLE 12.10 Differential diagnoses

Differential diagnosis PMR	Differential diagnosis GCA
Giant cell arteritis	Cervical spondylosis
Multiple myeloma (*see* p. 223)	Sinus problems (*see* pp. 136–9)
Fibromyalgia (*see* pp. 228–30)	Cluster headaches (*see* p. 201)
Late-onset RA	Migraine headaches (*see* pp. 201–6)
Osteoarthritis with a systemic problem such as intercurrent infection can mimic PMR.[62]	*Herpes zoster* (*see* pp. 188–91)
Depression	Ear problems (*see* pp. 132–6)

Treatment

Treatment of PMR and GCA is shown in Table 12.11.

TABLE 12.11 Treatment of PMR and GCA

Treatment of polymyalgia rheumatica	Treatment of giant cell arteritis
Daily prednisolone 15 mg for 3 weeks[63]	40–60 mg prednisolone daily[63]
Then 12.5 mg for 3 weeks	Higher dose needed if there are ischaemic symptoms (jaw or tongue claudication or visual symptoms)[64]
Then 10 mg for 4–6 weeks	The initial oral dose of corticosteroids should continue for 1 month before dose reduction is considered[65]
Then reduction by 1 mg every 4–8 weeks or alternate day reductions (e.g. 10/7.5 mg alternate days)	Dose reduced by 10 mg every 2 weeks to 20 mg[66]
	Then reduce by 1 mg every 1–2 months as long as there is no relapse[64]

Prescribing tips

Long-term steroid use is associated with a number of adverse effects including:
- suppression of the immune system, leading to more frequent infections
- osteoporosis
- impaired glucose tolerance/diabetes
- GI symptoms
- electrolyte imbalance with raised sodium levels and low potassium levels
- long-term effects of taking prednisolone include an increased risk of cataracts, glaucoma, bone thinning, fractures, loss of muscle mass, abnormal hair growth, and thinning of the skin.[67]

CLINICAL ALERT!

- Long-term treatment for up to 2 years is often needed for PMR.[68]
- Treatment for 3–4 years may be needed for GCA.[63]
- Bone protection should be considered for long-term steroid use.

Complications

⚠ **BEWARE!**

- Exacerbations may occur if corticosteroids are tapered too rapidly, and relapse is common, affecting up to 25% of all treated patients.[61]
- Possible drug side-effects.
- Patients with PMR have a risk of developing GCA.
- Patients with GCA are at higher risk of death from aortic aneurysms, and thoracic aneurysms are 17 times more likely to occur in GCA patients and can occur at any time during the disease course.[65]
- Vision problems in GCA results from ischaemia and infarction of the optic nerve, and can occur in up to 20% of patients with GCA.[69]

Key messages

- Both conditions are poorly understood and may coexist
- Both are common in older adults
- GCA has more serious complications
- Often require long-term treatment
- Many side-effects with long-term drug treatment.

FIBROMYALGIA

Introduction

Fibromyalgia is a chronic condition, which is thought to be common. Although symptoms can develop at any age, it is most common in those aged 20–50 with a greater prevalence among females than males.[70] The condition is associated with unpleasant symptoms causing functional impairment and disruption to activities of daily living[71] and therefore has the potential to significantly impact on health and general well-being.

Clues to aid the diagnosis

Symptoms are many and varied and include:
- widespread pain affecting several sites
- frequent headaches
- memory problems
- general tiredness and fatigue
- feeling dizzy or lightheaded.

⚠ BEWARE!

- Many sufferers also have comorbid anxiety and depression.[72]
- The frequency of depression and anxiety among those affected suggests that stress may be an influential factor.

Pathophysiology

The pathophysiology of fibromyalgia is poorly understood, but it is thought to cluster in families, suggesting the possibility of a genetic influence.[73] Some of the key suggestions focus on the possibility of abnormalities of descending inhibitory pain pathways and dysfunction in brain centres (or the pathways from these centres) that normally down-regulate pain signalling in the spinal cord.[74] Serotonin levels have also been studied. Serotonin is believed to play a part in both mood modulation and response to pain and there is some indication that levels are low in patients with fibromyalgia.[75]

TABLE 12.12 Differential diagnosis

Condition	Additional pointers	When to consider
Medication related	Statin therapy.	Generalised muscle aches and pains can be a side-effect of statins.
Hypothyroidism	Patient presents with symptoms of fatigue, muscle aches and pains and muscle weakness.	There are additional symptoms including weight gain, intolerance of cold and constipation.
Myofascial pain	Pain is felt as deep, localised aching pain in a muscle.	May present with a history of acute trauma associated with persistent muscular pain.[76] Pain is not relieved by self-help measures and may cause sleep disturbance.
Low vitamin D levels	General aches and pains, feeling of tiredness.	Patient may complain of muscle weakness and possible problems with certain activities such as climbing stairs or getting up from a sitting position.
Chronic fatigue syndrome	General fatigue with persistent tiredness.	There are additional symptoms such as poor concentration, poor memory, generalised aches and pains and a poor sleep pattern.
PMR	*See* pp. 226–8.	*See* pp. 226–8.

Treatment

Available treatment options include both non-pharmacological and pharmacological options (*see* Tables 12.13 and 12.14).

TABLE 12.13 Non-pharmacological treatments

Treatment	Supporting evidence
Exercise	Exercise programmes, which include strength and flexibility training, have been shown to increase the body's production of endogenous opioids improving oxygenation and circulation to muscles, improving mood, reducing disability, and reducing pain.[77]
Aromatherapy	There is some evidence to suggest aromatherapy may be beneficial in relieving pain, with use of the topical application of a proprietary mixture containing camphor oil, rosemary oil, eucalyptus oil, peppermint oil, aloe vera oil, lemon oil, and orange oil potentially reducing fibromyalgia pain more effectively than placebo.[78]
TENS machine	High-frequency TENS may be useful in relieving pain, anxiety, fatigue and stiffness, and in improving ability to work; it may be used as a short-term complementary treatment of fibromyalgia.[79]
Hot baths	In a randomised controlled trial, women with severe fibromyalgia symptoms benefitted from therapy in a warm pool three times per week for 16 weeks.[80] Not only did this improve pain but it also improved adherence and willingness to participate in exercise programmes in study participants.
Mind–body forms of exercise (pilates, yoga, breathing exercises, tai chi)	These forms of exercise have been shown to improve quality of life and offer pain relief and when the findings of individual studies have been collated suggest use of these techniques may be beneficial in the treatment of fibromyalgia.[81]

TABLE 12.14 Pharmacological treatment options

Treatment	Supporting evidence
Antidepressants	Amitriptyline 25–50 mg/day reduces pain, fatigue and depression in patients with fibromyalgia, and improves sleep and quality of life.[82]
Pain relief	Simple analgesia (e.g. paracetamol) may be prescribed, but there is limited evidence to support their use.[77] Weak opioids (e.g. tramadol) may be more effective but use may be limited by risk of side-effects and possible addiction.
Anti-epileptic drugs (e.g. gabapentin)	Several studies have looked at the effectiveness of gabapentin for pain relief. Arnold *et al.* reported that taken for up to 12 weeks, gabapentin is effective and safe in the treatment of pain and other symptoms associated with fibromyalgia.[83]

Stress management

Many patients with fibromyalgia have increased levels of stress and feelings of depression, anxiety and frustration. Several treatment options are available such as cognitive behavioural therapy and relaxation training, which some patients may find helpful.

Complications

The condition is not associated with the onset of other medical conditions, with the exception of depression and anxiety brought on by the effect of sleep disturbance and reduced quality of life.

Key messages
- Chronic condition
- More common in females than males
- Numerous symptoms
- Strong association with depression and anxiety
- Associated with reduced quality of life.

REFERENCES

1. Woolf AD, Akesson K. Understanding the burden of musculoskeletal conditions. The burden is huge and not reflected in national health priorities. *BMJ.* 2001; **322**: 1079–80.
2. Terkeltaub RA. Clinical practice. Gout. *N Engl J Med.* 2003; **349**: 1647–55.
3. Mikuls TR, Farrar JT, Bikker WB, *et al.* Gout epidemiology: results from the UK General Practice Research Database, 1990–1999. *Ann Rheum Dis.* 2005; **64**: 267–72.
4. Choi HK, Mount DB, Reginato AM. Pathogenesis of gout. *Ann Intern Med.* 2005; **143**: 499–516.
5. Soriana LC, Rothenbacher D, Choi HK, *et al.* Contemporary epidemiology of gout in the UK general population. *Arth Res and Ther.* Available at: http://arthritis-research.com/content/13/2/R39 (accessed 6 August 2012).
6. Saag KG, Choi H. *Epidemiology, risk factors, and lifestyle modifications for gout.* Available at: http://arthritis-research.com/content/8/S1/S2#abs (accessed 19 August 2013).
7. Rider TG, Jordan KM. The modern management of gout. *Rheumatology.* 2010; **49**: 5–14.
8. Rubin BR, Burton R, Navarra S, *et al.* Efficacy and safety profile of treatment with etoricoxib 120 mg once daily compared with indomethacin 50 mg three times daily in acute gout: a randomized controlled trial. *Arthritis Rheum.* 2004; **50**(2): 598–606.
9. British National Formulary. 2012. Available at: www.bnf.org/bnf/index.htm
10. MeReC. *NSAIDs and Cardiovascular Risks: more evidence, but this shouldn't be new news.* 2011. Available at: www.npc.nhs.uk/rapidreview/?p=2451
11. Terkeltaub RA, Furst DE, Bennett K, *et al.* High versus low dosing of oral colchicine for early acute gout flare: twenty-four-hour outcome of the first multicenter, randomized, double-blind, placebo-controlled, parallel group, dose-comparison colchicine study. *Arthritis Rheum.* 2010; **62**: 1060–8.
12. Prasad S, Ewigman B. Acute gout: oral steroids work as well as NSAIDs. *J Fam Practice.* 2008; **57**(10): 655–7.
13. Rothschild B. *Gout and Pseudogout Treatment & Management.* Available at: http://emedicine.medscape.com/article/329958-treatment (accessed 3 August 2012).
14. Khanna D, Khanna PP, Fitzgerald JD, *et al.* American College of Rheumatology. Guideline for management of gout. Part 2. Therapy and anti-inflammatory prophylaxis of acute gouty arthritis. *Arth Care Res.* 2012; **64**(10): 1447–61.
15. Janssens HJ, Janssen M, Van de Lisdonk EH, *et al.* Use of oral prednisolone or naproxen for the treatment of gouty arthritis: a double-blind, randomised equivalence trial. *Lancet.* 2008; **371**: 1854–60.
16. Conway N, Schwartz S. Diagnosis and management of acute gout. *Medicine and Health.* 2009; **92**(11) 356–8.

17. Zang W, Doherty M, Bardin T, *et al.* EULAR evidence based recommendations for gout. Part II: Management. Report task force of the EULAR standing committee for international clinical studies including therapeutics (ESCISIT). *Ann Rheum Dis.* 2006; **65**: 1312–24.

18. Eggebeen A. Gout: an update. *Am Fam Physician.* 2007; **76**(6): 801–8.

19. BPAC. *The Medical Management of Gout Revisited.* Available at: www.bpac.org.nz/magazine/2011/august/gout.asp (accessed 9 September 2012).

20. National Institute for Health and Clinical Excellence. *Febuxostat for the Management of Hyperuricaemia in People with Gout: NICE guideline 164.* London: NICE; 2008. Available at: www.nice.org.uk/nicemedia/pdf/TA164Guidance.pdf

21. University of Maryland. *Gout: complications.* Available at: www.umm.edu/patiented/articles/what_lifestyle_measures_can_help_prevent_gout_000093_9.htm (accessed 5 August 2012).

22. Mayo Foundation for Medical Education and Research (MFMER). *Gout: complications.* Available at: www.mayoclinic.com/health/gout/DS00090/DSECTION=complications (accessed 5 September 2012).

23. Arthritis Research Campaign. *Arthritis: the big picture.* Available at: www.ipsos-mori.com/Assets/Docs/Archive/Polls/arthritis.pdf

24. Hootman JM, Helmick CG. Projections of US prevalence of arthritis and associated activity limitations. *Arthritis Rheum.* 2006; **54**(1): 226–9.

25. Brooks P. Inflammation as an important feature of osteoarthritis. *Bull World Health Organ.* 2003; **81**: 689–90.

26. Lozada CJ. *Osteoarthritis.* Available at: http://emedicine.medscape.com/article/330487-overview (accessed 15 August 2012).

27. Mainil-Varlet P, Aigner T, Brittberg M, *et al.* Histological assessment of cartilage repair: a report by the Histology Endpoint Committee of the International Cartilage Repair Society (ICRS). *J Bone J Surg Am.* 2003; **85A**(Suppl 2): 45–7.

28. BMJ. *Osteoarthritis.* Available at: http://bestpractice.bmj.com/best-practice/monograph/192/diagnosis/differential.html (accessed 18 August 2012).

29. National Institute for Health and Clinical Excellence. *Osteoarthritis: national clinical guideline for care and management in adults. NICE guideline 59.* London: NICE; 2008. Available at: www.nice.org.uk/nicemedia/pdf/CG59NICEguideline.pdf

30. Bosomworth NJ. Exercise and knee osteoarthritis: benefit or hazard? *Can Fam Physician.* 2009; **55**(9): 871–8.

31. Tanna S. *Osteoarthritis: 'Opportunities to Address Pharmaceutical Gaps'.* Available at: http://archives.who.int/prioritymeds/report/background/osteoarthritis.doc (accessed 9 August 2012).

32. Denegar CR, Dougherty DR, Friedman JE, *et al.* Preferences for heat, cold or contrast in patients with knee osteoarthritis affecting treatment response. *Clin Interventions in Aging.* 2010; **5**: 199–206.

33. Derry S, Moore RA, Rabbie R. Topical NSAIDs for chronic musculoskeletal pain in adults. *Cochrane Database Syst Rev.* 2012; **9**: CD007400.

34. National Institute for Health and Clinical Excellence. *Low back pain: early management of persistent non-specific low back pain. NICE guideline 88.* London: NIHCE; 2009. Available at: www.nice.org.uk/nicemedia/live/11887/44345/44345.pdf

35. Waknine Y. *International Drug Alerts: COX-2 Inhibitors and Co-proxamol.* Available at: www.medscape.com/viewarticle/500026

36. National Institute for Health and Clinical Excellence. *Low back pain: NICE guideline 88.* London: NIHCE; 2009. Available at: www.nice.org.uk/nicemedia/live/11887/44343/44343.pdf

37. Davies R. Low back pain. *InnovAiT.* 2008; **1**(6): 440–5.

38. Bono CM. Spectrum of spine infections in patients with HIV: a case report and review of the literature. *Clin Orthop Relat Res.* 2006; **444**: 83–91.

39. Janis KA. Diagnosis of osteoporosis and assessment of fracture risk. *The Lancet.* 2002; **359**: 1929–36.

40. Cleveland Clinic. *Spondylosis.* Available at: http://my.clevelandclinic.org/disorders/back_pain/hic_spondylolysis.aspx (accessed 10 August 2012).

41. Chuo CY, Fu YC, Lu YM. Spinal infection in intravenous drug abusers. *J Spinal Disord Tech.* 2007; **4**: 324–8.

42. Carragee EJ. Pyogenic vertebral osteomyelitis. *J Bone Joint Surg Am.* 1997; **79**: 874–80.

43. University of Maryland. *Osteomyelitis.* Available at: www.umm.edu/altmed/articles/osteomyelitis-000119.htm (accessed 19 August 2012).

44. NHS Choices. *Spondylolisthesis.* Available at: www.nhs.uk/conditions/spondylolisthesis/Pages/Introduction.aspx (accessed 25 September 2013).

45. Sama AA. *Spinal Tumours.* Available at: http://emedicine.medscape.com/article/1267223-overview#aw2aab6b3 (accessed 19 August 2012).

46. Cancer research UK. *Myeloma Symptoms.* Available at: www.cancerresearchuk.org/cancer-help/type/myeloma/about/myeloma-symptoms (accessed 13 February 2014).

47. Mayo Foundation for Medical Education and Research (MFMER). *Ankylosing Spondylitis.* 2011. Available at: www.mayoclinic.com/health/ankylosing-spondylitis/DS00483/DSECTION=symptoms (accessed 13 February 2014).

48. Lavy C, James A, Wilson-MacDonald J, *et al.* Cauda equina syndrome. *BMJ.* 2009; **338**: b936.

49. Dawodu ST. *Cauda Equine and Conus Medullaris Syndromes.* Available at: http://emedicine.medscape.com/article/1148690-clinical (accessed 9 August 2013).

50. National Institute of Neurological Disorders and Stroke. *Back Pain Information.* Available at: www.ninds.nih.gov/disorders/backpain/backpain.htm (accessed 10 August 2012).

51. Connelly C. Patients with low back pain: how to identify the few who need extra attention. *Post-grad Med.* 1996; **100**: 143–6.

52. Hayden J, van Tulder MW, Malmivaara A, *et al.* Exercise therapy for treatment of non-specific low back pain. *Cochrane Database Syst Rev.* 2010; **10**: CD000335.

53. Kuukkanen T, Malkia E, Kautiainen H, *et al.* Effectiveness of a home exercise programme in low back pain. *Physiother Res Int.* 2007; **12**(4): 213–24.

54. Aure OF, Nilsen JH, Vasseljen O. Manual therapy and exercise therapy in patients with chronic low back pain: a randomized, controlled trial with 1-year follow-up. *Spine.* 2003; **28**: 525–31.

55. Hutchinson AJ, Ball S, Andrews JC, *et al.* The effectiveness of acupuncture in treating chronic non-specific low back pain: a systematic review of the literature. *J Orthop Surg Res.* 2012; **7**: 36.

56. Staiger TO, Barak MD, Sullivan MD, *et al.* Systematic review of antidepressants in the treatment of chronic low back pain. *Spine.* 2003; **28**(22): 2540–5.

57. Barkin RL, Fawcett J. The management challenges of chronic pain: the role of antidepressants. *Am J Therapeutics.* 2000; **7**(1): 31–49.

58. Epperley T, Moore KE, Harrover JD. Polymyalgia rheumatic and temporal arteritis. *Am Fam Physician.* 2000; **62**: 789–96.

59. Sweeney K. Polymyalgia: easy to overlook. *Practitioner.* 1995; **239**: 382–6.

60. National Institute of Arthritis and musculoskeletal and skin diseases. *Polymyalgia Rheumatica and Giant Cell Arteritis.* Available at: www.niams.nih.gov/Health_Info/Polymyalgia/ (accessed 15 August 2012).

61. Popadopoulos PJ. *Polymyalgia Rheumatica.* Available at: http://emedicine.medscape.com/article/330815-overview (accessed 17 August 2012).

62. Sengupta R, Kyle V. Recognising polymyalgia rheumatica. *Practitioner.* 2006; **250**(1688): 40–7.

63. Dasgupta B, Borg F, Hassan N, *et al.* BSR and BHPR guidelines for the management of polymyalgia rheumatica. *Rheumatology.* 2009; **49**(1): 186–90.

64. Charlton R. Optimal management of giant cell arteritis and polymyalgia rheumatica. *Ther Clin Risk Manag.* 2012; **8**: 173–9.

65. Molloy E, Koening CL, Hoffman GS. *Polymyalgia Rheumatica and Giant Cell Arteritis.* Available at: www.clevelandclinicmeded.com/medicalpubs/diseasemanagement/rheuma tology/polymyalgia-rheumatica-and-giant-cell-arteritis/ (accessed 19 August 2012).

66. Hassan N, Dasgupta B, Barraclough K. Giant cell arteritis. *BMJ.* 2011; **342**: d3019.

67. American Cancer Society. *Prednisone.* Available at: www.cancer.org/treatment/treatment sandsideeffects/guidetocancerdrugs/prednisone (accessed 25 June 2013).

68. Kyle V, Hazleman BL. Treatment of polymyalgia rheumatic and giant cell arteritis: relation between steroid dosing and steroid associated side effects. *Ann Rheum Dis.* 1989; **48**: 662–6.

69. Unwin B, Williams CM, Gilliland W. Polymyalgia rheumatica and giant cell arteritis. *Am Fam Physician.* 2006; **74**(9): 1547–54.

70. Chakrabarty S, Zoorob R. Fibromyalgia. *Am Fam Physician.* 2007; **76**(2): 247–54.

71. Buckner Winfield J. *Fibromyalgia.* Available at: http://emedicine.medscape.com/article/329838-overview (accessed 17 August 2012).

72. Arnold LM, Hudson JI, Keck PE, *et al.* Comorbidity of fibromyalgia and psychiatric disorders. *J Clin Psychiatry.* 2006; **67**(8): 1219–25.

73. Jahan F, Nanji K, Qidwai W, *et al.* Fibromyalgia syndrome: an overview of pathophysiology, diagnosis and management. *Oman Med J.* 2012; **27**(3): 192–5.

74. Abeles AM, Pillinger MH, Solitar BM, *et al.* Narrative review: the pathophysiology of fibromyalgia. *Ann Intern Med.* 2007; **146**: 726–34.

75. Wolfe F, Russell IJ, Vipraio G. Serotonin levels, pain threshold, and fibromyalgia symptoms in the general population. *J Rheum.* 1997; **24**(3): 555–9.

76. Phillips DC. *Myofacial pain.* Available at: http://emedicine.medscape.com/article/305937-clinical (accessed 5 June 2012).

77. Dedhia JD, Bone ME. Pain and fibromyalgia. *Contin Educ Anaesth Crit Care Pain.* 2009; **9**(5): 162–6.

78. Ko GD, Hum A, Traites G, *et al.* Effects of topical 024 essential oils on patients with fibromyalgia syndrome: a randomised placebo controlled pilot study. *J Muscoskelet Pain.* 2007; **15**: 11–19.

79. Carbonario F, Matsutani LA, Yuan SL, *et al.* Effectiveness of high-frequency transcutaneous electrical nerve stimulation at tender points as adjuvant therapy for patients with fibromyalgia. *Eur J Phys Rehabil Med.* 2013; **49**(2): 197–204.

80. Munguía-Izquierdo D, Legaz-Arrese A. Assessment of the effects of aquatic therapy on global symptomatology in patients with fibromyalgia syndrome: a randomized controlled trial. *Arch Phys Med Rehabil.* 2008; **89**(12): 2250–7.

81. Busch AJ, Webber SC, Brachaniec A. Exercise therapy for fibromyalgia. *Curr Pain Headache Rep.* 2011; **15**(5): 358–67.

82. Uçeyler N, Häuser W, Sommer C. A systematic review on the effectiveness of treatment with antidepressants in fibromyalgia syndrome. *Arthritis Rheum.* 2008; **59**(9): 1279–98.

83. Arnold LM, Goldenberg DL, Stanford SB. Gabapentin in the treatment of fibromyalgia: a randomized, double-blind, placebo-controlled, multicenter trial. *Arthritis Rheum.* 2007; **56**(4): 1336–44.

CHAPTER 13

Blood disorders

INTRODUCTION

Blood disorders cover a wide and varied range of conditions and can affect people of any age. Some of these conditions are easily treatable, while others are more complex and their cause can be acquired, inherited or genetic or in some cases arise as a result of the presence of other comorbid conditions.

CONDITIONS COVERED IN THIS CHAPTER

- Anaemia (iron deficiency)
- B_{12} deficiency
- Anaemia of chronic disease
- Leukaemia.

COMMON PRESENTING SYMPTOMS

- Tiredness
- Lethargy
- Malaise
- Breathlessness
- Feeling faint.

TAKING THE HISTORY

Initial history as described in Chapter 3, followed by a focused enquiry relating to the symptoms experienced.

TABLE 13.1 Symptoms enquiry and further questioning for specific symptoms

Symptom	Further questioning
Tiredness	When did symptoms begin?
	Any associated symptoms, feeling faint or palpitations, or dizziness?
	Sleep patterns?
	Weight changes?
Lethargy	As above.
Breathlessness	Severity of symptoms and duration of symptoms?
	Associated symptoms?
	Any precipitating factors (known allergies, smoking history)?
	When does problem occur (worse on exertion, when lying flat or happening at rest)?
Dizziness	Is the dizziness episodic or constant?
	Any associated symptoms?
	How long do the dizzy spells last?
	Does anything make them worse or anything make them better?
Feeling faint	Duration of symptoms?
	Associated symptoms?
	Does the patient feel as if they are going to pass out?

Table 13.2 shows a summary of presenting signs and symptoms and the diseases they may suggest.

TABLE 13.2 Findings on examination and the diseases they may suggest

	Tiredness	Lethargy	Breathlessness	Dizziness	Feeling faint
Anaemia (iron deficiency)	Yes	Yes	Yes	Yes	Yes
Anaemia of chronic disease	Yes	Yes	Yes	Yes	Yes
B_{12} deficiency	Yes	Yes	Yes	Yes	Yes
Leukaemia (for additional symptoms specific to leukaemia type, *see* p. 248)	Yes	Yes	Yes	Possible	Possible

FURTHER INVESTIGATIONS

Investigations should be chosen on the basis of the history and symptoms, including the duration of symptoms and the overall clinical picture.

URGENT REFERRAL TO A HAEMATOLOGIST REQUIRED

- Bone pain and anaemia symptoms suspicious of multiple myeloma
- Lymphadenopathy and splenomegaly suspicious of Hodgkin's or non-Hodgkin's lymphoma
- Abnormal blood result suggesting leukaemia of any type.

IRON DEFICIENCY ANAEMIA

Iron deficiency anaemia can affect people of any age. It is one of the most common causes of anaemia worldwide and is frequently microcytic[1] (*see* pp. 267, 270). Statistics indicate that approximately 30% of the world's population is affected by the condition,[2] while the British Society for Gastroenterology suggests a prevalence rate of 2%–5% among adult men and postmenopausal women in the developed world.[3] The numbers of people affected is variable among different populations with prevalence rates influenced by age, ethnicity, gender and race.

Clues to aid the diagnosis

Where the degree of anaemia is mild, the patient may be relatively asymptomatic. However, when the problem is more severe, the patient will experience a number of non-specific signs and symptoms that include:

- pallor
- breathlessness on exertion
- palpitations
- hair loss
- fatigue and tiredness
- chest pain.

CLINICAL ALERT!

⚠ BEWARE!

Be alert to additional symptoms that may suggest a more serious underlying pathology, such as:

- altered bowel habit
- loss of appetite
- abdominal pain
- unexplained weight loss
- poor response to treatment.

Pathophysiology

Iron plays a vital role and is essential for multiple metabolic processes, including oxygen transport, DNA synthesis, and electron transport.[4] Iron levels are carefully regulated to maintain a stable environment so that any loss of iron from the body is compensated for by adequate absorption of iron, which serves to maintain a healthy balance. The regulation of iron absorption takes place in the small intestine and errors in this process can lead to either a deficiency in iron levels or an excess. Poor dietary intake is a frequent and common cause of inadequate iron levels, while haemorrhage or bleeding is often found to be the cause of excessive loss of body iron.[4] *See* Table 13.3 for other causes.

TABLE 13.3 Possible causes of anaemia

Common causes of blood loss from the gastrointestinal tract	Rarer causes of blood loss from the gastrointestinal tract	Other common causes	Other rarer causes
Aspirin or NSAID use	Tumours of the small bowel	Menorrhagia	Epistaxis
Gastric carcinoma	Carcinoma of the oesophagus	Coeliac disease	Haematuria
Gastric ulceration	Oesophagitis	Post gastrectomy	

Differential diagnosis

Table 13.4 presents differential diagnoses for anaemia.

TABLE 13.4 Differential diagnoses

Condition	Additional pointers	When to consider
Thalassaemia	Genetic condition which exists in several forms. *See* Chapter 15 for more information on interpreting the FBC result, but generally mean cell volume (MCV) and mean cell haemoglobin (MCH) are low and in more severe cases haemoglobin level (HB) is also low.	If person is of Mediterranean, Middle Eastern, Chinese origin or from India, Asia or Africa where prevalence rates of various types of thalassaemia are higher.
Anaemia of chronic disease	*See* pp. 242–4.	*See* pp. 242–4.
Sideroblastic anaemia	Can be congenital or acquired or of unknown cause.	Consider if there are secondary causes of sideroblastic anaemia such as prolonged exposure to certain toxic substances or drugs, or the patient has other conditions such as immune disorders, granulomatous disease, tumours, or metabolic diseases.[5]

Treatment

Oral iron therapy is usually first-line treatment for iron deficiency anaemia; however, if HB is very low or the patient is severely symptomatic a blood transfusion may be required. An increase in the haemoglobin level of 1 g per dL (10 g per L) should occur every 2–3 weeks on iron therapy, but it may take up to 4 months for the iron stores to return to normal after the haemoglobin has corrected.[6] However, oral medication is not without problems and side-effects such as constipation, nausea and epigastric discomfort are dose related[7] and may affect compliance in some patients.

Prescribing tips

- Constipation is common in patients taking iron therapy.
- Absorption of iron is enhanced if taken with orange juice and in children older than 6 years of age ferrous fumarate given with orange juice has been shown to increase iron absorption twofold.[8]
- Absorption can be reduced when taken with tea or coffee, milk, eggs and whole grains.[9]
- Absorption is also reduced in those taking gastric medications such as antacids and proton pump inhibitors and also with ciprofloxacin, norfloxacin and ofloxacin and bisphosphonates, while concurrent administration of iron with tetracyclines may impair absorption of both agents.[9]

Complications

⚠ **BEWARE!**

If left untreated anaemia can lead to a number of problems, while in those with certain comorbid conditions consequences can be more serious. *See* Table 13.5.

TABLE 13.5 Complications

Pregnant women	Iron deficiency anaemia is associated with an increased risk of preterm delivery when diagnosed in early or mid-pregnancy.[10]
Children and adolescents	Growth rates may be slowed, and a decreased capability to learn has been noted.[4]
Elderly	Anaemia in the elderly is associated with an increased risk of falls and reduced survival rates in patients who have had an MI.[11]
HF	Anaemia can lead to reduced exercise tolerance and is associated with a more rapid deterioration in HF, and increased mortality rates.[12]
Kidney disease	The condition is associated with higher mortality rates in patients with kidney disease.[11]
Cancer	Anaemia is recognised as an independent predictor of poor prognosis in cancer patients.[13]

Key reminders

- Can occur at any age
- Can present with vague signs and symptoms
- Common in pregnancy
- Multiple causes
- Referral needed if there are symptoms suggestive of more serious underlying causes (e.g. alteration in bowel habit or unexplained weight loss).

B$_{12}$ DEFICIENCY

Vitamin B$_{12}$ deficiency occurs in countries around the world and although often associated with the elderly, there are now more cases where the condition is detected in younger patients.[14] Among older patients the prevalence of vitamin B$_{12}$ deficiency has been reported at approximately 5% in people 65–74 years of age, and is found in more than 10% of those 75 years of age or older.[15]

Clues to aid the diagnosis

The following are commonly reported signs and symptoms:

- abnormal gait
- glossy tongue
- fatigue and tiredness
- loss of appetite
- weight loss
- cognitive impairment.

Pathophysiology

Obtained from dietary sources, vitamin B$_{12}$ is released from food by the gastric acid within the stomach. In healthy individuals, vitamin B$_{12}$ combines with intrinsic factor normally produced in the stomach by the parietal cells to enable the formation of a complex. Once formed the complex binds to receptors within the ileum, which then allow absorption to take place. Inadequate or reduced production of intrinsic factor leads to an autoimmune condition called pernicious anaemia, and this is reported to be the leading cause of B$_{12}$ deficiency.[16]

There are a number of other causes shown which have been classified as nutritional deficiency, malabsorption syndromes, and other gastrointestinal causes.[17] *See* Table 13.6.

TABLE 13.6 Causes of B$_{12}$ deficiency

Cause	Additional information
Nutritional causes	Those at risk of poor dietary intake include the elderly, chronic alcoholics and vegans.[18]
Malabsorption problems	Pernicious anaemia is an autoimmune condition in which destruction of the gastric parietal cells occurs, whose function in healthy individuals is to produce intrinsic factor needed for absorption of B$_{12}$.
GI causes	May occur following previous gastric surgery such as gastrectomy or gastric resection or in association with conditions such as Crohn's disease.

BEWARE OF

Patients with a history of long-term use of drugs that affect gastric acid production (e.g. H_2 blockers such as ranitidine and PPIs) who can have deficiency caused by lack of gastric acid that is needed to release vitamin B_{12} bound to proteins in the diet.[19]

Table 13.7 presents differential diagnoses for vitamin B_{12} deficiency.

TABLE 13.7 Differential diagnoses

Condition	Additional pointers	When to consider
Progressive bone marrow failure (myelodysplasia)	More common in older adults aged 60–80 and symptoms such as shortness of breath, fatigue, bruising and pallor may be mistaken for other causes.	Anaemia is common but occasionally there will be isolated thrombocytopenia, and, less commonly, isolated neutropenia with isolated thrombocytopenia possibly occurring 2–10 years prior to the development of symptoms.[20]
Severe thyroid deficiency	Common signs and symptoms include lethargy, dislike of cold, weight gain, constipation and breathlessness.	TFT test results are grossly abnormal. There may also be anaemia, and approximately 55% of patients with primary hypothyroidism can have a slightly raised serum creatinine level.[21]
Myeloma	Lethargy and tiredness, loss of appetite, backache and weight loss.	Consider if FBC shows reduced RCC, WCC and reduced platelets with raised ESR.[22]
Aplastic anaemia	Onset may be abrupt or insidious and again presents with symptoms such as breathlessness, pallor, headache, palpitations and fatigue that may again be mistaken for other causes. There may also be ankle oedema and visual disturbance which occurs as a result of retinal haemorrhage.[23]	Consider if HB, platelet count and neutrophils are all low.[23]

Treatment

Suggested guidance is based on the presence or absence of neurological symptoms

- Where neurological symptoms are absent, intramuscular injection of hydroxocobalamin 1 mg three times weekly for 2 weeks then three-monthly.[24]
- Or if neurological symptoms are present, 1 mg intramuscular hydroxocobalamin on alternate days until no further improvement then 1 mg every 2 months.[25]

Neurological symptoms present

COMPLICATIONS INCLUDE

- Visual disturbances
- Memory loss
- Paraesthesia
- Untreated B_{12} deficiency can lead to the development of serious neuropathies (including optic neuropathy), peripheral neuropathy, myelopathy and encephalopathy.[26]

CLINICAL ALERT!

⚠ **BEWARE!**

- Severe vitamin B_{12} deficiency in pregnancy produces a cluster of neurological symptoms in infants, including irritability, failure to thrive, apathy, anorexia and developmental regression.[27]
- In severe cases where treatment has been delayed for 6 months or longer since the onset of neurological involvement any neurological problems may become permanent, with the possibility of paralysis.[26]

Key reminders

- Common in the elderly
- If left untreated can cause neurological symptoms
- Easily treated
- Serious consequences in the newborn if severe deficiency occurs in pregnancy.

ANAEMIA OF CHRONIC DISEASE

Anaemia is common in patients with chronic conditions of inflammation, infection or malignancy and is reported to be the commonest side-effect of cancer and chemotherapy treatment.[28] The condition is frequently found in those with heart disease, rheumatoid arthritis and diabetes mellitus[29] and the presence of one or more of these additional problems places an extra burden on the health of patients already battling with a chronic condition.

Clues to aid the diagnosis

Any signs and symptoms are the same as for those of iron deficiency anaemia (*see* pp. 237–9).

Additional pointers

The presence of underlying infection, inflammation or neoplasm and/or chronic renal failure as the condition is more frequently found in association with one or more of these problems.[30]

Table 13.8 gives some diagnostic pointers to differentiating between iron deficiency anaemia and the anaemia of chronic disease.

TABLE 13.8 Differentiating between iron deficiency anaemia and anaemia of chronic disease

Anaemia type	Hb	Transferrin	Total iron binding capacity	Serum transfer receptor levels	Serum ferritin
Iron deficiency	Low	Elevated	High	High	Low
Anaemia of chronic disease	Low	Reduced	Low	Low to normal	Normal or raised

CLINICAL ALERT!

- The serum transferrin receptor is much less affected by inflammation than serum ferritin and is better able to distinguish anaemia of chronic disease from iron deficiency with elevated results seen in iron-deficiency anaemia and usually low to low-normal in anaemia of chronic disease.[31]
- Diagnosis may be hampered by coexisting blood loss, the effects of medications, or the presence of other conditions (such as thalassaemia) that can cause errors in haemoglobin synthesis.[32]

Pathophysiology

The pathophysiology is again highly complex. Disturbances of iron homeostasis develops, with an increased uptake and retention of iron within cells that leads to a diversion of iron from the circulation into storage sites of the reticuloendothelial system, with subsequent limited availability of iron and iron-restricted erythropoiesis.[32] The decreased availability of iron, and decreased levels of erythropoietin, are accompanied by a mild decrease in the lifespan of RBCs to 70–80 days (normally 120 days).[33] Any disease underlying anaemia of chronic disease can further affect erythropoiesis through the infiltration of tumour cells or of micro-organisms into bone marrow, which is seen in conditions such as HIV infection, hepatitis C, and malaria.[34]

Table 13.9 presents differential diagnoses for anaemia of chronic disease.

TABLE 13.9 Differential diagnoses

Cause	Additional pointers	When to consider
Medication induced	Risk of anaemia is increased with use of certain medications.	Increased risk in patients taking anti-retroviral therapy (HAART) for treatment of HIV or AIDS, in particular, the drug AZT.[35] Other medications that may contribute to anaemia include ACE inhibitors such as lisinopril, ARBs and certain anticonvulsants such as phenytoin.[36] Long-term use of aspirin and NSAIDs can cause significant bleeding from the digestive tract.[37]
Thalassaemia minor	Thalassemia minor is an inherited condition in which the affected person inherits a defective haemoglobin gene from one parent.[38]	The red cell distribution width (RDW) is usually elevated in iron deficiency anaemia but normal in thalassaemia.[39]

Treatment

Treatment is generally of the underlying cause where this is possible.

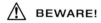
CLINICAL ALERT!

⚠ BEWARE!

- Oral iron is not recommended as the added iron can become free to nourish bacteria and cancer cells.[31]
- There is some indication that treatment of the anaemia of chronic disease with traditional iron therapy may worsen rather than improve clinical outcomes.[40]

Complications

In patients with CKD and diabetes, anaemia has been implicated as an independent risk factor for the development of CVD.[41]

CLINICAL ALERT!

⚠ BEWARE!

Patients with CKD and anaemia have double the risk of death from CVD and for those with a combination of anaemia, CKD and CVD the risk of death from CVD is tripled.[42]

Key messages

- Common in the elderly
- Associated with chronic comorbid health problems

- Symptoms same as those of iron deficiency anaemia
- Treatment of the underlying cause if possible rather than of the anaemia itself.

LEUKAEMIA

Leukaemia can occur in adults and children alike with acute and chronic leukaemias constituting about 2.5% of all newly diagnosed malignancies each year in the UK and resulting in the death of over 4000 people each year. [43] However, improved treatment and management has led to increased survival rates with 5-year survival rates for all types of childhood leukaemias rising from 33% to 79% between 1971 to 2000, and cure rates improving from 25% to 68% between 1971 and 1995.[44] In adults, estimates suggest a 5-year survival rate of about 40%, but with improvements in treatment the chances of surviving for 10 years or more are greater than ever.[45]

Classification of leukaemia
- Chronic myeloid leukaemia (CML)
- Acute myeloid leukaemia (AML)
- Chronic lymphocytic leukaemia (CLL)
- Acute lymphoblastic leukaemia (ALL).

CLINICAL ALERT!

- CML is most common in older people, with a slightly increased prevalence among males.[46]
- AML is the most common acute leukaemia in adults and although it can occur at any age the median age of onset is 70 years of age.[47]
- CLL is the most common type of leukaemia in the Western world, accounting for 40% of all leukaemias in individuals over the age of 65 years, with a median age of presentation between 65 and 70 years.[48]
- ALL is the most common cancer in children with a peak age of incidence occurring in 2–4 year olds, and 80% of cases are in this age group, becoming much rarer in adulthood.[49]

Clues to aid the diagnosis
See Table 13.10.

TABLE 13.10 Assisting diagnosis

Anaemia type	Symptoms	Additional information
CML	Tiredness Weight loss Bone pains Abdominal discomfort Night sweats	Up to half of patients with CML will be asymptomatic at the time of diagnosis; abnormality often detected on a routine blood test.[46]
AML	Fatigue and general weakness Frequent infections Breathlessness Bruising frequently Weight loss Fever	May present as a flu-like illness with non-specific and often vague symptoms.
CLL	Abdominal discomfort Anaemia Weight loss Frequent infections which are difficult to treat Swollen lymph glands	Again patient may be asymptomatic and abnormalities will be detected on a routine blood test.
ALL	Similar to those of acute myeloid leukaemia	May also have aching joints, swollen glands and bleeding from the gums or the nose.

CLINICAL ALERT!

⚠ BEWARE!

Leukaemia symptoms are often vague and non-specific, and in the early stages may resemble other common conditions or mimic flu symptoms.

Differentiating between the types of leukaemia

Table 13.11 shows variation in abnormalities on blood results.

TABLE 13.11 Variation in abnormalities on blood results

Leukaemia type	Blood results
CML	Elevated neutrophil and leucocyte count with low Hb, and raised platelets.[50]
AML	Characterised by anaemia and thrombocytopenia, but WCC may be high, normal or low.[51]
CLL	Neutrophil count may be normal or may decrease, but lymphocytes (B-cells) will increase, and platelets will be reduced.[52]
ALL	HB and neutrophil counts will be low but there will be large numbers of immature lymphocytes (lymphoblasts).[53]

Pathophysiology

The pathophysiology varies according to leukaemia type and is highly complex. A simplified explanation will therefore be given.

CML

This type tends to progress slowly and occurs in phases recognised as a chronic phase, an accelerated phase and a blastic phase.

- **Chronic phase**: During the initial chronic phase the patient may be asymptomatic and there are a few blast cells that are immature, abnormally large white blood cells, which can potentially block blood vessels, impeding oxygen supply to the tissues.[54]
- **Accelerated phase**: During the accelerated phase the number of blast cells is increasing with a reduced number of normal cells and during this phase the spleen may become enlarged.
- **Blastic phase**: More than 30% of cells in the blood or bone marrow are blast cells that may cause tumours outside of the bone marrow at other sites such as the bone or lymph nodes.[55]

AML

AML is characterised by an overproduction of immature white blood cells that circulate around the body via the bloodstream, but are unable to function correctly because of their immaturity, hence impeding the body's attempts to prevent or fight any infection.

CLL

CLL is usually a slow-growing type of leukaemia in which the lymphocytes are the cancerous cells. Abnormal cells invade the bloodstream, spreading to other parts of the body, although many patients may remain asymptomatic for several years before symptoms appear.

ALL

In acute lymphoblastic leukaemia large numbers of immature cells are produced that crowd the bone marrow, impeding production of normal blood cells. Because they are malformed they are ineffective in preventing or fighting infections. Abnormal cells multiply and divide rapidly so that this type of leukaemia usually progresses quickly if left untreated.

TABLE 13.12 Differential diagnoses

Leukaemia type	Differential diagnosis	Additional pointers	Consider if
CML	Essential thrombocytosis	Some patients are asymptomatic, others may experience vasomotor symptoms including headaches, visual disturbances, light-headedness, atypical chest pain, distal paraesthesias, and thrombotic or haemorrhagic disturbances.[56]	Platelet count is high. There may also be anaemia, leucocytosis and erythrocytosis.
	Myelodysplastic syndromes	May be asymptomatic in the early stages or may present with symptoms of shortness of breath, dizziness and tinnitus.[24]	Varying degrees of anaemia, neutropenia or thrombocytopenia.[20]
	Polycythaemia vera	Insidious onset with vague symptoms which can include headaches, dizziness, vertigo, tinnitus and visual disturbances.[58]	Blood results show an increased number of red cells and possibly increased platelets or white blood cells and elevated Hb and haematocrit levels.[57]
AML	Anaemia	*See* pp.237–9.	*See* pp.237–9.
	Aplastic anaemia	*See* p. 241. Onset often insidious with symptoms of anaemia, skin and mucosal haemorrhages and visual disturbances.[23]	RBC count, WCC and platelet levels may all be reduced.
	Bone marrow failure	Insidious onset with presenting symptoms of weakness and fatigue.	Possible anaemia with low reticulocyte and platelet counts, decreased neutrophils, eosinophils and basophils; decrease in monocytes.[20]
	Myelodysplastic syndrome	See above.	See above.
Chronic lymphocytic	Non-Hodgkin's lymphoma	May present with painless swelling in the groin, armpit or neck with symptoms of unexplained weight loss, intermittent fever and night sweats.	Blood results may show progressive anaemia, thrombocytopenia, leucopenia, and lymphocytosis.[59]
Acute lymphoblastic	Non-Hodgkin's lymphoma	See above.	See above.

CLINICAL ALERT!

All of the above require bone marrow biopsy to confirm the diagnosis; lymph node biopsy is also used to confirm non-Hodgkin's lymphoma.

Treatment

Treatment is with consultant guidance and depends on leukaemia type but may involve chemotherapy and radiotherapy.

Complications

All four types of leukaemia are associated with a weakened immune system that impedes the body's ability to fight invading organisms and makes the patient vulnerable to recurrent infections.

Key reminders

- Various types of leukaemia with all requiring bone marrow biopsy to confirm diagnosis
- Some types common in children, others more common in adults; blood results help determine type.

REFERENCES

1. Silver BJ. *Anaemia*. Cleveland Clinic Centre for Continuing Education. Available at: www. clevelandclinicmeded.com/medicalpubs/diseasemanagement/hematology-oncology/ anemia/ (accessed 4 March 2013).
2. Gasche C, Lomer MC, Cavill I, *et al*. Iron, anaemia, and inflammatory bowel diseases. *Gut*. 2004; **53**: 1190–7.
3. Goddard AF, James MW, McIntyre AS, *et al*. On behalf of the British Society for Gastroenterology. *Guidelines for the Management of Iron Deficiency Anaemia*. Available at: www.bsg.org.uk/pdf_word_docs/iron_def.pdf (accessed 4 March 2013).
4. Harper JL. *Iron Deficiency Anaemia*. Available at: http://emedicine.medscape.com/ article/202333-overview#a0104 (accessed 4 March 2013).
5. National Organisation for Rare Disorders, Inc. *Anaemias, Sideroblastic*. Available at: http:// icmmt.alere.com/kbase/nord/nord351.htm (accessed 19 August 2013).
6. Fairbanks VF. Laboratory testing for iron status. *Hosp Pract (Off Ed)*. 1991; **26**(Suppl. 3): S17–24.
7. Zhu A, Khaneshiro M, Kaunitz JD. Evaluation and treatment of iron deficiency anaemia: a gastroenterological perspective. *Dig Dis Sci*. 2010; **55**(3): 548–59.
8. Balay KS, Hawthorne KM, Hicks PD, *et al*. Orange but not apple juice enhances ferrous fumarate absorption in small children. *J Paediatr Gastroenterol Nutr*. 2010; **50**(5): 545–50.
9. Electronic Medicines Compendium. *Ferrous sulphate 200 mg*. Available at: www.medicines. org.uk/emc/medicine/26874/SPC#INTERACTIONS (accessed 2 May 2013).
10. Scholl TO. Iron status during pregnancy: setting the stage for mother and infant. *Am J Clin Nutr*. 2005; **81**(5): S1218–22.
11. University of Maryland Medical Centre. *Anaemia: complications*. Available at: www.umm. edu/patiented/articles/what_symptoms_of_anemia_000057_4.htm (accessed 7 March 2013).

12. Coats AJS. Anaemia and heart failure. *Heart.* 2004; **90**(9): 977–9.

13. Harper P, Littlewood T. Anaemia of cancer: impact on patient fatigue and long-term outcome. *Oncology.* 2005; **69**(Suppl. 2): 2–7.

14. Malizia RW, Baumann BM, Chansky ME, *et al.* Ambulatory dysfunction due to unrecognized pernicious anaemia. *J Emerg Med.* 2010; **38**(3): 302–7.

15. Clarke R, Grimley Evans J, Schneede J, *et al.* Vitamin B$_{12}$ and folate deficiency in later life. *Age & Ageing.* 2004; **33**(1): 34–41.

16. American Association for Clinical Chemistry. *Vitamin B12 Deficiency and Folate Deficiency.* Lab tests online. Available at: https://labtestsonline.org/understanding/conditions/vitaminb12/start/2 (accessed 19 March 2013).

17. Snow CF. Laboratory diagnosis of vitamin B$_{12}$ and folate deficiency: a guide for the primary care physician. *Arch Intern Med.* 1999; **159**: 1289–98.

18. Robert C, Brown DL. Vitamin B12 deficiency. *Am Fam Physician.* 2003; **67**(5): 979–86.

19. British Columbia Medical Association. *B12 Deficiency: investigation and management of vitamin B12 and folate deficiency.* Available at: www.bcguidelines.ca/pdf/cobalamin.pdf (accessed 10 March 2013).

20. Kouides PA, Bennett JM. Understanding myelodysplastic syndromes. *The Oncologist.* 1997; **2**(6): 389–401.

21. Montenegro J, Gonzalez O, Saracho R, *et al.* Changes in renal function in primary hypothyroidism. *Am J Kidney Dis.* 1996; **27**: 195–8.

22. Seiter K. *Multiple Myeloma.* Available at: http://emedicine.medscape.com/article/204369-workup#aw2aab6b5b2 (accessed 14 March 2013).

23. Marsh J, Ball SE, Cavanagh J, *et al.* Guidelines for the diagnosis and management of aplastic anaemia. *Brit J Haematol.* 2009; **147**: 43–7.

24. Simon S, Everitt H, van Dorp F. *Oxford Handbook of General Practice.* Oxford: Oxford University Press; 2010.

25. British National Formulary 2013. Available at: www.bnf.org/bnf/index.htm

26. Medical Disability Guidelines. *B12 Deficiency.* Available at: www.mdguidelines.com/vitamin-b12-deficiency (accessed 17 March 2013).

27. Dror DK, Allen LH. Effect of vitamin B12 deficiency on neurodevelopment in infants: current knowledge and possible mechanisms. *Nut Rev.* 2008; **66**(5): 250–5.

28. Caville I, Aueerbach M, Bailie GR. Iron and the anaemia of chronic disease: a review and strategic recommendations. *Curr Med Res Opin.* 2006; **22**(4): 731–7.

29. Lerma EV. *Anaemia of Chronic Disease and Renal Failure.* Available at: http://emedicine.medscape.com/article/1389854-overview#aw2aab6b4 (accessed 20 March 2012).

30. Fitzsimons EJ, Brock JH. The anaemia of chronic disease. *BMJ.* 2001; **322**(7290): 811–12.

31. Iron Disorders Institute. *Anaemia of Chronic Disease.* Available at: www.irondisorders.org/anemia-of-chronic-disease (accessed 17 March 2012).

32. Weiss G, Goodnough LT. Anaemia of chronic disease. *N Engl J Med.* 2005; **352**: 1011–23.

33. Besarab A, Levin A. Defining a renal anaemia management period. *Am J Kidney Dis.* 2000; **36**(Suppl. 3): S13–23.

34. Gordeuk VR, Delanghe JR, Langlois MR, *et al.* Iron status and the outcome of HIV infection: an overview. *J Clin Virol.* 2001; **20**: 111–15.

35. University of Maryland Medical Centre. *Anaemia Causes.* Available at: www.umm.edu/patiented/articles/who_becomes_anemic_000057_2.htm (accessed 24 March 2013).

36. Cleveland Clinic. *Aging and Anaemia.* Available at: http://my.clevelandclinic.org/disorders/anemia/hic_aging_and_anemia.aspx (accessed 22 March 2012).

37. Iron Disorders Institute. *Iron out of Balance in the Elderly.* Available at: www.irondisorders.org/elderly (accessed 17 July 2013).

38. Medline Plus. *Thalassaemia*. Available at: www.nlm.nih.gov/medlineplus/ency/article/000587.htm (accessed 25 March 2012).

39. Eivazi-Ziaei J, Dastgiri S, Pourebrahim S, *et al*. Usefulness of red blood cell flags in diagnosing and differentiating thalassemia trait from iron-deficiency anaemia. *Haematology*. 2008; **13**(4): 253–6.

40. Zarychanski R, Houston DS. Anaemia of chronic disease: a harmful disorder or an adaptive, beneficial response? *CMAJ*. 2008; **179**(4): 333–7.

41. Vlagopoulos PT, Tighiouart H, Weiner DE, *et al*. Anaemia as a risk factor for cardiovascular disease and all-cause mortality in diabetes: the impact of chronic kidney disease. *J Am Soc Nephrol*. 2005; **16**: 3403–10.

42. Silverberg D, Wexler D, Blum M, *et al*. The cardio-renal anaemia syndrome: does it exist? *Nephrol Dial Transplant*. 2003; **18**(Suppl. 8): Sviii, 7–12.

43. Bhayat F, Das-Gupta E, Smith C, *et al*. The incidence and mortality from leukaemias in the UK: a general population based study. *BMC Cancer*. 2009; **9**: 252.

44. Shah A, Stiller CA, Kenward MG, *et al*. Childhood leukaemia: long-term excess mortality and the proportion 'cured'. *Br J Cancer*. 2008; **99**(1): 219–23.

45. Cancer Research UK. *Cancer Stats Key Facts: leukaemia*. Available at: www.cancerresearchuk.org/cancer-info/cancerstats/keyfacts/leukaemia-key-facts/uk-leukaemia-statistics (accessed 20 February 2013).

46. Cancer Research UK. *Chronic Myeloid Leukaemia: risks and causes*. Available at: www.cancerresearchuk.org/cancer-help/type/cml/about/chronic-myeloid-leukaemia-risks-and-causes (accessed 22 February 2013).

47. Estey E, Dohner H. Acute myeloid leukaemia. *Lancet*. 2006; **368**(9550): 1894–907.

48. BJH guideline. Guidelines on the diagnosis and management of chronic lymphocytic leukaemia. *Brit J Haematol*. 2004; **125**: 294–317.

49. Redaelli A, Laskin BL, Stephens JM, *et al*. A systematic literature review of the clinical and epidemiological burden of acute lymphoblastic leukaemia (ALL). *Eur J Cancer Care*. 2005; **14**(1): 53.

50. Sobecks RM, Theil K. *Chronic Leukaemias*. Available at: www.clevelandclinicmeded.com/medicalpubs/diseasemanagement/hematology-oncology/chronic-leukemias/ (accessed 22 February 2013).

51. Seiter K. *Acute Myelogenous Leukaemia*. Available at: http://emedicine.medscape.com/article/197802-workup#aw2aab6b5b2 (accessed 25 May 2013).

52. Chronic Lymphocytic Leukaemia Support Association. *Understanding your Blood Results*. Available at: www.cllsupport.org.uk/uybresults.htm (accessed 21 February 2013).

53. Seiter K. *Acute Lymphoblastic Leukaemia*. Available at: http://emedicine.medscape.com/article/207631-overview (accessed 28 May 2013).

54. American Cancer Society. *Leukemia: Chronic Myeloid (Myelogenous)*. Available at: www.cancer.org/cancer/leukemia-chronicmyeloidcml/detailedguide/index (accessed 27 May 2013).

55. Cancer Research UK. *Staging for Acute Myeloid Leukaemia*. Available at: www.cancerresearchuk.org/cancer-help/type/cml/treatment/staging-for-chronic-myeloid-leukaemia#cml (accessed 22 February 2013).

56. Briere JB. *Essential Thrombocytopaenia*. Available at: www.ojrd.com/content/2/1/3 (accessed 24 February 2013).

57. Kumar P, Clark M. *Clinical Medicine*. 8th ed. London: Elsevier; 2009.

58. Mayo Foundation for Medical Education and Research (MMFER). *Polycythaemia Vera*. Available at: www.mayoclinic.com/health/polycythemia-vera/DS00919/DSECTION=tests-and-diagnosis (accessed 22 February 2013).

59. Zelenetz AD, Abramson JS, Advani RH, *et al.* Non Hodgkin's lymphomas. *J Natl Comp Can Netw.* 2011; **9**: 484–560.

CHAPTER 14

The elderly: common infections

ILLNESSES COVERED IN THIS CHAPTER

- UTI
- Pneumonia
- Influenza.

INTRODUCTION

With improvements in healthcare and medical treatments the number of people living to 65 years and over is rising, and it is predicted that by 2033 a quarter of the population will fall into this age group, with more than a fifth reaching the age of 85 years or older.[1] Advancing age brings with it a higher risk of illness, which may be either acute or chronic, and older adults' assessment and diagnosis presents a challenge for several reasons. Problems such as impaired mobility, falls and incontinence are easy to recognise; however, when these problems occur in addition to an infectious disease, symptoms are frequently more difficult to assess and presenting features may be atypical in the older adult. In addition to the normal signs of ageing, such as memory loss, poor mobility and poor sleep patterns, the development of an acute illness in older adults can often be further complicated by the presence of other known comorbid health problems or the intake of multiple medications. Although treatment and management is frequently the same irrespective of the age of the person, presentation is often not.

INFECTIOUS DISEASES IN THE ELDERLY

Infectious diseases account for one third of all deaths in people aged 65 and over[2] and some of the most common infections reported in the elderly population are UTIs, pneumonia and influenza. The signs and symptoms of these common conditions vary considerably between older and younger persons (*see* Table 14.1 and Table 14.4, pp. 255, 259).

Unusual symptoms, such as incontinence, fatigue and poorer appetite may be attributed by the patient to growing older, which can result in failure to report new symptoms during the early stages of the disease. This may potentially lead to a delay in diagnosis that can then result in potentially serious consequences, most importantly, increased severity putting the patient at an increased risk of more serious outcomes and in some cases death.[3]

REDUCED IMMUNE RESPONSE AND IMPAIRED ABILITY TO FIGHT DISEASE

One of the main reasons for the increase in infections observed in the elderly is believed to be a process termed immunosenescence, which is a term used to describe the immune system's diminished function with age,[4] and one which leads to an impaired response to infection.

CLINICAL ALERT!

⚠ **BEWARE!**

- Up to 50% of older infected patients will not develop a total WBC outside the normal range, further confusing the clinical picture once assessment and investigations begin.[5]
- An ageing and poorly functioning immune system, in association with poor nutritional intake and other age-related physiological changes in the body, increases the susceptibility to infections.
- A poorly functioning immune system will result in an inability to contain the infection, which increases the risk of increased disease severity and poorer outcomes.
- Ageing causes the defence mechanisms of the airways to decrease, with reduced efficiency of the mucociliary clearance system and a decrease in the efficacy of the cough reflex,[6] making the older person more susceptible to airborne infections that invade via the respiratory route.

COMORBID ILLNESSES

Normal host defences are further compromised in the elderly patient where other comorbid health problems also exist, such as COPD, diabetes and CHD, which are often found in this age group. In some cases, these conditions can worsen during infection, adding another dimension to the illness. Patients with diabetes have an increased susceptibility to various types of infections and in those with microvascular and macrovascular complications there is an additional resultant poor tissue perfusion that further increases the risk of infection.[7] Impairment of the normal defence mechanisms may lead to delayed phagocytosis and delayed clearance of any invading bacteria.[3]

URINARY TRACT INFECTION (UTI)

UTI in older persons can be symptomatic or asymptomatic. Both types are common in the elderly, their prevalence increasing with older age, but occurring more frequently in females than males.

Asymptomatic bacteriuria

Asymptomatic bacteriuria is characterised by the presence of a significant quantity of bacteria in a urine specimen from a person without symptoms or signs of a UTI.[8] Statistics suggest that bacteriuria affects approximately 20% of people aged 65–75, rising to 20%–50% in women aged 80 and over, while prevalence in men is estimated to be approximately 3% at age 65–70, rising to around 20% at age 80 and above.[9]

> **CLINICAL ALERT!**

One of the commonest organisms found in asymptomatic bacteriuria is E. Coli,[10] which generally lives in the GI tract of healthy persons.

Clues to aid the diagnosis

> **CLINICAL ALERT!**

 BEWARE OF NON-SPECIFIC SYMPTOMS!

In the presence of any mental impairment, it may be the patient's carer or family reporting symptoms such as falls, immobility and confusion. The lower urinary tract symptoms usually associated with a UTI may be absent or altered in older patients, presenting instead with mental changes, nausea or vomiting, and possible abdominal pain.

Table 14.1 shows differences in the presentation between older and younger people.

TABLE 14.1 Presentation differences between older and younger people

Presentation in younger adults	Presentation in older adults
Dysuria	Incontinence
Frequency	Confusion
Urgency	Anorexia
Lower abdominal pain	Falls
Loin pain	Nausea and vomiting

Pathophysiology

In the elderly, the female to male ratio of incidence of UTI narrows. This is a result of elderly men with bladder outlet obstruction frequently caused by benign prostatic hyperplasia, which is thought to predispose to the development of UTIs.[11] In healthy individuals urine is sterile, and UTIs occur because of invasion of the bladder by an unwanted organism. Any condition that allows stagnation of urine in the bladder can lead to chronic bacteriuria, such as neurogenic bladder, an obstruction, or the presence of a urinary catheter.[5] Infection occurs when organisms have entered the urethra and spread upwards to the bladder. Elderly females are thought to be at an increased risk of UTI because of hormonal changes affecting the vaginal flora. In younger women, a low pH is maintained in the vagina, which serves to prevent bacterial invasion and this is achieved by the action of oestrogen, which stimulates colonisation of the vagina by lactobacilli. In post-menopausal women, this function becomes impaired when the production of oestrogen ceases. Oestrogen deficiency and subsequent disappearance of lactobacilli leads to increased colonisation of the vagina by micro-organisms and it is thought that this increased colonisation by enteric bacteria may be at least partly responsible for the increased frequency of UTIs in older women.[12]

Age-specific predisposing factors

- In males an enlarged prostate is associated with a higher risk of UTI.
- In females an increase in vaginal pH, vaginal atrophy caused by oestrogen depletion after the menopause, and incomplete emptying of the bladder all have an impact on predisposition to UTIs.
- Indwelling catheters can also be a source of infection as they can become colonised with bacteria. Urethral catheters encourage organisms into the bladder and promote colonisation by providing a surface for bacterial adhesion and causing mucosal irritation.[13]

TABLE 14.2 Differential diagnoses

Condition	Additional information
Pyelonephritis	Consider as a possibility when there is acute pain in the lower abdominal and loin region.
Cystitis	Urine culture shows no bacteriuria.
Atrophic vaginitis	Vaginal atrophy and women with prolapsed uterus or bladder may have poor emptying of the bladder that predisposes to cystitis.
Drug-induced cystitis	Can occur as a result of treatment with cyclophosphamide, or allopurinol.[14]
Urological cancer	Urgent referral required for painless macroscopic haematuria or unexplained microscopic haematuria.

Treatment

- Local guidelines may suggest treatment options but generally a 3-day course of trimethoprim is recommended for women and a 7-day course for men.[15]
- An alternative is nitrofurantoin and may be suggested by laboratory if resistance to trimethoprim is found when analysing the urine sample.

Prescribing tips

Nitrofurantoin is not recommended in those with renal impairment because of problems achieving appropriate concentrations in the urine.[16]

 CLINICAL ALERT!

 BEWARE!

- In the presence of asymptomatic infections, controversy exists as to whether treatment should be prescribed or not. Ultimately, this decision lies with the clinician.
- As asymptomatic bacteriuria is common, caution is needed when treating the elderly as a result of evidence that treatment may be more harmful than beneficial with an increased risk of adverse effects in the elderly.[17]
- Urine culture provides useful information as it helps to identify the causative organism and suggest a suitable antibiotic. In patients with atypical symptoms, a positive urinary nitrate test is an immediate and reliable indicator of the presence of UTIs with 100% specificity and 90% sensitivity.[18]
- First infections are typically caused by E. coli and are not usually caused by resistant strains; however, recurrent infections are more likely to be caused by organisms with increased resistance.[17]

Complications

 BEWARE!

- In diabetic patients UTIs can lead to diabetic complications such as ketoacidosis.[19]
- Progression to more serious pyelonephritis is possible.
- UTI leading to kidney infection can cause permanent damage, including scarring of the kidneys and reduced renal function.[20]
- Rarely an acute kidney infection may lead to septicaemia, increasing mortality risk.

Prevention of UTIs

- Adequate fluid intake is important and adults should consume between six and eight glasses of fluid a day.
- Fluid intake may need to be more closely monitored in patients with dementia and those with mobility problems who may be at a greater risk of dehydration.
- Good hygiene is important to reduce the risk of transfer of bacteria after defaecation.
- Constipation should be avoided.

Key reminders

- May be symptomatic or asymptomatic
- Presentation may be entirely different to that seen in younger adults, with mental confusion and falls common symptoms
- Treating asymptomatic bacteriuria is controversial as treatment may cause more problems in terms of adverse drug reactions
- Where an MSU can be obtained the causative organism, if identified will guide treatment options.

PNEUMONIA

Pneumonia can affect people of any age, and in the US pneumonia and influenza combined are the sixth leading causes of death;[2] and in the UK alone, estimates indicate that approximately 90% of pneumonia-related deaths occur in people over the age of 65. In older people the incidence of community-acquired pneumonia (CAP) is almost four times higher than the number of cases seen in younger people, increasing stepwise with every decade, culminating in a 30% higher mortality rate in the elderly.[3] Death rates may rise even higher among patients who contract pneumonia in healthcare facilities. This has been attributed to the presence of comorbidities, the development of hypotension, worsening hypoxaemia, urinary incontinence of recent onset, and apyrexia.[21]

CLINICAL ALERT!

- *Streptococcus pneumoniae* is by far the predominant pathogen isolated in hospital-based studies of elderly patients with CAP, accounting for up to 58% of cases, with *Haemophilus influenzae* also a frequently reported pathogen.[22]
- Pneumonia caused by streptococcal pneumonia tends to occur more frequently in patients with coexisting lung disease, liver disorders, or in alcohol abusers.[23]

Predisposing factors

CLINICAL ALERT!

⚠ BEWARE!

- Comorbidity, UTI and influenza are reported to be the main predisposing factors.
- Those with a malignant disease are also thought to be at greater risk.
- Smoking and alcohol abuse are common risk factors for the development of pneumonia in elderly patients.[6]
- Further possible associations thought to further increase risk are the mental status of the person, physical activity levels and the presence of depression.[24]

Age-specific predisposing factors

Susceptibility to pneumonia increases with increasing age and this is a result of decreased mucociliary clearance, poorer alveolar ventilation, and a diminished cough reflex.[2]

TABLE 14.3 Age-related changes and their effects

Problem	Effect	Cause
Impaired ability to clear the airways of foreign bodies.	Vulnerability to any invading organisms.	Destruction and inefficient functioning of the cilia, particularly in smokers and ex-smokers.
Weaker muscles and loss of the elasticity of the alveoli and muscles.	Impaired ventilation adds to the risk of contracting respiratory infections.	Age-related changes.
Diminished cough reflex.	Inability to expel any irritant invading organisms.	Age-related changes.

CLINICAL ALERT!

 BEWARE!

Signs and symptoms are often non-specific.

Table 14.4 shows a comparison between classic symptoms seen in younger subjects and those seen in the elderly that can mimic a whole host of other conditions and make assessment and diagnosis difficult.

TABLE 14.4 Classic symptoms seen in younger subjects and the elderly

Younger people	Elderly
Rapid onset of symptoms	Insidious onset
Fever	Less productive cough
Productive cough	Mental impairment and confusion
Breathlessness	Anorexia and malaise
Rusty-coloured sputum	Possible absence of fever

Pathophysiology

For pathophysiology *see* p. 27.

Differential diagnosis

⚠ **BEWARE!**

- Lung cancer (*see* p. 24).
- Exacerbation of COPD (*see* pp. 22–5).
- PE (*see* p. 20).

CLINICAL ALERT!

There are also some medications which can induce lung disease. *See* Table 14.5.

TABLE 14.5 Drugs which can cause lung disease

Cytotoxic drugs
NSAIDs
Sulphonamides
Amiodarone
Methotrexate

Treatment

Treatment is the same as for younger subjects, but care should be taken in relation to risk of interactions with other medications, the greater risk of side-effects and risk of *C. difficile* with antibiotic use (*see* pp. 297–8).

The decision to treat at home or refer to hospital is based on the severity of the patient's symptoms. Any patient presenting with mental confusion, rapid respiratory rate, low blood pressure and deterioration of other comorbid illnesses will require hospital treatment, as these features are associated with a poorer prognosis in elderly patients.[25]

Antibiotic choices

Guidance suggests amoxicillin or in combination with clarithromycin for more severe infections or clarithromycin or doxycycline used alone if allergic to penicillin for 7 days.[26]

Complications

These include:

- pleural effusion
- empyema
- respiratory failure
- lung abscess
- invasive pneumococcal disease includes septicaemia and meningitis, and these complications are more likely to occur in those with decreased immune

function either from disease or drugs, in those with chronic heart or lung diseases, smokers and in those with liver or renal diseases.[27]

CLINICAL ALERT!

Empyema is associated with significant morbidity rates.[28]

Key reminders
- Although pneumonia deaths can occur at any age, the majority occur in the over 65 age group.
- Risk of death increases with advanced age.
- Again, symptoms may differ from those seen in younger adults.
- Risk of developing pneumonia is more likely in those with comorbidities such as COPD.
- Vaccination is available to all over the age of 65 and younger people with comorbidities.

INFLUENZA

Influenza in the elderly is a potentially life-threatening illness and carries a high mortality rate, with estimates indicating that the mortality rate for persons aged 85 years or older is 16 times greater than that of persons aged 65 to 69 years of age.[29] Although there is little difference in the signs and symptoms of influenza across the ages, the condition is often more serious in the elderly as it carries the potential to worsen existing medical conditions such as asthma, chronic lung disease and HF.

Age-specific signs and symptoms

In the elderly the fever response is often blunted even in the presence of bacteraemia.[30] Although the reasons for this absence are not clearly understood, several theories have been suggested. It is thought possible that thermoregulatory responses are diminished, and there may be abnormalities in both the production of and response to endogenous pyrogens, and a reduced response by the hypothalamus to any invading organism.[31]

Pathophysiology

Pathophysiology of influenza has been discussed in Chapter 4 (*see* p. 15).

Predisposing factors

The predisposing factors for influenza are the same as for pneumonia and in the elderly comorbid illnesses are thought to have an influence on the risk of contracting the disease, particularly diabetes, chronic lung diseases, renal disease, CHD and those who are immunocompromised.

Differential diagnosis

⚠ BEWARE OF

- The common cold (*see* pp. 14–15)
- Pneumonia (*see* pp. 25–8)
- Acute or chronic bronchitis (*see* pp. 27–8).

Treatment

General self-help measures to ease symptoms include advice to increase fluid intake, stay at home, take regular analgesia and eat a light diet. Antiviral drugs are available, but adverse effects are more prominent in the elderly.[32]

Complications

The commonest complications include:

- pneumonia (viral or secondary bacterial)
- exacerbation of COPD or other chronic lung diseases
- exacerbation of underlying heart problems, such as HF and/or IHD.

CLINICAL ALERT!

⚠ BEWARE!

- Recovery time may be longer, with symptoms lasting for many weeks because of the body's reduced ability to fight infection. This increases the risk of developing the complications shown above.
- Elderly current and ex-smokers have been found to have higher mortality rates than non-smokers.[33]
- Infection with *Staphylococcus aureus*, including methicillin-resistant strains, is an important cause of secondary bacterial pneumonia with high mortality rates.[34]

Key reminders

- Presentation of some infections may be unusual and vague.
- A change in mental capacity is a common finding.
- Non-specific symptoms such as anorexia or nausea may be mistaken for a variety of other diseases.
- Symptoms may be complicated by other comorbid conditions.
- Infections can cause worsening of comorbid conditions.

REFERENCES

1. Cumisky A. *Consultation Skills: consulting with elderly patients.* Available at: www.gponline. com/Education/article/1013804/Consultation-skills---Consulting (accessed 2 April 2013).
2. Mouton CP, Bazaldua OV, Pierce B, *et al.* Common infections in older adults. *Am Fam Physician.* 2001; **63**(2): 257–69.
3. Bellmann-Weiler R, Weiss G. Pitfalls in the diagnosis and therapy of infections in elderly patients. *Gerontology.* 2009; **55**(3): 241–9.
4. McElhaney JE. Overcoming the challenges of immunosenescence in the prevention of acute respiratory illness in older people. *Conn Med.* 2003; **67**: 469–74.
5. Koronkowski MJ. *Infectious Diseases and Host Response in Older Persons.* Available at: www. uic.edu/classes/pmpr/pmpr652/Final/Koronkowski/infect.html (accessed 9 April 2013).
6. Pejčić T, Ivanka Đorđević I, Stanković I. Prognostic mortality factors of community acquired pneumonia in the elderly. *Scientific J Fac of Med in Niš.* 2011; **28**(2): 71–6.
7. Khardora R. *Infection in Patients with Diabetes Mellitus.* Available at: http://emedicine. medscape.com/article/2122072-overview (accessed 20 April 2013).
8. Rubin RH, Shapiro ED, Andriole VT, *et al.* Evaluation of new anti-infective drugs for the treatment of urinary tract infection. *Clin Inf Dis.* 1992; **15**(Suppl. 1): S216–27.
9. Gray RP, Malone–Lee J. Review: urinary tract infection in elderly people: time to review management? *Age and Ageing.* 1995; **24**(4): 341–5.
10. Jurivich DA, Webster JR. *Infectious Diseases.* Available at: www.galter.northwestern.edu/ geriatrics/chapters/infectious_diseases.cfm (accessed 10 April 2013).
11. Lieber MM, Jacobsen SJ, Roberts RO, *et al.* Prostate volume and prostate-specific antigen in the absence of prostate cancer: a review of the relationship and prediction of long-term outcomes. *Prostate.* 2001; **49**: 208–12.
12. Staykova S. *Urinary Tract Infections in Geriatric Patients.* Available at: www.webmedcentral. com/article_view/3968 (accessed 30 September 2013).
13. Vergidis P, Patel R. Novel approaches to the diagnosis, prevention, and treatment of medical device-associated infections. *Infect Dis Clin North Am.* 2012; **26**(1): 73–86.
14. Bramble FJ, Morley R. Drug induced cystitis: the need for vigilance. *Br J Urology.* 1997; **79**: 3–7.
15. Beveridge LA, Davey PG, Phillips G, *et al.* Optimal management of urinary tract infections in older people. *Clin Inter Aging.* 2011; **6**: 173–80.
16. Scottish Intercollegiate Guidelines Network. *Management of Suspected Bacterial Urinary Tract Infection in Adults: a national clinical guideline. SIGN guideline 88.* Edinburgh: SIGN; updated July 2012. Available at: www.sign.ac.uk/pdf/sign88.pdf
17. Nicolle L. Urinary tract pathogens in complicated infection and in elderly individuals. *J Inf Dis.* 2001; **183**(Suppl. 1): S5–8.
18. Evans PJ, Leaker BR, McNabb WR, *et al.* Accuracy of reagent strips for urinary tract infection in the elderly. *J Roy Soc Med.* 1991; **84**: 558–9.
19. Nicolle LE. Update in adult urinary tract infection. *Curr Infect Dis Rep.* 2011; **13**(6): 552–60.
20. National Kidney and Urologic Diseases Information Clearinghouse (NKUDIC). *Urinary Tract Infection in Adults.* Available at: http://kidney.niddk.nih.gov/kudiseases/pubs/ utiadult/#prevention (accessed 1 October 2013).
21. El Sohl AA, Sikka P, Rasmadan F, *et al.* Aetiology of severe pneumonia in the very elderly. *Am J Resp Crit Care Med.* 2001; **163**: 645–51.
22. Lim WS, Macfarlane JT. A prospective comparison of nursing home acquired pneumonia with community acquired pneumonia. *Eur Respir J.* 2001; **18**: 362–8.

23. Ruiz M, Ewig S, Torres A, *et al.* Severe community acquired pneumonia. Risk factors and follow-up epidemiology. *Am J Respir Crit Care Med.* 1999; **160**: 923–9.

24. Kostka T, Praczko K. Interrelationship between physical activity, symptomology of upper respiratory tract infections and depression in elderly people. *Gerontology.* 2007; **53**: 187–93.

25. Seppa Y, Bloigu A, Honkanen PO, *et al.* Severity assessment of lower respiratory tract infection in elderly patients in primary care. *Arch Intern Med.* 2001; **161**: 2709–13.

26. British National Formulary 2013. Available at: www.bnf.org/bnf/index.htm

27. Centres for Disease Control and Prevention. *Pneumococcal Disease.* Available at: www.cdc.gov/vaccines/pubs/pinkbook/downloads/pneumo.pdf (accessed 9 August 2013).

28. Reynolds JH, McDonald G, Alton H. Pneumonia in the immunocompetent patient. *Brit J of Radiology.* 2010; **83**: 998–1009.

29. Thompson WW, Shay DK, Weintraub E, *et al.* Influenza-associated hospitalizations in the United States. *JAMA.* 2004; **292**: 1333–40.

30. Werner H, Kuntsche J. Infection in the elderly: what is different? *Gerontol Geriatr.* 2000; **33**(5): 350–6.

31. Norman DC. Fever in the elderly. *Clin Inf Dis.* 2000; **31**: 148–51.

32. Nicholson KG. Use of antiviral in influenza in the elderly: prophylaxis and therapy. *Gerontology.* 1996; **42**(5): 280–9.

33. Wong CM, Yang L, Chan KP, *et al. Cigarette Smoking as a Risk Factor for Influenza-associated Mortality: evidence from an elderly cohort.* Available at: www.ncbi.nlm.nih.gov/pubmed/22813463 (accessed 19 July 2013).

34. Rothberg MB, Haessler SD, Brown RB. Complications of viral influenza. *Am J Med.* 2008; **121**: 258–64.

CHAPTER 15

Understanding blood results

TOPICS COVERED IN THE CHAPTER

- FBC
- U&Es
- LFTs
- TFTs
- CRP and ESR.

THE FULL BLOOD COUNT (FBC)

An FBC is requested for a number of reasons and is useful both as a diagnostic tool and for monitoring of certain conditions. Abnormal parameters may in some instances resolve without intervention or treatment.

Measurements and normal values

Table 15.1 shows the normal values.

TABLE 15.1 FBC normal values

Parameter	Value in males	Value in females
Hb	13.5–18.0 g/dL	11.5–16.0 g/dL
WCC (total)	4.00–11.00 × 10^9/L	4.00–11.00 × 10^9/L
Platelets	150–400 × 10^9/L	150–400 × 10^9/L
MCV	78–100 fL	78–100 fL
MCH	27.0–32.0 pg	27.0–32.0 pg
RCC	4.5–6.5 × 10^{12}/dL	3.8–5.8 × 10^{12}/dL
PCV	0.40–0.52 L/L	0.37–0.47 L/L
MCHC	31.0–37.0 g/dL	31.0–37.0 g/dL

(continued)

Parameter	Value in males	Value in females
RDW	11.5–15.0 fL	11.5–15.0 fL
Neutrophils	$2.0–7.5 \times 10^9$/L	$2.0–7.5 \times 10^9$/L
Lymphocytes	$1.0–4.5 \times 10^9$/L	$1.0–4.5 \times 10^9$/L
Monocytes	$0.2–0.8 \times 10^9$/L	$0.2–0.8 \times 10^9$/L
Eosinophils	$0.04–0.40 \times 10^9$/L	$0.04–0.40 \times 10^9$/L
Basophils	$< 0.1 \times 10^9$/L	$< 0.1 \times 10^9$/L

There is a slight difference in values for males and females. The normal range represents the predicted values for 95% of the population, with the remaining 5% falling outside of the 'normal range'. Care is needed when assessing those who fall into this category as they may also be normal. One example is the patient who has had a splenectomy where transient elevations of the WCC and platelet count (PC) are normal physiologic responses[1] but may easily be misinterpreted. Normal ranges should be regarded as a guide, and any abnormalities should always be considered as part of a complete picture.

CLINICAL ALERT!

⚠ BEWARE!

There are instances when results appear abnormal but when considered alongside medical history they are acceptable for that particular patient. One example of this would be a raised lymphocyte count following splenectomy, which would appear abnormal when evaluating the patient's results but considered normal for the patient in those circumstances.

Understanding the components and abnormal values
Hb

Haemoglobin is a protein that forms part of the red blood cell and is measured in grams per decilitre (g/dL). Its primary function is to transport oxygen from the lungs to the cells and tissues of the body, and to carry carbon dioxide back to the lungs so that it can be exhaled. There are many causes of abnormal values and where abnormalities are only slightly outside of the normal range, the patient may be asymptomatic and no treatment will be required. When interpreting the results it is important to consider the values alongside one another, which will be explained later in the chapter.

Assessing HB values alongside MCV, MCH and MCHC values

MCH, MCHC and MCV form part of the FBC and are an indication of the size of the cells and the concentration of Hb, and assessment of these parameters can be used to categorise and differentiate between anaemia types.

MCV

MCV gives an indication of the average volume of red cells in a specimen and is elevated or reduced in accordance with the size of the red cell. Low MCV indicates a small average RBC size (microcytic), normal MCV indicates normal average RBC size (normocytic), while high MCV indicates a large average RBC size (macrocytic).[2]

⚠ **BEWARE!**

MCV is particularly difficult to interpret in the elderly and can be misinterpreted because although microcytosis occurs in iron deficiency anaemia, microcytosis is a late finding and typically occurs only after chronic iron deficiency, leading to an Hb value of less than $10\,g/dL$[3], while macrocytosis (raised MCV) can be caused by alcoholism, vitamin B_{12} and folate deficiencies, certain medications, hypothyroidism, liver disease, and primary bone marrow dysplasias.[4]

MCH

MCH is a calculation of the average amount of oxygen-carrying haemoglobin inside a red blood cell.[5] In general, MCH and MCV values usually follow a similar pattern in that when the MCV is raised so is MCH, or alternatively low MCV is mimicked by a low MCH.

MCHC

MCHC provides a measure of the average concentration of haemoglobin inside red blood cells. When this value is reduced (hypochromia) it reflects abnormally diluted haemoglobin inside the cell, which may be a finding in iron deficiency anaemia, or thalassaemia, suggesting abnormally concentrated haemoglobin within red cells, seen in people with artificial heart valves, or plaques in the blood vessels from high cholesterol, or spherocytosis.[6]

PCV (HAEMATOCRIT)

Haematocrit (or PCV) indicates the percentage of RBCs in a volume of whole blood.[7] There are many causes of both elevated and reduced levels, which are shown in Table 15.2.

TABLE 15.2 Causes of elevated and reduced PCV levels

Elevated PCV	Reduced PCV
Severe burns	Leukaemia
Polycythaemia	Liver disease
Severe dehydration	Hyperthyroidism
Erythrocytosis	Elderly
Males	Females
Severe shock	Pregnancy
Severe diarrhoea	Multiple myeloma

RDW

RDW is a red blood cell parameter that measures variability of red cell volume/size[2] and is therefore indicative of the size and shape of red cells. Increased levels are found in certain anaemias where there is variation in cell size and shape. This parameter has also been shown to be an independent predictor of mortality in patients with HF and CHD, with increased mortality risk found among subjects with a high RDW regardless of Hb levels and anaemia status.[8]

RBC

These cells are produced by the bone marrow and the RBC count is a measure of the number of red cells per litre of blood.[9] Defective functioning of the bone marrow will result in low values that may occur in the presence of iron deficiency or blood loss, or abnormal destruction of red blood cells, while high values can be found in association with the presence of lung conditions such as COPD, dehydration and kidney disease.[10]

PLATELETS

Platelets are the smallest of all the blood cells and play an important role in the clotting process. When bleeding occurs platelets act to form a plug at the site, which they achieve by swelling and clumping together. Low platelet counts can occur with a number of diseases, and common causes include infections (including HIV), drugs (frequently chemotherapeutic agents), alcohol, vitamin deficiencies (e.g. folate, vitamin B_{12}), marrow infiltration by tumours, or bone marrow failure.[11] Conditions where bone marrow function is defective can lead to overproduction of platelets, which will give rise to elevated platelet counts; this can occur as a result of advanced or metastatic malignancy.[12]

BEWARE!

Excessive numbers of platelets may cause clot formation inside blood vessels, potentially leading to a DVT or embolism.

Other measurements

Serum ferritin

Ferritin is a protein found within cells and is responsible for storing iron for later use; the serum ferritin level is therefore directly related to the amount of iron stored in the body.[13] Ferritin levels are a reflection of total iron stores. However, its value when measuring iron stores is limited by the fact that it is an acute-phase protein so levels will increase in situations where there is acute or chronic inflammation,[14] therefore making evaluation difficult where inflammatory conditions are present. Ferritin levels are low in long-term iron deficiency, and are useful for assessing patients with suspected iron deficiency.[15] Levels are also commonly raised with excess alcohol intake and obesity, and raised levels are often seen in obese patients with type-2 diabetes, hypertriglyceridaemia or fatty liver.[16]

- Subnormal ferritin levels can be detected when iron stores are exhausted but before the serum iron level is affected; levels are therefore a sensitive indicator of early iron deficiency.[17]
- Serum ferritin levels are raised in inflammatory conditions such as rheumatoid arthritis and are also raised in infection and malignancy.[18]

Total iron binding capacity (TIBC)

TIBC indicates the maximum amount of iron needed to saturate plasma or serum transferrin (TRF), which is the primary iron-transport protein.[19] High TIBC usually indicates iron deficiency, while a low TIBC may occur if there is an excess of stored iron (haemochromatosis), which may occur as a result of infection, chronic disease, malnutrition, cirrhosis or nephrotic syndrome (a kidney disease that causes loss of protein in urine).[20]

Transferrin (TRF)

Transferrin is a transport protein and saturation levels reflect the ratio of serum iron to total iron-binding capacity, and measurements are an indication of how much of the TRF that is available to bind is actually bound to iron (e.g. 30% means that 30% of free iron is being carried by TRF).[21] When serum iron concentrations fall below the normal level, TRF levels rise.

⚠ **BEWARE!**

- A subnormal iron level in association with high TRF levels is highly suggestive of iron deficiency.[17]
- TRF levels can be falsely elevated in patients taking vitamin C or dietary supplements, with iron therapy and oestrogen preparations, while they may be lowered in patients with colds, inflammatory conditions, liver disease and malignancies.[21]

TABLE 15.3 Anaemia types with suggested causes

Type	Hb	MCV	MCH	MCHC	RDW	Causes
Microcytic	Low	Low	Low	Low	Raised	Iron deficiency
						Thalassaemia
Normocytic	Low	Normal	Normal	Normal	Raised	Bleeding
						B_{12} folate deficiencies
						Bone marrow disorders
						Anaemia of chronic disease
Macrocytic	Low	Raised MCV	Normal MCH	Normal MCHC	Raised	B_{12} and folate deficiency
						Drug-induced (e.g. methotrexate and trimethoprim)[22]
						Hypothyroidism
						Excessive alcohol intake
					Normal	Aplastic anaemia

WCC

The WCC measures the total number of white cells and is made up of a number of parameters, each of which has its own role to play in keeping the body healthy. Evaluation of the test result requires analysis of each of the white cell differentials in order to help make a diagnosis.

Neutrophils

Neutrophils are the most numerous of the white cells and their function is to engulf bacteria and cellular debris. Their numbers are therefore increased in acute infections, and also in certain malignant neoplastic diseases.

Lymphocytes

Lymphocytes account for 20%–45% of the total WCC.[23] There are two forms of leucocytes. B cells function to produce antibodies, while T cells are active in the recognition of foreign bodies and the subsequent process that takes place to remove them from the body.

Monocytes

Monocytes function in the ingestion of bacteria and other foreign particles and make up approximately 5%–10% of the total white cell count.[24]

Eosinophils

Eosinophils play an important role in allergic reactions and parasitic infections. Typically, eosinophils make up less than 5% of circulating white blood cells in healthy individuals and their presence increases in certain infections (caused by parasites), eosinophil-associated gastrointestinal disorders, leukaemia and other conditions.[25]

Basophils

These cells contain large amounts of histamine and release this as part of the body's response when an allergic reaction occurs.

P blood film

A P blood film (otherwise called a peripheral blood film or blood smear) may be requested by the clinician or carried out by the laboratory when abnormalities are found on either the full blood count and/or white cell differential count. It provides useful information in relation to cells that are poorly developed, or abnormal in appearance. The test is useful as an aid to diagnosis of some infections, or in the differential diagnosis of anaemia and thrombocytopenia, and also in the identification and characterisation of leukaemia and lymphoma.[26]

Table 15.4 looks at the white cell count and white cell differentials and possible causes of abnormal results.

TABLE 15.4 White cell count, white cell differentials and possible causes of abnormal results

WCC	Elevated in:	Signs and symptoms
	Infection	Specific symptoms differ in accordance to the site of infection.
	Leukaemias	*See* pp. 245–8.
WCC	**Reduced in:**	**Signs and symptoms**
	During chemotherapy and radiotherapy	Swollen lymph nodes, fever and sore throat.
	HIV	
Neutrophils	**Elevated in:**	**Signs and symptoms**
	Acute infection	Again differ with the site of infection.
	Inflammatory conditions	Common symptoms include malaise, fever, loss of appetite.
		Other symptoms vary with the cause.

(*continued*)

Neutrophils	Reduced in:	Signs and symptoms
	Neutropenia	May be asymptomatic or cause signs of infection.
	Leukaemia	*See* pp. 245–8.
	Aplastic anaemia	*See* p. 241.
	Bone marrow dysfunction	Bone and joint pains, weight loss, enlarged lymph nodes, pallor, weakness and fatigue, enlarged liver and spleen, frequent infections.
Lymphocytes	Elevated in:	Signs and symptoms
	Leukaemia	*See* pp. 245–8.
	Mononucleosis	Fever, fatigue, sore throat, swollen glands.
	Hepatitis	May be asymptomatic or may cause fatigue, muscle aches and pains, nausea and vomiting and loss of appetite.
Lymphocytes	Reduced in:	Signs and symptoms
	Aplastic anaemia	*See* p. 241.
	AIDS	Tiredness, fever, muscle pains, sore throat.
	Multiple sclerosis	Balance problems, tingling sensation in the limbs, mobility problems, blurred vision.
Monocytes	Elevated	Signs and symptoms
	TB	*See* p. 29.
	Hodgkin's lymphoma	This type is a rarer form of lymphoma and involves proliferation of lymphoid cells predominantly involving lymphoid tissues.
	Malaria	Presents with fever, muscle aches and pains and episodes of sweating.
	Infective endocarditis	Pallor, weakness, joint pains, fever, weight loss, muscle and joint pains.
Monocytes	Reduced in:	
	Bone marrow problems	*See* pp. 241, 248
	Some leukaemias	*See* pp. 245–8.
Eosinophils	Elevated in:	
	Hay fever	*See* pp. 140–3.
	Asthma	*See* pp. 18–21.
	Allergic reactions	Rash, sneezing, wheezing, shortness of breath, swelling.
	Reduced in:	
	Corticosteroid therapy	Moon face, diabetes, insomnia, fatigue, acne.
Basophils	Raised in:	
	Allergic reactions	As above.
	Acute infections	As above.
	Hodgkin's disease	See above.
	Reduced in:	
	Leukaemia	*See* pp. 245–8.

Key reminders

- Consider the whole picture (history, signs and symptoms) alongside any abnormal measurements.
- Abnormalities may indicate a need for further investigations and if grossly abnormal urgent investigation may be needed.
- Excess alcohol intake and certain medications may affect results.
- Malignancy and chemotherapy can both affect parameters.

UREA AND ELECTROLYTES (U&Es)

Assessment of U&Es is frequently used to detect abnormalities in renal function and in common with other blood tests there are several components that need to be assessed, each having its own role to play in keeping the body functioning efficiently.

Measurements and normal values

Table 15.5 shows the normal values.

TABLE 15.5 U&Es normal values

Parameter	Value in males and females
Potassium	3.5–5.3 mmol/L
Sodium	133–146 mmol/L
Urea	2.5–7.8 mmol/L
Creatinine	44–133 mmol/L
eGFR	*See* pp. 276–8

As with other laboratory tests, there are always instances when results appear to be abnormal but when considered in relation to other medical information they may be entirely acceptable for that particular patient. This situation may be seen in patients with HF and impaired renal function who frequently have impaired creatinine and urea levels, or in patients taking diuretics, which may also affect results.[27] Age and gender can also impact on individual parameters.

Potassium

Serum potassium is the major electrolyte within cells, but its concentration in the serum is minimal. However, relatively minor alterations to the balance can have significant consequences.[28] High levels of potassium are referred to as hyperkalaemia, while hypokalaemia is the term used for low levels. Dietary sources of potassium are shown in Table 15.6.

TABLE 15.6 Dietary sources of potassium

Salmon
Cod
Chicken
Bananas
Citrus fruits and juices
Tomatoes
Avocados

Symptoms of mild hypokalemia are weakness, fatigue, paralysis, respiratory difficulty, constipation, paralytic ileus and leg cramps, whilst hyperkalaemia causes weakness, ascending paralysis and respiratory failure.[29]

Sodium

Sodium is the major extracellular electrolyte and in order to ensure a healthy level of sodium in the bloodstream is maintained there is a balance between dietary intake and renal excretion. The majority of salt in Western diets is obtained from packaged, processed, store-bought and restaurants foods.[30] Very little is thought to be obtained by salt added during the cooking process or at the table. At healthy levels salt plays a vital part in maintaining fluid balance, and ensuring the healthy functioning of nerve cells and muscles. However, a diet high in salt is known to be linked to a number of health problems and may be partially or wholly the cause of certain conditions such as hypertension, stroke, kidney stones, osteoporosis, as well as gastrointestinal tract cancers, asthma, exercise-induced asthma and insomnia.[31] Symptoms experienced with high and low sodium levels are shown in Table 15.7.

TABLE 15.7 Symptoms of high and low sodium levels

Hyponatraemia	Hypernatraemia
Nausea	Anorexia
Anorexia	Nausea
Lethargy	Vomiting
Difficulty concentrating	Thirst
Seizures	Twitching and tremor

Urea

Urea is produced during the process of breakdown of protein. During this process nitrogen in the form of ammonia is produced in the liver, which then combines with other chemicals to produce urea that is excreted via the urine as a waste product. In healthy persons, approximately 90% of the urea produced by the body is excreted via the kidneys, making assessment of blood urea levels useful in assessing how efficiently the kidneys are working. High urea levels can cause a number of symptoms including fatigue, nausea, poor sleep patterns and dry or itchy skin, while low levels may indicate liver disease or damage, or malnutrition.[32]

Creatinine

Creatine, an amino acid, is obtained from meat and fish in the diet, but it is also produced by the liver, kidneys and pancreas.[33] It is stored in the muscles after conversion to creatinine phosphate where it remains until it is needed to provide energy. In the initial stages when levels are minimally raised the patient may be asymptomatic, but as levels rise further numerous symptoms can develop (*see* Table 15.8).

TABLE 15.8 Symptoms of raised creatinine levels

Mild fever
Lethargy
Headaches
Loss of appetite
Reduced urine output
Malaise
Breathing difficulties
Weight changes

CLINICAL ALERT!

⚠ **BEWARE!**

- Creatinine levels do not begin to rise until approximately 40% of kidney function has been lost so are not useful in detecting early kidney disease.[34]
- Creatinine levels are linked to muscle mass so will be low in frail elderly and those debilitated by illness but are higher in those with a large muscle mass.[35]
- Low levels are rare but can occasionally be found in advanced liver diseases.
- Because renal function may be substantially reduced before creatinine levels rise eGFR is a useful indicator of renal failure.[36]

TABLE 15.9 Causes of high and low levels

Parameter	Causes of high levels	Causes of low levels
Potassium	Renal disease Tissue injury Infection Addison's disease	Diarrhoea Vomiting Very rarely poor dietary potassium intake
Sodium	Excessive loss of fluid without adequate fluid replacement Kidney disease Cirrhosis of the liver	Excessive fluid loss, which may occur with diarrhoea and vomiting Excessive sweating Diuretic use
Urea	Impaired renal function Reduced blood flow (e.g. HF) Severe burns and dehydration	Severe liver disease
Creatinine	Renal disease	Low body weight and decreased muscle mass

eGFR

eGFR is an abbreviation of estimated glomerular filtration rate. It is calculated from the serum creatinine level, taking into account other factors such as the age, sex and race of the person. eGFR is an indicator of how well the kidneys are functioning, providing useful information on their filtering capacity; however, the calculation used in providing results is not suitable for all. Race is an important consideration when assessing results, and in black patients estimates should be increased by 20%.[37]

CLINICAL ALERT!

⚠ **BEWARE!**

- eGFR is only an estimate and may be inaccurate, particularly in extremes of body type (e.g. malnourished patients or the severely obese).
- A low or falling eGFR is a good indicator of CKD, and an eGFR of less than 45 mL/min in older people is at the very least a marker for vulnerability and combined with assessment of the albumin creatinine ratio (ACR) is a strong independent predictor of mortality and serious morbidity.[38]
- Deteriorating eGFR leads to a number of symptoms including lethargy, reduced urine output, nausea and vomiting.

TABLE 15.10 Stages of CKD in relation to eGFR values

CKD stage	Description	GFR	Management
One	Kidney damage with normal or increased eGFR	≥ 90	Treatment of any comorbid conditions, and reduction in CVD risk if possible.
Two	Kidney damage with mild reduction in eGFR	60–89	As above.
Three	Moderate decrease in eGFR	30–59	Management of comorbid conditions. Evaluation and treatment where possible of complications, which may include appetite loss, muscle cramps, swollen feet and ankles, dry skin, poor sleep pattern and lethargy.
Four	Severe decrease in eGFR	15–29	Preparation for kidney transplant if appropriate.
Five	Kidney failure	< 15	Kidney transplant if deemed appropriate.

CLINICAL ALERT!

Non-modifiable risk factors for development of CKD include age, gender, race, diabetes and genetic make-up, while modifiable risk factors include elevated BP and raised blood glucose levels, proteinuria, anaemia and dyslipidaemia, with risk factors such as hypertension, proteinuria, anaemia, dyslipidaemia and diabetes common to both cardiac and kidney disease.[39]

Risk factors for progression of CKD

⚠ **BEWARE!**

- Inadequately controlled diabetes and hypertension increase the risk of progression of CKD to kidney failure.[40]
- Repeated episodes of acute kidney injury from a variety of causes such as infections, drugs or toxins, can also contribute to progression of CKD to kidney failure, especially in the elderly.[40]

Table 15.11 shows measures to prevent worsening of CKD and deterioration of eGFR.

TABLE 15.11 Measures to prevent worsening of CKD and deterioration of eGFR

Intervention	Supporting evidence
Tight BP control	The progression of CKD is strongly linked to the control of hypertension.[41] ACE inhibitors and ARBs are widely used for BP control in patients with CKD with or without diabetes. They are the preferred choice because of their multiple benefits, which include reducing proteinuria, slowing the progression of kidney disease, and possibly reducing CVD risk by mechanisms in addition to lowering BP.[42]
Diabetes	Improved diabetes control is linked to a reduction in risk for microvascular complications and any reduction in HBAIC is believed to reduce risk of complications with greatest benefits seen in those with HBA1C below 7% or 53 mmol/L.[43]

⚠ BEWARE!

Commonly prescribed medications can affect renal function (*see* Table 15.12).

TABLE 15.12 Commonly used drugs which can affect renal function

Lithium

Analgesics

Antiviral agents

Beta-blockers

Vasodilators

Aminoglycosides

ACE inhibitors

NSAIDs

Diuretics

Key reminders

- High levels of alcohol intake can compromise kidney function.
- Abnormalities may be asymptomatic.
- Elderly patients on several drugs may have abnormal urea and electrolyte results.
- Progression of CKD can be reduced by controlling BP and blood glucose levels.

LIVER FUNCTION TESTS (LFTs)

The LFT is another of the commonly requested tests and again the test has several components. Liver diseases are common, but although LFTs can be useful in assisting with the diagnosis of liver diseases there are also instances where parameters are abnormal but further investigations fail to find evidence of liver disease.

Measurements and normal values

Table 15.13 shows the normal values.

TABLE 15.13 LFT normal values

Parameter	Reference range
ALT	5–45 u/L
AST	5–45 u/L
Alkaline phosphatase (ALP)	245–110 u/L
Bilirubin	1–20 mmol/L
Albumin	33–49 g/L
Gamma-glutamyltransferase (gamma GT)	< 65

Understanding the components

Alanine transaminase (ALT)

ALT is a sensitive indicator of liver cell injury, with increased levels occurring in response to any type of liver cell damage.[44] ALT and aspartate aminotransferase (AST) should be analysed together as the two go hand in hand as indicators of liver cell malfunction. ALT is found primarily in the liver, and is therefore more specific for liver damage, whereas AST is found at several other sites including cardiac muscle, skeletal muscle, kidneys, brain, pancreas, lungs, leucocytes and red cells;[36] therefore, abnormalities are less sensitive and specific for the liver and may be altered by disease at other sites.

CLINICAL ALERT!

The decision to arrange further investigation and the urgency at which this is required should be guided by the level of ALT. A serum level less than five times the upper limit of normal should be reassessed before further intervention is commenced.[45]

AST

AST is an enzyme found primarily in the liver and the heart, but it can also be found in the kidney, brain, pancreas, muscle tissue and red blood cells.[46] Any damage to any of these organs, or to the process of haemolysis, stimulates release of the enzyme into the bloodstream, which results in elevated blood levels. AST has a high level of activity in muscle, so any damage to cardiac or skeletal muscle will result in elevated levels. When this occurs the abnormal LFT has a cause unrelated to liver function.

TABLE 15.14 Causes of abnormal AST and ALT values

Parameter	Causes
Mildly raised AST and ALT	Drug toxicity, fatty liver, liver cirrhosis and myositis.
Moderately raised AST and ALT	Acute and chronic hepatitis, alcoholic hepatitis and biliary obstruction.
Severely raised AST and ALT	Severe viral hepatitis, and drug or toxin-induced liver necrosis.

CLINICAL ALERT!

AST/ALT RATIO

- The ratio of AST to ALT can be useful in determining the presence of alcohol-induced liver disease and is often greater than two when this is present.[47]
- Accuracy of both ALT and AST levels is dependent on adequate vitamin B6 levels, which if low or depleted will result in artificially low levels.[48]

Alkaline phosphatase

In healthy adults most of the alkaline phosphatase activity in the serum originates from liver and bone,[45] so any disease originating from either of these two sites will result in abnormal test results. If the cause of the abnormality is biliary obstruction, alkaline phosphatase levels take 1–2 days to rise, and once the obstruction is corrected levels may take several days to revert to normal, a factor attributed to its long half life.[49]

Gamma GT

Gamma GT is an enzyme found in the cells of the pancreas, the intestine, renal tubules, liver hepatocytes and biliary epithelial cells. Results are elevated in about 75% of those with a chronic alcohol problem.[50] The test is therefore useful as a screening tool for chronic alcohol abuse, but it can also be used to monitor liver function and improvements in patients undergoing treatment for an alcohol-related liver disease.

CLINICAL ALERT!

⚠ BEWARE!

- Gamma GT test is raised in liver disease but not in bone diseases[50] and is therefore useful in determining the source of the disease.
- A rise in gamma GT accompanied by an elevated alkaline phosphatase makes a liver cause more likely.[51]
- If bone disease has been excluded, other possible causes include biliary

obstruction, injury to the bile duct epithelium, a problem with bile formation or obstruction to the flow of bile.[52]

- A gamma GT level of twice the normal level is indicative of alcohol abuse, but it is not specific to alcohol and may be raised in several non-liver diseases including renal failure, COPD, diabetes, pancreatic disease, and following an MI.[36]

Bilirubin

Bilirubin is formed from the breakdown of haemoglobin by the liver and is excreted into bile ready for elimination, having been converted to a water-soluble substance, conjugated bilirubin. In health, excretion of conjugated bilirubin into bile is a rapid process, so that only minimal quantities are detectable in the urine, but in liver disease the secretion of conjugated bilirubin into the bile is impaired, which results in a rapid filtration into the urine where it can be detected on dipstick testing.[53] Elevated bilirubin levels manifests itself as the typical jaundiced appearance associated with liver disease as infiltration into the sclera of the eyes, the skin and mucous membranes occurs.

CLINICAL ALERT!

 BEWARE!

Serum levels of conjugated bilirubin do not rise until the liver has lost at least half of its excretory capacity.[53]

Albumin

Albumin is a plasma protein synthesised in the liver and secreted on a daily basis and when liver function is deteriorating, synthesis of albumin is impaired, resulting in a fall in levels detected in the serum. When this happens the liver attempts to compensate by increasing the rate of synthesis to twice the healthy basal rate. Albumin has a long half life, leading to a longer time for serum levels to alter to reflect changes in rates of synthesis. Low albumin levels can also arise as a result of damage to the kidneys (causing leakage of albumin into the urine) and can also occur as a result of inflammation, malnutrition and in diseases where the absorption of protein is impaired such as Crohn's disease or coeliac disease.[54]

CLINICAL ALERT!

 BEWARE!

One of the key problems when interpreting LFT results is that the test lacks sensitivity because results can remain normal in certain liver diseases (such as cirrhosis), and it lacks specificity because alterations to individual parameters are not specific for any particular disease and can be affected by problems outside of the liver.

Referral needed
- Grossly abnormal parameters need further investigation, or when abnormalities persist.
- Consider referral of asymptomatic patient with abnormal results because many individuals with chronic liver disease have non-specific or no symptoms.[54]

Key reminders
- The history can sometimes point towards a possible cause (e.g. excessive alcohol intake or IV drug use).
- Abnormalities are not always a result of liver disease.
- Patients with abnormal liver function may be asymptomatic.
- Medications can alter test results.
- Isolated abnormalities may revert to normal when rechecked.

THYROID FUNCTION TESTS (TFTs)
Thyroid disorders are among the most common medical problems and as a result TFTs are the most commonly used endocrine test, with approximately 10 million tests ordered annually in the UK alone at a cost of over £30 million.[55] Hyperthyroidism is a cause of short-term morbidity and long-term mortality, while hypothyroidism is also associated with long-term morbidity but its often non-specific symptoms are frequently mistaken for other conditions.[56]

Measurements and normal values
Table 15.15 shows the normal values.

TABLE 15.15 TFT normal values

Parameter	Reference range
Thyroid stimulating hormone (TSH)	0.4–4.5 mu/L
Total thyroxine (T4)	60–160 nmol/L
Free thyroxine (FT4)	9.0–25 pmol/L
Total triiodothyronine (T3)	1.2–2.6 nmol/L
Free triiodothyronine (FT3)	3.5–7.8 pmol/L

Normal thyroid function
The thyroid gland produces two main thyroid hormones, T4 and T3, which are produced by the thyroid gland after stimulation by thyroid stimulating hormone (TSH) that is produced by the anterior pituitary gland. Once released into the bloodstream, T3 and T4 control TSH secretion by a negative feedback mechanism. This means

that when there are increased levels of T4 and T3 TSH synthesis and secretion is inhibited, whereas when levels of T3 and T4 are low TSH secretion increases. TSH secretion is also influenced by thyrotropin-releasing hormone (TRH), which is synthesised in the hypothalamus, although the precise mechanisms regulating TRH synthesis and release are unclear.[57]

Components and abnormal values
TSH
When circulating blood levels of thyroid hormones are low (hypothyroidism), TSH secretion increases so that high levels of TSH are detected in the bloodstream. When there is excess thyroid hormone (hyperthyroidism) secretion of TSH from the pituitary is reduced, leading to low levels of TSH.

CLINICAL ALERT!

⚠ **BEWARE!**

- Although TSH is considered a valuable indicator of thyroid function, results can be misleading because the response to either increased or decreased levels of thyroid hormone is a gradual process, and it can take several weeks for TSH levels to alter to reflect the true status of thyroid hormones in the blood.[58]
- The TSH and T4 levels are often low in severe illness.[59]

Total T4 and Free T4
Both T3 and T4 are mostly bound to protein in the plasma with a small portion remaining free, and it is this free portion which is active and can act on cells to alter metabolism.

Measurement of total T4 includes both bound and free fractions, whereas measurement of free T4 excludes the portion that is bound to protein. Looking at the thyroid hormone levels (T4 and T3) as well as TSH accurately determines how well the thyroid is functioning.[60]

CLINICAL ALERT!

- Occasionally, abnormalities in total T4 levels can occur as a result of elevated or low concentrations of the protein that binds T4.
- Abnormalities may be caused by several factors and can be confusing. Increased levels of binding protein and high T4 levels may be found in association with pregnancy, and in patients using oral contraceptives, while severe illness or use of corticosteroids decreases levels of binding protein, resulting in low T4 levels, but the person does not have hypothyroidism.[60]

Total T3 and free T3

As with T4, total T3 measures both bound and free fractions, while free T3 excludes the portion bound to protein. Only about 20% of the T3 circulating in the blood-stream comes from the thyroid gland; the remaining 80% is derived from various cells all over the body where T4 is converted to T3. However, it is not useful in diag-nosing hypothyroidism because levels are not reduced until the hypothyroidism is severe.[61] FT3 levels, however, may be useful when hyperthyroidism is suspected, which will be reflected by a reduced TSH level, a normal or raised FT4 and a raised T3 level.[62]

TABLE 15.16 Meaning of low or high values

TSH	T4	T3	Interpretation	Additional information
High	Normal	Normal	Hypothyroidism (mild)	TSH may revert to normal without intervention Patient may have mild symptoms of cold intolerance, tiredness and dry skin
High	Low	Low or normal	Hypothyroidism	May present with symptoms as above but also experience slow speech, constipation, pallor, coarse hair, forgetfulness and reduced sweating
Low	Normal	Normal	Hyperthyroidism (mild)	Restlessness Irritability Palpitations Weight loss Increased appetite Poor sleep pattern Tiredness Menstrual disturbance Tremor
Low	Raised	Raised	Hyperthyroidism	As above

CLINICAL ALERT!

⚠ **BEWARE!**

- Symptoms may have an insidious onset developing over several weeks.
- Symptoms often non-specific and all can have other causes.
- Patient may not exhibit textbook signs and symptoms and may only have one or two of those described.

Thyroid peroxidise antibodies

Thyroid antibody testing may be requested to help determine whether the cause of the patient's symptoms is an autoimmune thyroid disease (e.g. Graves' disease). Eighty per cent of Graves' disease patients have high levels of anti-TPO antibodies and about 4% of patients with subclinical hypothyroid disease and positive TPO antibodies subsequently develop clinical hypothyroidism.[63] Patients with known autoimmune disease such as SLE, rheumatoid arthritis or pernicious anaemia should be assessed, as the prevalence of thyroid antibodies in patients with autoimmune disease who develop thyroid problems has been estimated at 1%– 40%.[64]

Key reminders

- Symptoms of thyroid dysfunction can be mistaken for other causes.
- It may have an insidious onset.
- Thyroid function can be altered in the presence of other medical conditions.
- Once treatment is commenced monitoring is continuous.
- Medication is for life.

C-REACTIVE PROTEIN (CRP) AND ERYTHROCYTE SEDIMENTATION RATE (ESR)

These two tests are commonly referred to as acute phase proteins (or inflammatory markers) whose levels fluctuate in response to tissue injury of a variety of kinds including trauma, myocardial infarction, acute infections, chronic inflammation, malignancies, rheumatoid arthritis and burns.[65] They are therefore used as an aid to diagnosis of certain diseases but can also be useful in monitoring conditions and whether treatment for a particular condition is effective. A recent study has indicated that after the age of 40, there is an age-related elevation of both ESR and CRP, increasing steadily, especially after age 60 years, but with CRP increasing to a lesser extent than ESR.[66] Both appear to be equally useful and reliable as a screening test, but when required as a clinical test in the management of patients with specific diseases both tests should be carried out in tandem.[66]

CRP

The test measures the levels of a particular protein in the bloodstream and is deemed non-specific as elevated results give no indication of where the underlying problem may be. It is therefore used in conjunction with signs, symptoms and other test results to assist in making a diagnosis.

Measurements and normal values

Normal values would be detected in the plasma at less than 5.

What do abnormal values suggest?

Elevated results are suggestive of inflammation or infection somewhere in the body. CRP is reported to be more effective than ESR for monitoring fast changes as it does not depend on fibrinogen or immunoglobulin levels, and is unaffected by any changes to red blood cells.[67]

CLINICAL ALERT!

- Useful in determining whether infection is viral or bacterial with higher levels detected in bacterial infections than those detected in viral infections.[68]
- May be used to monitor known diseases such as rheumatoid arthritis.
- Also useful as a guide to the severity of the inflammation in pancreatitis and has been found useful in accurately differentiating between mild and severe attacks.[69]
- Monitoring disease activity in other conditions such as infections or malignancies.
- CRP has also been cited as a strong predictor for CHD and stroke and is considered to be a more accurate predictor than low-density lipoprotein (LDL) cholesterol levels.[70]
- In those over 70 years of age raised CRP is associated with increased risk of mortality as well as a risk of cardiovascular diseases, diabetes and RA.[71]

ESR

ESR measures the rate at which red blood cells settle when anticoagulated whole blood is allowed to stand.

Normal values are shown in Table 15.17.

TABLE 15.17 ESR normal values

Men aged 18–65	10 mm/hr
Women aged 18–65	20 mm/hr
Over 65 years of age	Can increase by 5–10 mm/hr

Useful in assisting the diagnosis of conditions associated with acute and chronic inflammation, including infections, cancers and autoimmune diseases, the test can also be used for monitoring conditions such as GCA and PMR[72] (*see* pp. 226–8). Results, however, are non-specific and give no indication of the underlying cause of any abnormality. An extreme elevation of the ESR may occur with inflammation, infection or malignancy and is also a prognostic factor in other conditions such as CHD, stroke, HF and prostate cancer.[73]

TABLE 15.18 Causes of elevated ESR

Anaemia
Malignancy
Osteomyelitis
Renal disease
Thyroid disease
Systemic infections
Tuberculosis

⚠ **BEWARE!**

- The ESR rises with age, but this increase may be associated with a higher disease prevalence of chronic disease in the elderly.[74]
- ESR is raised in the presence of infection, inflammatory diseases and malignancy.[75]
- ESR can also be affected by certain drugs such as methyldopa oral contraceptives, theophylline and vitamin A, while aspirin, steroids and quinine may decrease it.[76]
- Raised ESR in men aged 40–60 has been identified as a strong predictor of mortality from CHD, and appears to be a marker of aggressive forms of this disease.[77]

Decreased ESR

A decreased ESR is associated with a number of blood diseases in which red blood cells have an irregular or smaller shape, and this causes slower settling.[78]

Causes of decreased ESR are shown in Table 15.19.

TABLE 15.19 Causes of decreased ESR

Polycythaemia
Sickle cell anaemia
HF
Leucocytosis

Key reminders

- Both ESR and CRP are inflammatory markers and are therefore raised in any condition where inflammation is present.
- Both ESR and CRP are raised in the elderly.
- They are useful to exclude certain diseases (e.g. PMR).
- When results are elevated they do not give any indication of the underlying problem.
- ESR and CRP can be used to aid the diagnosis and also to monitor disease activity.

REFERENCES

1. Weng J, Brown CV, *et al.* White blood cell and platelet counts can be used to differentiate between infection and the normal response after splenectomy for trauma: prospective validation. *J Trauma.* 2005; **59**(5): 1076–80.
2. Curry VC. *Mean Corpuscular Volume (MCV).* Available at: http://emedicine.medscape.com/article/2085770-overview#showall (accessed 5 May 2013).

3. Arzt A. *Anaemia in Elderly Persons*. Available at: http://emedicine.medscape.com/article/1339998-overview#aw2aab6c12 (accessed 27 July 2013).

4. Kaferle J, Strzoda CE. Evaluation of macrocytosis. *Am Fam Physician.* 2009; **79**(3): 203–8.

5. Lab Test Help. *Red Blood Cell Indices*. Available at: www.labtesthelp.com/test/Red_Blood_Cell_Indices (accessed 14 August 2013).

6. Braden CD. *Chronic Anaemia*. Available at: http://emedicine.medscape.com/article/780176-workup#showall (accessed 4 May 2013).

7. Pascal-Figal DA, Bonaque JV, Redondo B, *et al.* Red blood cell distribution width predicts long-term outcome regardless of anaemia status in acute heart failure patients. *Eur J Heart Fail.* 2009; **11**(9): 840–6.

8. RnCeus. *Red Blood Cell Count*. Available at: www.rnceus.com/cbc/cbcrbc.html (accessed 27 July 2013).

9. American Association for Clinical Chemistry. *Red Blood Cell Count*. Available at: www.labtestsonline.org.uk/understanding/analytes/rbc/tab/test (accessed 15 May 2013).

10. Baz R, Mekhail T. *Disorders of Platelet Function and Number*. Available at: www.clevelandclinicmeded.com/medicalpubs/diseasemanagement/hematology-oncology/disorders-platelet-function/ (accessed 19 August 2013).

11. RNCeus. *Platelet Count*. Available at: www.rnceus.com/coag/coagplate.html (accessed 25 August 2013).

12. Iron Health Alliance. *Transferrin Saturation Measurement*. Available at: www.ironhealthalliance.com/diagnostics/transferrin-saturation-measurement.jsp (accessed 25 August 2013).

13. WHO/UNICEF/UNU. *Iron Deficiency Anaemia: assessment, prevention and control, a guide for programme managers*. Available at: www.who.int/nutrition/publications/micronutrients/anaemia_iron_deficiency/WHO_NHD_01.3/en/index.html (accessed 25 August 2013).

14. Galloway M. *Raised Ferritin*. GP online. Available at: www.gponline.com/Clinical/article/984023 (accessed 19 October 2013).

15. Lecube A, Hernandez C, Pelegri D, *et al.* Factors accounting for high ferritin levels in obesity. *Int J Obes.* 2008; **32**: 1665–9.

16. Firkin F. Interpretation of biochemical tests for iron deficiency: diagnostic difficulties related to limitations of individual tests. *Aust Presc.* 1997; **20**: 74–6.

17. Berkhan L. Interpretation of an elevated serum ferritin. *NZFP.* 2002; **29**(1): 45–8.

18. Yamanishi H, Iyama S, Yamaguchi Y. Total iron-binding capacity calculated from serum transferrin concentration or serum iron concentration and unsaturated iron-binding capacity. *Clin Chem.* 2003; **49**(1): 175–8.

19. American Association for Clinical Chemistry. *TIBC, UIBC and Transferrin*. Available at: www.labtestsonline.org.uk/understanding/analytes/tibc/tab/test (accessed 20 July 2013).

20. Centres for Disease Control and Prevention. *Haemochromatosis (Iron Storage Disease)*. Available at: www.cdc.gov/ncbddd/hemochromatosis/training/diagnostic_testing/testing_protocol.html (accessed 19 August 2013).

21. Tefferi A. Anaemia in adults: a contemporary approach to diagnosis. *Mayo Clin Proc.* 2003; **78**: 1274–80.

22. Simon S, Everitt H, van Dorp F. *Oxford Handbook of General Practice*. Oxford: Oxford University Press; 2010.

23. Longmore M, Wilkinson I, Turmezei T, *et al. Oxford Handbook of Clinical Medicine*. 7th ed. Oxford: Oxford University Press; 2007.

24. Collins M. *What is an Eosinophil?* Available at: http://apfed.org/drupal/drupal/what_is_eosinophil (accessed 24 July 2013).

25. Bain B. Diagnosis from the blood smear. *New Eng J Med.* 2005; **353**: 498–507.

26. Klein L, Massie BM, Leimberger JD, *et al.* Admission or changes in renal function during hospitalization for worsening heart failure predict post discharge survival. *Circ Heart Fail.* 2008; **1**(1): 25–33.

27. Pagana KD, Pagana TJ. *Manual of Diagnostic and Laboratory Tests.* 4th ed. St Louis, MO: Mosby Elsevier; 2010.

28. Mayo Foundation for Medical Education and Research (MFMER). *High Blood Pressure (Hypertension).* Available at: www.mayoclinic.com/health/blood-pressure/AN00352 (accessed 12 August 2013).

29. American Heart Association Guidelines for Cardiopulmonary Resuscitation and Emergency Cardiovascular Care. Part 10.1: Life-Threatening Electrolyte Abnormalities. *Circulation.* 2005. Available at: http://circ.ahajournals.org/content/112/24_suppl/IV-121.full (accessed 16 January 2014).

30. Centres for Disease Control and Prevention. *Sodium and Food Sources.* Available at: www.cdc.gov/salt/food (accessed 19 July 2013).

31. Antonio TF, MacGregor GA. Salt – more adverse effects. *Lancet.* 1996; **348**: 250–1.

32. Mayo Foundation for Medical Education and Research (MMFER). *Blood Urea Nitrogen Test.* Available at: www.mayoclinic.com/health/blood-urea-nitrogen/MY00373 (accessed 25 July 2013).

33. University of Maryland. Creatinine. Available at: http://umm.edu/health/medical/altmed/supplement/creatine (accessed 17 January 2014).

34. Murphree DD. Thelen SM. Chronic kidney disease in primary care. *J Am Board Fam Med.* 2010; **23**: 4542–50.

35. Smith AF, Beckett GJ, Walker SW, *et al. Clinical Biochemistry.* 6th ed. Oxford: Blackwell Science; 1998.

36. McGhee M. *A Guide to Laboratory Investigations.* 5th ed. Oxford: Radcliffe Publishing; 2008.

37. The Renal Association. About egfr. Available at: www.renal.org/information-resources/the-uk-eckd-guide/about-egfr#sthash.e5AfY3Yj.dpbs (accessed 19 January 2014).

38. Roderick PJ. Chronic kidney disease in older people: a cause for concern? *Nephrol Dial Transplant.* 2011; **26**(10): 3083–6.

39. Levin A. Identification of patients and risk factors in chronic kidney disease: evaluating risk factors and therapeutic strategies. *Nephrol Dial Transplant.* 2001; **16**(Suppl. 7): S57–60.

40. Centres for Disease Control and Prevention. *National Chronic Kidney Disease Fact Sheet.* Available at: www.cdc.gov/diabetes/pubs/factsheets/kidney.htm (accessed 23 July 2013).

41. Lascano ME, Schreiber MJ, Nurko S. *Chronic Kidney Disease.* Available at: www.clevelandclinicmeded.com/medicalpubs/diseasemanagement/nephrology/chronic-kidney-disease/ (accessed 1 August 2013).

42. National Kidney Foundation. NKF K/DOQI guidelines. *K/DOQI Clinical Practice Guidelines on Hypertension and Antihypertensive Agents in Chronic Kidney Disease.* 2002. Available at: www.kidney.org/professionals/kdoqi/guidelines_bp/guide_11.htm (accessed 29 July 2013).

43. Stratton IM, Adler AI, Neil HAW. Association of glycaemia with macrovascular and microvascular complications of type 2 diabetes (UKPDS 35): prospective observational study. *BMJ.* 2000; **321**: 405.

44. Kaplan MM. Alanine aminotransferase levels: what's normal? *Ann Intern Med.* 2002; **137**(1): 49–51.

45. Limdi JK, Hyde GM. Evaluation of normal liver function tests. *Postgrad Med.* 2003; **79**: 307–12.

46. Pratt DS, Kaplan MM. Evaluation of abnormal liver enzyme results in asymptomatic patients. *N Engl J Med.* 2000; **342**: 1266–71.

47. Sorbi D, Boynton J, Lindor KD. The ratio of aspartate aminotransferase to alanine

aminotransferase: potential value in differentiating non alcoholic steatohepatitis from alcoholic liver disease. *Am J Gastroenterol.* 1999; **94**: 1018–22.

48. Devaraj S. *Aspartate Amino Transferase.* Available at: http://emedicine.medscape.com/article/2087224-overview#showall (accessed 2 August 2013).

49. Giannini EG, Testa R, Savarino V. Liver enzyme alteration a guide for clinicians. *Can Med Ass J.* 2005; **172**(3): 367–9.

50. American Association for Clinical Chemistry. *GGT.* Available at: http://labtestsonline.org/understanding/analytes/ggt/tab/ (accessed 30 July 2013).

51. BPAC. *Liver Function Testing in Primary Care.* Available at: www.bpac.org.nz/resources/campaign/lft/bpac_lfts_poem_pf.pdf (accessed 20 August 2013).

52. Aragon G, Younossi ZM. When and how to evaluate mildly elevated liver enzymes in apparently healthy patients. *Cleveland Clin J Med.* 2010; **77**(3): 195–204.

53. Johnston DE. Special considerations in interpreting liver function tests. *Am Fam Physician.* 1999; **59**(8): 2223–30.

54. George GK, Ryder S, Collier J, *et al.* Management of abnormal liver function tests in asymptomatic patients. *Brit Soc Gastroenterology.* 2005. Available at: www.bsg.org.uk/pdf_word_docs/ablft_draft05.doc (accessed 3 August 2013).

55. Lawrence D. Thyroid problems in primary care. *InnovAiT.* 2008; **1**(12): 788–92.

56. Boelaert K, Franklyn JA. Thyroid hormone in health and disease. *J Endocrinol.* **187**(1): 1–15.

57. The Merck Manual. *Overview of Thyroid Function.* Available at: www.merckmanuals.com/professional/endocrine_and_metabolic_disorders/thyroid_disorders/overview_of_thyroid_function.html (accessed 7 December 2012).

58. Moore E. *Drugs and Tests: laboratory tests for thyroid function.* Available at: www.ithyroid.com/thyroid_test_interpretation.htm (accessed 7 December 2012).

59. Young R, Worthly LI. Diagnosis and management of thyroid disease and the critically ill patient. *Crit Care Resusc.* 2004; **6**(4): 295–305.

60. American Association for Clinical Chemistry. *FT4.* Available at: www.labtestsonline.org.uk/understanding/analytes/ft4/ (accessed 9 December 2012).

61. National Institute of Diabetes and Digestive and Kidney Diseases. *Thyroid Function Tests.* Available at: http://endocrine.niddk.nih.gov/pubs/thyroidtests/thyroidtests_508.pdf (accessed 17 May 2013).

62. Reid JR, Wheeler SF. Hyperthyroidism: diagnosis and treatment. *Am Fam Physician.* 2005; **72**(4): 623–30.

63. Kandi S, Rao P. Anti-thyroid peroxidase antibodies: its effect on thyroid gland and breast tissue. *Ann Trop Med Pub Health.* 2012; **5**(1): 1–2.

64. Benvenga S, Bartolone L, Squadrito S, *et al.* Thyroid hormone antibodies elicited by fine needle biopsy. *J Clin Endocrinol Metab.* 1997; **82**: 4217–23.

65. GP Notebook. *Acute Phase Proteins.* Available at: www.gpnotebook.co.uk/simplepage.cfm?ID=1026883606 (accessed 14 December 2012).

66. Osei Bimpong A, Meek JH, Lewis SM. ESR or CRP? A comparison of their clinical utility. *Haematology.* 2007; **12**(4): 353–7.

67. Black S, Kushner I, Samols D. C-reactive protein. *J Biol Chem.* 2004; **279**(47): 48487–90.

68. Sasaki K, Fujita I, Hamasaki Y, *et al.* Differentiating between bacterial and viral infection by measuring both C-reactive protein and 2'-5'-oligoadenylate synthetase as inflammatory markers. *Infect Chemother.* 2002; **8**(1): 76–80.

69. Mayer AD, McMahon MJ, Bowen M, *et al.* C-reactive protein: an aid to assessment and monitoring of acute pancreatitis. *J Clin Pathol.* 1984; **37**(2): 207–11.

70. Albert CM, Ma J, Rifai N, *et al.* Prospective study of C-reactive protein, homocysteine, and plasma lipid levels as predictors of sudden cardiac death. *Circulation.* 2002; **105**(22): 2595–9.

71. Evrin PE, Nilsson SE, Oberg T, *et al.* Serum C-reactive protein in elderly men and women: association with mortality, morbidity and various biochemical values. *Scand J Clin Lab Invest.* 2005; **65**(1): 23–31.

72. Bridgen M. Clinical utility of the erythrocyte sedimentation rate. *Am Fam Physician.* 1999; **60**(5): 1443–50.

73. Bochen K, Krasoska A, Milaniuk S. Erythrocyte sedimentation rate: an old marker with new applications. *J Pre Clin Clin Res.* 2011; **5**(2): 50–5.

74. Olshaker JS, Jerrard DA. The erythrocyte sedimentation rate. *J Em Med.* 1997; **15**(6) 869–74.

75. Monig H, Marquardt D, Arendt T, *et al.* Limited value of elevated erythrocyte sedimentation rate as an indicator of malignancy. *Fam Pract.* 2002; **19**: 436–8.

76. American Association for Clinical Chemistry. *ESR.* Available at: www.labtestsonline.org.uk/understanding/analytes/esr/tab/related (accessed 15 December 2012).

77. Erikssen G, Liestol K, Bornholt JV, *et al.* Erythrocyte sedimentation rate: a possible marker of atherosclerosis and a strong predictor of coronary heart disease mortality. *Eur Heart J.* 2000; **21**(19): 1614–20.

78. Saadeh C. The erythrocyte sedimentation rate: old and new clinical applications. *South Med J.* 1998; **3**: 220–5.

CHAPTER 16

Choosing the right antibiotic

INTRODUCTION

The discovery of penicillin and subsequent development of antibiotics revolution-ised medicine, and their use has played an active part in reducing morbidity and mortality rates from infectious diseases around the world. Since their original dis-covery many more antibiotics have been developed to deal with a wide range of disease-causing bacteria. In recent times the problem of antibiotic resistance has caused concern with some micro-organisms developing resistance to antimicrobial agents to which they were previously sensitive. In clinical practice it can be very dif-ficult to determine whether the patient is suffering from a viral or a bacterial illness, particularly when there are shared or similar signs and symptoms for either type. However, when the decision to treat with antibiotics is made there is potentially a range from which to choose.

ANTIBIOTIC TYPES

Antibiotics are either:
- bactericidal, which means they are able to kill the bacteria directly, or
- bacteriostatic, which means they are able to prevent the bacteria from reproducing (*see* Table 16.1).

TABLE 16.1 Antibiotic types

Type	Drug type	Example
Bactericidal	Penicillins	Benzyl penicillin
	Cephalosporins	Cephalexin
	Aminoglycosides	Streptomycin
	Beta-lactams	Amoxicillin
Bacteriostatic	Tetracyclines	Oxytetracycline
	Macrolides	Erythromycin
	Trimethoprim	

Broad-spectrum antibiotics

These are effective against a wide range of organisms and are able to target a structure or process shared by several bacteria and can therefore successfully treat a number of bacterial infections. Antibiotics of this type include penicillin, tetracyclines and ciprofloxacin. They are useful if the causative organism is not known.

Narrow-spectrum antibiotics

These act on a specific molecule or process in the metabolism of particular bacteria that is unique to that species and are therefore more appropriate if the causative organism is known. Examples include nitrofurantoin and metronidazole.

Gram-negative and gram-positive organisms

This refers to the ability of the bacterium to retain or repel the violet stain used in a process developed many years ago. The ability to do this depends on the structure of the cell. Gram-negative organisms have additional proteins, polysaccharides and phospholipids in the make-up of their structure, making it difficult for some antibiotics to penetrate this layer.

CLINICAL ALERT!

Is an antibiotic needed at all?

Viral infections

Viral infections are common (*see* Table 16.2) and are usually self-limiting and should resolve without treatment. Concerns relating to inappropriate use of antibiotics have been prevalent for several years and in the US it has been estimated that more than a fifth of all antibiotic prescriptions for children and adults are written for a variety of common conditions (such as coughs, colds, sore throats) that almost always have a viral cause.[1] Similar concerns for unnecessary prescribing have been issued in the UK, with concern that misuse of antibiotics is now known to play a part in the development of bacteria that are resistant to antibiotics, which is particularly worrying because resistant infections cost more to treat and can prolong healthcare use[2] and in some cases may have potentially fatal outcomes.

TABLE 16.2 Common viral infections

Common viral illnesses
Common cold
Laryngitis
Sore throat
Most ear infections
Acute bronchitis
Viral pneumonia

If an antibiotic is required how do they achieve their effects?

Penicillins

Antibiotics of this type target cell walls. The cell wall of bacteria contains peptidoglycan, which provides rigid stability to the cell wall. The peptidoglycan is composed of glycan chains that are cemented together by the action of enzymes situated on the cell wall. Penicillins bind to and inhibit the action of these enzymes so that they cannot function and are therefore ineffective.

Cephalosporins

These have a similar mode of action to the beta-lactams and penicillins and achieve their effect by inhibiting synthesis of the cell wall.

Aminoglycosides

These primarily prevent bacteria from making proteins. They bind to ribosomes that are responsible for synthesis of proteins, preventing the bacteria from synthesising proteins necessary for growth. They are also thought to displace portions of the cell wall, which may kill the bacteria before the drug acts on the ribosome itself.

Tetracyclines

These prevent ribonucleic acid (RNA) molecules from binding to the ribosome of the bacteria and therefore inhibiting protein synthesis needed for further growth of the bacteria.

Macrolides

These work by binding to a different sub-unit of the ribosomes, preventing the production of proteins necessary for continued growth of the bacteria.

Trimethoprim

This works by inhibiting the enzyme needed for the production of tetrahydrofolate, which starves the bacteria of the nucleotides needed for DNA replication and further growth of the bacteria.

⚠ BEWARE!

Viruses have no cellular structure and no metabolic processes, which means that antibiotics are completely ineffective if used for treatment of viral illnesses.

If an antibiotic is needed which antibiotic for which infection?

Table 16.3 shows antibiotic choice, mode of action and which organism each antibiotic can treat.

TABLE 16.3 Choosing antibiotics

Drug name	Examples	Effective against gram-positive or gram-negative?	Which bacteria?	Possible infections
Penicillins	Amoxicillin Flucloxacillin	Gram-positive	Streptococci E. coli Staphylococcus Helicobacter *Haemophilus influenza* Pneumococcal *Neisseria gonorrhoeae* *Proteus mirabilis*	Ear, nose and throat infections. Pneumonia. UTIs. Gonorrhoea.
Cephalosporins	Cefaclor Cephalexin	Gram-positive and gram-negative	*Staphylococcus aureus* *Streptococcus pneumoniae* *E. coli.* *Klebsiella* *P. mirabilis*	Skin infections. Respiratory tract infections. Sinus infections. Ear infections and UTIs. PID.
Aminoglycosides	Streptomycin Neomycin	Gram-positive and gram-negative	Staphylococci Streptococci *E. coli.* *Klebsiella* Proteus *Pseudomonas aeruginosa*	Ear infections. Eye infections. Skin infections.

(continued)

Drug name	Examples	Effective against gram-positive or gram-negative?	Which bacteria?	Possible infections
Tetracyclines	Oxytetracycline	Gram-positive and gram-negative	*Haemophilus influenzae* *E. coli* *Streptococcus pneumoniae* Staphylococci Mycoplasma pneumonia *Chlamydia psittaci* *Chlamydia trachomatis* *Neisseria gonorrhoeae*	UTIs. Respiratory infections. Acne and other soft tissue infections.
Macrolides	Erythromycin Clarithromycin Streptomycin	Gram-positive and gram-negative	Streptococcus *Staphylococcus pneumococcus* Chlamydia Mycoplasma Gonorrhoea Legionella	Alternative to penicillin for those allergic to this drug. Respiratory tract infections. UTIs. Part of triple therapy for *Helicobacter* infections.
Trimethoprim		Gram-positive and gram-negative	Staphylococcus *E. coli.* *Klebsiella* Proteus Enterobacter	UTIs.

Prescribing tips

- Local guidelines may suggest choice of antibiotic.
- Check any previous sensitivities before prescribing.
- Penicillins including co-amoxiclav are unsuitable if there is any history of penicillin allergy.
- Patient should complete the whole course.
- Some antibiotics are best taken with food, some on an empty stomach (check leaflet for advice).
- Interaction with statins and certain antibiotics (e.g. simvastatin and erythromycin) give increased risk of myopathy.

- Increased risk of muscle effects with macrolides (e.g. erythromycin or clarithromycin) in patients taking statins.
- Erythromycin has limited activity if causative organism is haemophilus influenza.[3]
- Gastrointestinal side-effects are common but can be reduced by taking with or after food.
- Alcohol avoidance with metronidazole.

ANTIBIOTIC RESISTANCE

Antibiotic resistance is defined as the resistance of a micro-organism to an antimicrobial agent to which it was previously sensitive.[4]

How does the problem develop?

For any antibiotic to successfully treat an infection it must be able to either kill the bacteria or stop it from reproducing as described above. Some bacteria have been resistant to particular antibiotics for many years, but many more are becoming resistant, which occurs via a number of processes.

- Mutations to the bacteria's genetic material can occur. Some mutations enable the bacteria to produce enzymes that inactivate the antibiotic, or the cell target that the antibiotic attacks is eliminated.[5]
- Other possible mechanisms include denying the antibiotic entry to the cell by closing entry routes so that it becomes ineffective.
- Bacteria can also acquire resistant genes through exchanging genes with other bacteria, which occurs when rapid reproduction takes place, allowing resistant traits to quickly spread to future generations of bacteria so that resistance can spread from one species of bacteria to other species, enabling them to develop multiple resistance to different classes of antibiotics.[6]

CLOSTRIDIUM DIFFICILE (C. DIFF)

C. diff is an anaerobic gram-positive bacillus present in the gut of up to 3% of healthy adults and 66% of infants,[7] rarely causing problems in healthy subjects as its activity is normally kept under control by other bacteria that reside in the intestine. However, when things go wrong C. diff can cause considerable disease, including diarrhoea, colitis and septicaemia,[8] and in some cases can result in death. The opportunity for the bacteria to multiply and produce toxins arises when the balance of bacteria in the gut is disturbed as a result of antibiotic use. The resulting diarrhoea can vary in severity, ranging from mild to severe. Risk of infection is highest among patients treated with broad-spectrum antibiotics, patients with serious comorbidities and the elderly. The number of deaths involving C. diff also increases with increasing age,[9] and more than 80% of C. diff infections occur in those over the age of 65.[7]

Pathophysiology

Infection with C. diff is associated with recent use of antibiotics and the majority of infections are acquired in healthcare settings.[8] Antibiotics alter the normal levels of protective bacteria found in the intestines and colon, and when there are fewer of these C. diff bacteria have the chance to thrive and produce toxins that can damage the bowel and cause diarrhoea.[10]

CLINICAL ALERT!

⚠ **BEWARE!**

- Risk of infection varies for different antimicrobial agents. In general, the risk of infection increases if the C. diff strain is resistant to the antimicrobial agent, and it is now known that C. diff is resistant to all cephalosporins.[11] Risk of developing the infection is therefore higher with cephalosporin use.
- Other high-risk antibiotics frequently implicated include broad-spectrum antibiotics such as clindamycin, and broad-spectrum penicillins.[12]
- Newer fluoroquinolones, such as moxifloxacin, have a greater spectrum of anaerobic activity and hence cause significant disruption of the gut flora. A newer strain of C. diff, identified in 2004, appears to be more virulent, with the ability to produce greater quantities of toxins, and in addition it is more resistant to the antibiotic group known as fluoroquinolones.[13]
- Factors in addition to antibiotic use predisposing patients to the development of symptomatic C. diff-associated diarrhoea include advanced age, number and severity of underlying diseases, and a faulty immune response to the toxins produced during infections.[14]
- Duration of the antibiotic course also appears to be important with the risk of developing antibiotic-associated diarrhoea more than doubling when treatment is for longer than 3 days.[15]

Treatment

When symptoms are mild, stopping the antibiotics is usually sufficient to cause cessation of symptoms, but more severe cases require treatment with metronidazole or vancomycin and supportive therapy with fluid and electrolyte replacement.[16]

Key messages

- When antibiotic treatment is needed, the antibiotic should be tailored to the patient, the site of infection and the causative organism whenever possible.
- Patients prescribed antibiotics should receive the right drug, at the right dose, given at the right time for the right duration and via the appropriate route if the desired effect is to be achieved.
- Unnecessary lengthy duration of antibiotic treatment and inappropriate use of broad-spectrum antibiotics should be avoided.

- Avoid prescribing if infection is likely viral.
- Delayed prescriptions can be issued for use if symptoms appear to be getting worse and where there is clinical uncertainty.
- Communication is key.
- Self-care and advice on how to self-treat may be sufficient in many cases.

REFERENCES

1. Gonzales R, Steiner JF, Sande MA. Antibiotic prescribing for adults with colds, upper respiratory tract infections, and bronchitis by ambulatory care physicians. *JAMA*. 1997; **278**: 901–4.
2. Centres for Disease Control and Prevention. *Antibiotics aren't always the Answer*. Available at: www.cdc.gov/features/getsmart/ (accessed 6 June 2013).
3. British National Formulary. 2013. Available at: www.bnf.org/bnf/index.htm
4. World Health Organization. *Antimicrobial Resistance Factsheet no 4*. Available at: www.cdc.gov/features/getsmart/ (accessed 9 November 2012).
5. Alliance for the Prudent Use of Antibiotics. *General Background: about antibiotic resistance*. Available at: www.tufts.edu/med/apua/about_issue/about_antibioticres.shtml (accessed 19 June 2013).
6. US Food and Drug Administration. *Battle of the Bugs: fighting antibiotic resistance*. Available at: www.fda.gov/drugs/resourcesforyou/consumers/ucm143568.htm (accessed 28 June 2013).
7. Health Protection Agency. *Clostridium difficile*. Available at: www.hpa.org.uk/Topics/InfectiousDiseases/InfectionsAZ/ClostridiumDifficile/ (accessed 18 November 2012).
8. Kelly CP, Pothoulakis C, LaMont TJ. Clostridium difficile colitis. *N Engl J Med*. 1994; **330**: 257–62.
9. Office for National Statistics. *Statistical Bulletin: deaths involving clostridium difficile, England and Wales 2011*. Available at: www.ons.gov.uk/ons/rel/subnational-health2/deaths-involving-clostridium-difficile/2011/stb-deaths-involving-clostridium-difficile-2011.html (accessed 7 November 2012).
10. Public Health Agency of Canada. *Fact Sheet – Clostridium difficile (C. difficile)*. Available at: www.phac-aspc.gc.ca/id-mi/cdiff-eng.php (accessed 9 September 2012).
11. Moudgal V, Sobel JD. Clostridium difficile colitis: a review. *Hosp Pract*. 2012; **40**(1): 139–48.
12. Owens RC, Donskey CJ, Gaynes RP, *et al*. Antimicrobial-associated risk factors for Clostridium difficile infection. *Clin Infect Dis*. 2008; **46**(Suppl. 1): S19–31.
13. Centres for Disease Control and Prevention. *Information about the Current Strain of C difficile*. Available at: www.cdc.gov/HAI/organisms/cdiff/Cdiff-current-strain.html (accessed 25 October 2012).
14. Schroeder MS. Clostridium difficile associated diarrhoea. *Am Fam Physician*. 2005; **71**(5): 921–8.
15. Wistrom J, Norrby SR, Myhre EB, *et al*. Frequency of antibiotic-associated diarrhoea in 2462 antibiotic-treated hospitalized patients: a prospective study. *J Antimicrob Chemother*. 2001; **47**: 43–50.
16. Mcfarland L. Alternative treatments for Clostridium difficile. *J Med Microbiol*. 2005; **54**: 101–11.

CHAPTER 17

Prescribing

PRESCRIBING CONSIDERATIONS

Drugs are selected and prescribed with consideration for their effectiveness at treating a particular condition after taking into account a number of factors such as the age and sex of the patient, ethnicity, and whether pregnant or breastfeeding. Additional consideration is given to the efficacy and safety of the drug, the best route of administration for the patient, side-effects, known drug sensitivities, interaction with other medications and any contraindications to its use.

HOW DRUGS ACHIEVE THEIR EFFECTS

To produce an adequate effect a drug must be at the right concentration and able to work at the site of action so that it can target the problem with maximum benefit. Pharmacokinetics is the way the body acts on the drug once it is administered and is the measure of the rate (kinetics) of absorption, distribution, metabolism and excretion.[1] Pharmacodynamics is the study of the way the drug affects the body.

Approximately 80% of drugs prescribed are given orally,[2] making this the most commonly used method of administering medication. Other routes of delivery are shown in Table 17.1.

TABLE 17.1 Routes of drug delivery

Orally
Intravenously
Inhaled
Intramuscularly
Rectally
Sublingually
Subcutaneously

ABSORPTION

The process of absorption involves the passage of the drug through the gastrointestinal tract, until it is absorbed into the bloodstream. For drugs to be able to pass satisfactorily along the tract they must be capable of surviving attack from both gastric acid and enzymes. Most drugs are absorbed primarily in the small intestine, largely because the small intestine has the greatest surface area for drug absorption in the GI tract, and its membranes are more permeable than those in the stomach.[3] Once absorbed, the drug enters the systemic circulation and passes into the portal circulation[4] where it is transported by the liver into the portal system.

BIOAVAILABILITY

The bioavailability of an administered substance is that fraction of the dose that reaches the general circulation unchanged.[5] Bioavailability is affected by many factors, including insufficient time for absorption in the GI tract, or failure to dissolve readily, or difficulty penetrating the epithelial membrane leading to insufficient time at the absorption site resulting in low or variable bioavailability.[6] Many of the factors that influence the bioavailability of oral medication can also be changed by food, the presence of which can affect drug absorption as a result of either physiological changes in the GI tract, or physical or chemical interactions between particular food components and drug molecules.[7] Any of these factors can therefore have the effect that absorption of drugs may be reduced or increased, delayed or remain the same.

DISTRIBUTION

Once absorbed, in order for drugs to produce the desired effect they have to be distributed to the site where their action is required. This may take place in a number of ways.

- Distribution into the body fluids, which may be via the interstitial fluid, intracellular fluid or the plasma. Some drugs are water soluble and tend to remain in the blood plasma or the interstitial fluid, while others are fat soluble and will concentrate in fatty tissue. In general, any fat-soluble drug will pass through tissues more quickly than water-soluble drugs can.[8]
- Some drugs are also able to target specific tissues (one example is iodine and the thyroid gland).
- Binding of the drug to plasma proteins is the means of distribution for some drugs and when this is the case, only the unbound or 'free' part of the drug is active. Extensive plasma protein binding will increase the amount of drug that has to be absorbed before effective therapeutic levels of unbound drug are reached.[9]

METABOLISM

Metabolism is the conversion of one chemical compound into another and most drug metabolism occurs in the liver, although some processes occur in the gut wall, lungs and blood plasma.[10] Some drugs are metabolised to form metabolites that once converted may be inactive, the same as, or different in terms of their activity levels and therapeutic activity. Some drugs called pro drugs are inactive until they have undergone change by the liver and have been metabolised into their active form.

Metabolism is often divided into two phases usually described as phase 1 and phase 2, both of which are complex processes necessary for correct processing of the medication. Phase 1 reactions are the initial process where the drug undergoes modification, and there is breaking up of unstable chemical bonds and formation of new ones with the formation of end products that may be more active than the parent drug.[11] Phase 2 reactions involve further change to a more water-soluble, generally inactive compound so that excretion via the kidneys will be possible.[12] Some drugs may undergo just one of these phases; others will undergo both. The liver's primary mechanism for metabolising drugs is via a specific group of cytochrome P-450 enzymes contained within the hepatocytes of the liver cells[13] and they are important in reducing or altering the pharmacologic activity of many drugs and facilitating their elimination.[14]

DRUG HALF LIFE

This is the duration of action of a drug and refers to the period of time it takes for the amount of drug in the body or its concentration to be reduced by one-half.

ELIMINATION

Elimination of drugs can occur via sweat, saliva, bile, breath and faeces, but elimination via the kidneys is the commonest route. To be excreted via the urine the drug needs to be water soluble, and may be excreted through glomerular filtration, a process where drugs are secreted into the proximal tubule. In patients with renal impairment the ability of the kidneys to filter out drugs may be impaired, so that drugs excreted via the kidneys may accumulate in the bloodstream, leading to toxicity. A lower dose may therefore be needed to avoid the risk of adverse effects.

ADVERSE DRUG REACTIONS

WHO defines adverse drug reactions (ADRs) as unintended reactions to medicines that occur at doses normally used for treatment.[15] ADRs are among the leading causes of death in many countries and can occur in patients of any age. Unpleasant reactions to medications arise for a number of reasons, some preventable but some not. Preventable causes of adverse effects are shown in Table 17.2.

TABLE 17.2 Preventable causes of adverse drug effects

Patient prescribed incorrect dose of medication

Patient misunderstanding and taking the drug incorrectly

Incorrect diagnosis, hence wrong treatment prescribed

Past history of reaction to same or similar drug

Interaction with other medications

Other potential factors thought to increase risk include any past history of allergy, comorbid illnesses, age (elderly or very young), and impaired renal or liver function.[16]

DRUGS AND THE ELDERLY

Drug absorption

CLINICAL ALERT!

In older subjects a number of age-related changes are thought to affect drug absorption. Increased gastric pH and reduced gastric blood flow may cause reduced drug absorption, whereas reduced GI motility may result in more of the drug(s) being absorbed.[17] Changes to the pH of the gastric acid can also be influenced by certain medications. PPIs are one example and their use can affect the bioavailability of some medications. Studies have shown that the initiation of omeprazole can increase the absorption of digoxin, resulting in toxic digoxin levels[18] but can have the opposite effect and decrease metabolism of warfarin.[19]

Drug distribution

Distribution of most medications is related to body weight and composition and can therefore be affected by the changes that occur with the ageing process, which are often an increase in body fat, a decrease in muscle mass and a reduction in the amount of body water. When drugs are distributed in the body these changes are important because they potentially impact on the volume of distribution. This relates to the amount of drug in the body and the concentration of the drug measured in body fluid, and with an increase in body fat, fat-soluble drugs will have a greater volume of distribution, while drugs distributed in muscle will have a reduced volume of distribution.[17]

Drug metabolism

CLINICAL ALERT!

⚠ BEWARE!

- Metabolism by the liver may be impaired, thought to be caused by a combination of reduced hepatic blood flow (approximate 35% reduction in hepatic blood flow in the elderly) and reduced hepatic volume (hepatic volume is reduced by 28% in men and 44% in women by the age of 91).[20]
- Impaired hepatic metabolism in the elderly affects both bioavailability and hepatic clearance of drugs.[21] A decrease in liver mass and perfusion can lead to an increase in the bioavailability of some drugs,[22] leading to an increased risk of adverse effects.
- A reduction in albumin production means less protein available for binding, which leads to an increased amount of free drug, with more drug available to reach receptors and a subsequent increased risk of adverse effects.[23]

Drug elimination

CLINICAL ALERT!

⚠ BEWARE!

Older people are thought to be particularly at risk of medication-related side-effects, largely because age-related changes affect the way in which drugs are metabolised.
- Efficiency of the kidneys is impaired in the elderly with glomerular function reducing by 6%–10% per decade after the age of 40, which together with reduced tubular function means that by the age of 90 there may be a 30%–40% reduction in overall renal function.[24]
- Renal function may also be adversely affected by the presence of coexisting disease, e.g. hypertension, diabetes, congestive cardiac failure, or acute illnesses.
- A number of drugs including warfarin, propranolol, ibuprofen, diltiazem, verapamil and theophylline that are metabolised by phase 1 pathways have reduced clearance in older people.[25]
- The half life of drugs is increased as renal function deteriorates,[17] which means that drugs stay around for longer with greater risk of adverse effects.

Prescribing tips

TABLE 17.3 Prescribing suggestions

Suggested advice	Potential problems
Clinical assessment and accurate diagnosis before prescribing.	Unnecessary prescribing.
Low doses where possible.	Greater risk of side-effects.
Beware of adverse reactions.	Any side-effects may be atypical: confusion is a common side-effect.
Keep drug regime as simple as possible (written instructions may be needed). Once daily may aid compliance rather than three or four times daily.	The greater number of medications the patient is taking the greater the risk of drug interactions.
Avoid prolonged courses of antibiotics.	Risk of *C. difficile* (*see* pp. 297–8).

PRESCRIBING FOR CHILDREN

Prescribing for children follows the same principles that would be followed when prescribing for adults, but there are differences in the way drugs are dealt with by children.

Drug absorption

Absorption of oral medications in children differs from adults. In young children there is delayed gastric emptying and slower GI transit, which means that drugs taken orally stay in the stomach for a longer time. In neonates, gastric emptying time can be delayed for approximately 6–8 hours and does not reach adult rates until the age of 6–8 months.[26] The pH of gastric acid is also different in young children to that seen in adults. It is generally higher, which interferes with the bioavailability of some drugs, leading to increased bioavailability of those affected; this includes drugs such as penicillin and erythromycin when taken by the oral route.[26]

Distribution

Plasma protein levels are reduced in neonates, which increases the amount of free drug circulating, with the potential to cause drug reactions and adverse effects.

The volume of distribution of many drugs is often markedly increased in new-born babies partly because of reduced plasma protein levels but also because of an increased volume of extracellular fluid relative to total body water.[27]

Metabolism

Further problems may arise as a result of reduced levels of plasma proteins so that binding of drugs is reduced as a result. With reduced levels of protein, there is an increase in the amount of active drug, again potentially leading to adverse effects. Metabolic rate increases dramatically in children and is often greater than in adults so that compared with adults, children may require more frequent dosing or higher doses on a mg/kg basis.

Excretion

Renal function is reduced during infancy.[28] This causes decreased clearance of drugs and prolonged half life, potentially leading to drug toxicity.[11]

Prescribing tips

TABLE 17.4 Prescribing suggestions

Suggested advice	Potential problems
Clinical assessment and accurate diagnosis before prescribing.	Risks and benefits should be assessed before prescribing to ensure benefits outweigh risks.
Liquid form if needed.	Unpleasant taste may impede willingness to take prescribed medication.
Beware of adverse reactions.	Parents should be advised to report any adverse effects should they occur.
Written instructions may be needed for parents/carers.	Simplified regimes, e.g. once daily or twice daily, may help avoid the need for medication to be taken at school.
Accurate calculation of drug dose.	Usually calculated by mg/kg of body weight up to the dose which would be applicable for adults.

REFERENCES

1. Lim S. *Pharmacokinetics Basics – absorption, distribution, metabolism and excretion.* Available at: http://pharmaxchange.info/press/2011/04/pharmacokinetics-basics-absorption-distribution-metabolism-and-excretion/ (accessed 4 October 2013).
2. Shephard M. Administration of drugs 1: oral route. *Nursing Times.* 2011; **107**: 32–3.
3. Merck Manual. *Drug Absorption.* Available at: www.merckmanuals.com/professional/clinical_pharmacology/pharmacokinetics/drug_absorption.html (accessed 6 October 2013).
4. Winstanley PA, Orme ML. The effects of food on drug bioavailability. *Br J Clin Pharmacol.* 28(6): 621–8.
5. Kwan KC. Oral bioavailability and first pass effects. *DMD.* 1997; **25**(12): 1329–36.
6. Merck Manual. *Drug Bioavailability.* Available at: www.merckmanuals.com/professional/clinical_pharmacology/pharmacokinetics/drug_bioavailability.html (accessed 7 October 2013).
7. Toothaker RD, Welling PG. The effect of food on drug bioavailability. *Ann Rev Pharmacol Toxicol.* 1980; **20**: 173–99.
8. Barber P, Robertson D. *Essentials of Pharmacology for Nurses.* Maidenhead: Open University Press; 2009.
9. University of Nottingham. *School of Nursing and Academic Division of Midwifery Plasma Proteins and Drug Distribution.* Available at: www.nottingham.ac.uk/nmp/sonet/rlos/bioproc/plasma_proteins/5.html (accessed 15 October 2013).

10. Rolfe V. *The Liver and Drug Metabolism*. University of Nottingham. Available at: www.nottingham.ac.uk/nmp/sonet/rlos/bioproc/liverdrug/ (accessed 12 October 2013).

11. Kanneh A. Paediatric pharmacological principles: an update. Part 3. Pharmacokinetics: metabolism and excretion. *Paed Nursing*. 2002; **14**(10): 39–43.

12. Prosser S, Worster B, Macgregor J, *et al*. *Applied Pharmacology*. Italy: Harcourt Publishers Limited; 2002.

13. Bibi Z. Role of cytochrome P450 in drug interactions. *Nut Metabol*. 2008; **5**: 27.

14. Williamson GR. Drug metabolism and variability among patients in drug response. *N Engl J Med*. 2005; **352**: 21.

15. World Health Organization. *Medicines: safety of medicines – adverse drug reactions*. Fact sheet No. 293. Available at: www.who.int/mediacentre/factsheets/fs293/en/ (accessed 19 September 2013).

16. Kelly WN. Can the frequency and risks of fatal adverse drug events be determined? *Pharmacotherapy*. 2001; **21**(5): 521–7. Available at: www.medscape.com/viewarticle/409711_7 (accessed 20 September 2013).

17. Wooten JM. Pharmacotherapy considerations in elderly adults. *South Med J*. 2012; **105**(8): 437–45.

18. Kiley CA, Cragin DJ, Roth BJ. Omeprazole-associated digoxin toxicity. *South Med J*. 2007; **100**(4): 400–2.

19. Sutfin T, Balmer K, Boström H, *et al*. Stereoselective interaction of omeprazole with warfarin in healthy men. *Ther Drug Monit*. 1989; **11**: 176–84.

20. Woodhouse KW, James OF. Hepatic drug metabolism and ageing. *Brit Med Bull*. 1990; **46**(1): 22–35.

21. Hilmer SN, Shenfield GM, Le Couteur DG. Clinical implications of changes in hepatic drug metabolism in older people. *Ther Clin Risk Manag*. 2005; **1**(2): 151–6.

22. Klotz U. *Drug Metab Rev*. Pharmacokinetics and drug metabolism in the elderly. 2009; **41**(2): 67–76.

23. Hutchinson LC, O'Brien CE. Changes in pharmacokinetics and dynamics in the elderly patient. *J Pharm Prac*. 2007; **20**: 4–12.

24. Hughes SG. Prescribing for the elderly patient: why do we need to exercise caution? *Brit J Clin Pharm*. 1998; **46**(6): 531–3.

25. Le Couteur DG, McLean AJ. The aging liver. Drug clearance and an oxygen diffusion barrier hypothesis. *Clin Pharmacokinet*. 1998; **34**: 359–73.

26. Morselli PL. Clinical pharmacology of the perinatal period in early infancy. *Clin Pharacokinet*. 1989; **17**(Suppl. 1): 13–28.

27. Routledge PA. Pharmacokinetics in children. *J Antimicrob Chemother*. 1994; **34**(Suppl. A): S19–24.

28. Milsap RL, Jusko WJ. Pharmacokinetics in the infant. *Environ Health Perspect*. 1994; **102**(Suppl. 11): 107–10.

Index

Entries in **bold** refer to tables.

CPD with Radcliffe

You can now use a selection of our books to achieve CPD (Continuing Professional Development) points through directed reading.

We provide a free online form and downloadable certificate for your appraisal portfolio. Look for the CPD logo and register with us at: www.radcliffehealth.com/cpd

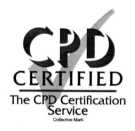